T&T Clark Reader in Abortion and Religion

T&T Clark Reader in Abortion and Religion

Jewish, Christian, and Muslim Perspectives

Edited by
Rebecca Todd Peters and Margaret D. Kamitsuka

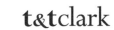

LONDON · NEW YORK · OXFORD · NEW DELHI · SYDNEY

T&T CLARK
Bloomsbury Publishing Plc
50 Bedford Square, London, WC1B 3DP, UK
1385 Broadway, New York, NY 10018, USA
29 Earlsfort Terrace, Dublin 2, Ireland

BLOOMSBURY, T&T CLARK and the T&T Clark logo are trademarks of Bloomsbury
Publishing Plc

First published in Great Britain 2023

A catalogue record for this book is available from the British Library.

A catalog record for this book is available from the Library of Congress.

ISBN: HB: 978-0-5676-9472-0
PB: 978-0-5676-9471-3
ePDF: 978-0-5676-9474-4
eBook: 978-0-5676-9473-7

Typeset by Deanta Global Publishing Services, Chennai, India
Printed and bound in Great Britain

To find out more about our authors and books visit www.bloomsbury.com and sign up
for our newsletters.

We dedicate this volume to all the people who face difficult reproductive decisions with courage drawn from deep faith and to students and people everywhere who seek to think in more nuanced and meaningful ways about abortion and religion.

Credit Lines

"Muslim women having abortions in Canada: Attitudes, beliefs, and experiences" by Wiebe, Ellen, Roya Najafi, Naghma Soheil, and Alya Kamani. Reprinted by permission of Canadian Family Physician.

Teman, Elly, Tsipy Ivry, and Barbara A. Bernhardt. 2011. "Pregnancy as a Proclamation of Faith: Ultra-Orthodox Jewish Women Navigating the Uncertainty of Pregnancy and Prenatal Diagnosis." *American Journal of Medical Genetics* Part A 155.1: 69–80. Reprinted with permission.

Jones, Robert P., Natalie Jackson, Maxine Najle, Oyindamola Bola, and Daniel Greenberg. 2019. "The State of Abortion and Contraception Attitudes in All 50 States." Public Religion Research Institute (March 26): 1–32. Reprinted by permission.

Bartkowski, John P., Aida I. Ramos-Wada, Chris G. Ellison, and Gabriel A. Acevedo. 2012. "Faith, Race-ethnicity, and Public Policy Preferences: Religious Schemas and Abortion Attitudes among US Latinos." *Journal for the Scientific Study of Religion* 51.2: 343–358. Reprinted by permission.

Excerpt from Wu, Bohsiu, and Aya Kimura Ida. "Ethnic diversity, religion, and opinions toward legalizing abortion: The case of Asian Americans." Journal of Ethnic and Cultural Studies 5, no. 1 (2018). Reprinted with permission of the publisher.

Excerpt from Murphy, A. James. "Undesired Offspring and Child Endangerment in Jewish Antiquity." Journal of Childhood and Religion Volume 5, no. 3 (2014). Reprinted with permission of the publisher.

"Our Right to Choose" by Beverly Harrison Copyright 1983. Reprinted by permission of Beacon Press, Boston

Mistry, Zubin. "Unnatural Symbol: Imagining Abortivi in the Early Middle Ages," 262–295. In Abortion in the Early Middle Ages, C.500–900. Boydell & Brewer, 2015. Reproduced with permission of the Licensor through PLSclear.

Ghaly, Mohammed. 2014. "Pre-modern Islamic Medical Ethics and Graeco-Islamic-Jewish Embryology." Bioethics 28.2: 49–58 by permission of John Wiley and Sons.

Al-Matary, Abdulrahman and Jaffar Ali. 2014. "Controversies and Considerations Regarding the Termination of Pregnancy for Foetal Anomalies in Islam." *BMC Medical Ethics* 15.1: 1–10. Reprinted by permission.

"The problem of abortion in classical Sunni fiqh" by Marion Holmes Katz, first published in the book Islamic Ethics of Life: Abortion, War, and Euthanasia edited by Jonathan E. Brockopp and published by the University of South Carolina Press.

Shaikh, Sa'diyya. "Family Planning, Contraception and Abortion in Islam: Undertaking Kalifah." In Sacred Rights: The case for contraception and abortion in world religions, edited by Daniel Maguire (Oxford University Press, 2003). Reproduced with permission of the Licensor through PLSclear.

From *To Offer Compassion* by Doris Andrea Dirks and Patricia A. Relf © 2017 by the Board of Regents of the University of Wisconsin System. Reprinted by permission of the University of Wisconsin Press.

Miller, Patricia. 2014. Good Catholics: The Battle over Abortion in the Catholic Church. Berkeley: Univ of California Press by permission of University of California Press.

Excerpt from Scaldo, Stacy A. "Life, Death & the God Complex: The Effectiveness of Incorporating Religion-Based Arguments into the Pro-Choice Perspective on Abortion." N. Ky. L. Review 39 (2012). Reprinted with permission of the publisher.

Kranson, Rachel. 2018. "From Women's Rights to Religious Freedom: The Women's League for Conservative Judaism and the Politics of Abortion, 1970-1982." From *Devotions and Desires: Histories of Sexuality and Religion in the Twentieth-Century United States*, edited by Gillian Frank, Bethany Moreton, and Heather R. White. Copyright © 2018 by the University of North Carolina Press. Used by permission of the publisher.

Excerpt from Winter, Aaron. 'Anti-Abortion Extremism and Violence in the United States.' In Extremism in America, ed. G. Michael, Gainesville: University Press Florida, 2013. Reprinted with permission of the publisher.

Contents

Author Information

Margaret D. Kamitsuka is the Francis W. and Lydia L. Davis Professor Emeritus of Religion at Oberlin College, Ohio. Her research, writing, and public speaking offer a theological perspective on reproductive issues, bioethics, gender and sexuality, and mothering. She is the author of *Abortion and the Christian Tradition: A Pro-choice Theological Ethic* (2019) and *Feminist Theology and the Challenge of Difference* (2007) and the editor of *The Embrace of Eros: Bodies, Desires, and Sexuality in Christianity* (2010). She has published essays widely, including in *Journal of Religious Ethics, Journal for the Feminist Study of Religion, Theology Today,* and *Christianity and Literature.* Kamitsuka serves as the book editor for the American Academy of Religion's Academy Series.

Rebecca Todd Peters is Professor of Religious Studies at Elon University, North Carolina. Her work as a feminist social ethicist focuses on globalization, economic, environmental, and reproductive justice. She is the author or editor of eight books and more than twenty-five peer-reviewed publications, including *Trust Women: A Progressive Christian Argument for Reproductive Justice* (2018). She received the 2018 Walter Wink Scholar-Activist Award from Auburn Seminary in recognition of her work on reproductive justice and poverty and economic justice and served as a Public Fellow at the Public Religion Research Institute (PRRI) from 2018 to 2021. She is a member of Planned Parenthood's Clergy Advocacy Board and serves as an expert witness on abortion and religion with the Lawyering Project.

Acknowledgments

We wish to acknowledge all those who assisted us in bringing this massive and important project to completion. First and foremost, we thank the authors who provided the stellar scholarship on abortion in Jewish, Christian, and Muslim traditions and on reproductive realities in the US context. We are immensely grateful to our editor Anna Turton for her support from the start of the idea to the finished product. Sinead O'Connor at Bloomsbury was persistent in chasing elusive permissions for reprints. Darsev Kaur and Alaa Suleiman, students at Elon, provided invaluable editing and other assistance. The expert indexing by Kathleen Stratton contributes greatly to this book's effectiveness for researchers.

A special thank-you to Michal Raucher, Zahra Ayubi, Perry Hamalis, and Telly Papanikolaou, whom we consulted in developing the scope and content of this volume. Thanks, also, to Sophia Todd Hatcher Peters, who offered feedback on various versions of chapters and served as a helpful sounding board (for her mom) in developing the volume.

We are grateful for the financial support that made this project possible. Maggi acknowledges Oberlin College for the Senior Research Scholar Award. Toddie thanks Elon University for a teaching sabbatical in the fall of 2021, and her thanks also go to the following for arranging financial support for publisher permissions for this project: Gabie Smith, Kirby Wahl, and Elon College of Arts and Sciences; Brian Pennington and the Elon Center for the Study of Religion, Culture and Society; and Geoff Claussen and the Elon Religious Studies Department.

We offer our immense gratitude to our library colleagues at the Mary Church Terrell Library at Oberlin College and to Lynn Melchor, Patrick Rudd, Doris Davis at the Belk Library at Elon. Their timely and gracious support, particularly during the challenges of Covid, helped make our research possible.

Toddie is deeply grateful to Maggi for inviting me into this project. I have been delighted to discover the many ways our skills and knowledge base complement one another, ultimately making this a stronger volume. Maggi acknowledges her heartfelt thanks to Toddie. We began as academic co-editors and complete this project as friends.

A Note from the Editors

The excerpts in this volume were chosen with great care to represent a broad range of arguments, positions, historical figures and periods, and ideas. To facilitate usefulness in the classroom, we limited the excerpts to 1,000–3,000 words. We sought to ensure that each excerpt represents the integrity of author's intention, even if the excerpt does not represent the whole of the argument from any given piece. We strongly encourage students and researchers to seek out the original articles or book chapters in full. Each excerpt reflects the citation style of the original essay or chapter, with some minor alterations. Footnotes have been converted to endnotes and amended for brevity or clarity when needed. Ellipses and brackets are used to indicate where the editors have made deletions or changes to the body of the text or the endnotes.

Introduction

Abortion is a complicated and multifaceted reality about which Jews, Christians, and Muslims have endeavored in the past and the present day to address ethically and theologically. The dominant public conversation suggests that religions (and, by association, religious people) are morally opposed to abortion; however, the reality is much more complicated. Religious attitudes, teachings, and beliefs are certainly mobilized in contemporary discussions about abortion, but too often these attitudes are dehistoricized, taken out of context, or used to manipulate emotions. Developing a more careful and critical understanding of abortion requires studying the topic from a range of perspectives and disciplinary lenses. The articles in this *Reader on Abortion and Religion*, which offers a wide range of positions, voices, and scholarly perspectives, demonstrate the importance of examining how religion intersects with the topic of abortion both in the practice of religion and in the study of religion.

Pregnancy—Then and Now

We begin with reflecting on pregnancy—a biological reality that affects many people with female reproductive systems and is the context in which the question of abortion arises at all. Pregnancy and childbirth are central to the human experience and foundational to human culture and survival. Given the ubiquity of human reproduction throughout history and across culture, as well as the essential value and importance placed on children, families, and the continuity of tribe, community, and species, it is not surprising that knowledge about pregnancy and childbirth is documented in many historical and cultural accounts and material artifacts. There is also ample evidence from the earliest documentation of civilizations that women's desire to control their fertility has been a perennial concern.

Wanting to end a dangerous, ill-timed, or an unwanted pregnancy is as old as human civilization. One of the earliest known references to abortion comes from a Sumerian tablet that contains a fragment of an abortifacient recipe, but the instructions have been lost.[1] A 4,000-year-old Egyptian papyrus that bears the title "Recipe Not to Become Pregnant" describes how to mix crocodile dung with fermented dough and place it in the vagina.[2] Silphium, one of many plants with well-known contraceptive and abortifacient properties, was so crucial to the Cyrenian export economy in ancient North Africa that it appeared on their coins. Demand for silphium was so widespread throughout the Greco-Roman world that it was eventually driven to extinction.[3] There is also evidence that male and female medical practitioners and writers in the medieval and early modern period had knowledge of medicinal plants for use in fertility, contraception, abortion, birthing, and regulating their "flowers" or menstrual cycles.[4]

Given the reality of obstructed labor, infection and sepsis, eclampsia, excessive bleeding, short interpregnancy intervals, and other serious health risks, pregnancy and childbirth have often been the leading cause of death within populations of fertile women. So, for many women, pregnancy marked not only risks for their prenate but for their own lives as well. Maternal mortality has impacted women from all social classes, including the most privileged, as was the case with Mary Wollstonecraft, the late-eighteenth-century British philosopher and author of *A Vindication of the Rights of Woman*. Wollstonecraft died after childbirth as a result of the inept treatment of a male physician, who disregarded the care offered by Wollstonecraft's chosen attendant, a midwife.[5]

However, the risks to women's health posed by pregnancy and childbirth have clearly been exacerbated by patriarchy and white supremacy, and women's reproductive decision-making has never happened outside of the context of authoritarian social structures. Enslaved women not only endured riskier birthing experiences, but their bodies were used and abused by slavers, conquerors, and disreputable physicians, among others. In fact, a great deal of contemporary gynecological knowledge is the result of profoundly unethical and abusive research conducted by nineteenth-century physician Marion Sims on the unanesthetized bodies of enslaved women.[6] Abortion and sterilization have also been forced on women against their will, as a result of fathers, husbands, masters, or governments exerting control over the bodies of women and girls within their sphere of power. Often under the guise of "eugenics," state-sponsored sterilization abuse targeted vulnerable groups of women, including Native American women, Puerto Rican women, people with developmental disabilities, poor women, Black women, and immigrant women.[7]

Pregnancy, childbirth, and parenting in the modern world are both similar and different from human experience of them through much of history. Advancements in medical science have brought increased knowledge and understanding about processes of gestation. The discovery of penicillin, anesthesia, surgical techniques, and other medical advances have provided increased ability to address some of the more dangerous aspects of childbearing. However, the fact that the maternal mortality rate for Black and Native women in the United States continues to be two to three times that of white women also demonstrates the urgent need to address the persistent reality of structural racism within our culture and our healthcare system.[8]

In the modern era, the development of progressive notions of women's rights, along with medical advances, combined to promote women's reproductive management not as a private or shameful matter but as a necessary part of a moral agent's life well lived. The shift from agricultural to capitalist economies, knowledge of the limits of the carrying capacity of the planet, and medical advancements in birth control and contraception—all these have transformed the meaning and experience of pregnancy, childbirth, and parenting. In developed countries, childbearing and parenting have become increasingly limited and intentional rather than simply a consequence of heterosexual sexual experience. With 99 percent of US women using some form of contraception in their lifetimes,[9] most people have rejected the traditional Christian position that the purpose of sex is primarily procreation.

Despite advances in contraception, 45 percent of the six million annual pregnancies in the United States are unplanned.[10] While unplanned does not always mean unwanted, consistently, about 40 percent of unplanned pregnancies are terminated. Additionally, we now know that 30 percent of fertilized eggs never implant in a uterus, another 30 percent are spontaneously aborted before a menstrual cycle is missed, and another 10–15 percent spontaneously abort after implantation. This means that 70–75 percent of all fertilized eggs do not progress for various reasons.[11] While Christianity has historically cast women in the presumptive role of a natural Eve, the "mother of all living" (Gen. 1.20), women's experience challenges this notion. Bodies reject more fertilized eggs than they gestate, and some women struggle with repeated reproductive loss; increasingly, women who do not feel called to motherhood are highlighting that maternity is a calling that not all women share.[12]

Increased medical knowledge and skill have also created an environment where it is possible to end pregnancies more easily and safely than ever before in human history. Medical statistics show that legal abortions today in countries with developed healthcare systems are safe medical procedures, posing less risk than a colonoscopy.[13] Contrary to claims circulated both in prolife circles and state-mandated information shared with women before a pregnancy termination, abortion is not correlated with subsequent infertility, breast cancer, or posttraumatic stress.[14] Moreover, studies also show that denying a woman an abortion can have adverse outcomes for the mother and the child.[15] Given the increased safety of abortion and changing cultural norms and expectations of motherhood, one-quarter of women will have an abortion by the age of forty-five in the United States, making abortion an increasingly common part of women's reproductive experience, at least until the reversal of *Roe v. Wade* in 2022.[16]

Abortion and Religion

Matters pertaining to significant life transitions are often marked within religious communities through ritual or rites of passage. Experiences that occur on the boundaries of life and death or ones that shift social power or status are often labeled by religious studies scholars as "liminal." The category of liminality can help to identify and discuss life experiences, many particular to female bodies—puberty and menarche, marriage and pregnancy, and so on—that have been especially viewed in many religious traditions as existing outside of "ordinary" time and hence possibly profane.[17] While not always practiced today, Judaism, Christianity, and Islam have postpartum rituals that mark the ritual cleansing and reentry of the newly delivered mother into the worshipping community.[18] Religions have always made pronouncements related to family structures, marriage protocols, paternal obligations, and women's domestic duties as a means of maintaining orderly communal life and safeguarding sacred times and spaces.

Abortion is occasionally addressed in the historical documents, legal canons, theological texts, and ethical teachings of Islam, Christianity, and Judaism; however, neither the Hebrew Bible, the New Testament, nor the Quran mentions abortion. Moreover, any reference to women's bodies in scripture and other revered religious writings must be evaluated as a part of the patriarchal historical contexts within which these religions arose and spread. The androcentrism typical of all global religions has a particular manifestation in monotheisms such as Judaism, Islam, and Christianity, where God is referred to with male pronouns. And as Mary Daly argued, "if

God is male, then the male is God."[19] Women, even when honored as pious wives, mothers, and daughters, have traditionally been seen also as inciting lust and as having porous, leaking, and often bloody bodies, which need to be regulated and purified. Matters related to sex, pregnancy, and birthing have always come under the watchful eye of male religious authority.

Correlatively, religious women have sometimes found ways to challenge male control over their fertility and to circumvent other aspects of women's subordination. It is not coincidental that the rise of women's demand for access to contraception in the United States in the early twentieth century occurred in the same era that women got the vote, Christian women began to gain access to ordination in some branches of Christianity, and Jewish women began organizing synagogue sisterhoods for more involvement in religious matters outside the domestic sphere. Even if abortion is only marginally discussed in formative texts and traditions of Islam, Judaism, and Christianity, pregnancy and abortion remain key issues that religious scholars endeavor to address ethically and theologically.

Until recently in human history, the process of gestation has quite literally been hidden from human view. One might say that abortion is an increasingly central and complicated issue for theologians, ethicists, and ordinary believers today, in part because of how science is bringing the intricacies of pregnancy and fetal development to light. Abortion is also theologically complicated because modern female-bodied persons—including pious ones—are insisting on having a say in reproductive matters, at the same time that increasing numbers of people are challenging traditional gender binaries and gender expression.

Abortion is also a contentious issue because of how religion plays a role in the public square of American pluralistic society. Pregnancy terminations have historically been private decisions, even if people sometimes consulted religious authorities. Today conservative religious opponents of legalized abortion have made abortion a thoroughly combative issue in places of worship and the public square. While legal access to abortion is widely supported by the majority of people (61 percent), it is vehemently opposed by others (37 percent). Recent polling by Pew—which found that 46 percent of people thought abortion is morally wrong in all or most cases, 31 percent of people thought it morally acceptable, and 21 percent of people do not think abortion is a moral issue at all[20]—seems to indicate both the complexity of attitudes about abortion as well a hesitancy to impose those beliefs on others through the legislation.

Abortion has become a dominant and perplexing social ethical issue in our culture, deeply shaped by both religious beliefs and patriarchal and misogynist attitudes about women and sexuality—attitudes that have often been inspired or promoted by religious doctrine. Ethical questions about terminating a pregnancy arise in two distinct spaces in US society: the legal sphere and the religious sphere. The question of whether abortion should be legal is most often related to and influenced by religious attitudes and beliefs about the moral status of the *prenate*, a term Peters uses to refer to the developing products of conception as long as it remains inside the body or uterus. We can see this dynamic of privileging fetal status reflected in the contemporary US conversations about abortion, which Peters has argued are shaped by a framework of justification that assumes women who get pregnant are obligated to have a baby and that the prenate is a person. From this starting point, pregnant women are required to justify their abortions.[21] Evidence of domination of the justification framework is apparent in the PRIM (**P**renatal diagnosis, **R**ape, **I**ncest, **M**other's life) reasons for abortion, which are largely deemed the only morally acceptable reasons to end a pregnancy.[22] This assumption that the prenate has value, however, can ultimately be traced to religious teachings and traditions, not scientific consensus. Furthermore, framing abortion as requiring justification has fundamentally distorted the conversation about reproductive rights in this country into an artificial binary by focusing on the abstract moral question of whether abortion is right or wrong. Too often, prolife arguments seek to demonstrate that abortion is not justifiable while prochoice arguments seek to justify abortion decisions. However, abortion, is a particular answer to a different ethical question: "What should I do when faced with an unplanned, unwanted, or medically compromised pregnancy?" This is the concrete moral question that many people face in the course of their reproductive lives; focusing on this question could helpfully reshape the public discussion about abortion.

In Kamitsuka's approach to the maternal-fetal relationship, she has argued that the fetal being has value independent of the pregnant person's assent to pregnancy, but the pregnant person must be acknowledged as nevertheless retaining reproductive self-determination throughout the gestation process. While some reproductive rights thinkers have tried to justify some abortions based on the claim that an early fetus is an organism of negligible value, Kamitsuka takes a theological approach that affirms both fetal value and the gestating woman's moral authority (*coram Deo*) throughout a pregnancy. This position speaks to the spiritual sensibilities of religiously devout women, many of whom prayerfully decide to terminate their pregnancy, based on their sense of God having called them to other responsibilities and commitments.[23]

Abortion Battles in the United States

Debating abortion and religion in the United States is complicated. The moral arguments and attitudes of Christianity have historically played a deep and abiding role in shaping negative moral attitudes toward abortion and in supporting the imposition of legal restrictions on abortion—affecting all people, religious or not—in the United States since its founding.[24] In today's pluralistic, multireligious cultural climate, however, it is increasingly important to pay attention to the history, beliefs, and practices of a secular citizenry and people who practice minority religious traditions. At times, certain sets of religious teachings have been imposed on the broader populace in the name of morality, as is currently the case with conservative Christian claims about fetal personhood. In democracies with a separation of church and state and a constitutional mandate not to abridge the free exercise of religion, religious points of views are welcome in the public square; however, a theocracy of any single religion would be out of order in the United States, where the secular population is growing and the religious demographics are increasingly diverse.

Despite declining numbers in the pews, Christianity remains the most populous religion in the United States; however, the face of Christianity in America is literally changing. The Catholic Church, which was predominantly white twenty-five years ago, is only 55 percent white today, with rapidly increasing numbers of Hispanic members.[25] Muslims are a minority in the United States; however, Islam is the fastest-growing American religion, and the Pew Research Center predicts that in the next thirty years Muslims will outnumber Jews in America.[26] The American Jewish community is pivotal within Judaism, since the largest percentage of Jews globally live in North America.[27]

These three monotheisms are sometimes referred to as the three Abrahamic traditions because of their shared worship of the God of the Hebrew patriarch (Abraham/Ibrahim). One might say that there is a common ancestral mythos that led to the founding of three different religions, of which the religion of the ancient Hebrew people is the oldest. Christianity consolidated at the same period as the rise of rabbinic Judaism, from which all branches of present-day Judaism are traced. While Islam follows chronologically, it considers itself as having bestowed God's final true revelation through the Prophet Mohammed. This volume does not privilege either chronology or theological claims to culminating revelation, and readers will note that we vary the order in which we refer to these three religions. At various historical periods, adherents of Judaism, Christianity, and Islam have sometimes found themselves in opposition to each other in various parts of the globe. Nevertheless, in the North American context, it is appropriate to think of them as a "confraternity of three communities" living as neighbors within American pluralistic democracy.[28]

There exists a wide divergence of religious viewpoints on abortion in the theological and ethical teachings within and among Islam, Christianity, and Judaism, which affects the religious landscape of abortion for adherents living in the United States. In Islam, differences exist between Sunni and Shiite branches and in Judaism between Orthodox and more progressive branches. Evangelical Protestants, conservative Roman Catholics, and Eastern Orthodox believers make common cause on protecting the unborn child from conception, but they diverge on a number of moral issues, including contraception and nonprocreative sex. Islam, Judaism, Orthodox Christianity, and Protestantism affirm the morality of abortion to save a woman's life, but Roman Catholic moral teachings allow only certain forms of pregnancy termination and only in certain circumstances, even when the woman's life is threatened. Historically mainline Protestant denominations support retaining legal access to abortion, though their individual statements about abortion reflect a variety of positions and perspectives about the details. In recent decades, feminist scholars of Judaism, Islam, and Christianity have generated their own theological arguments in support of women's moral agency and fundamental gender equality within their traditions; these efforts have also included attention to women's reproductive moral authority. All these various alliances and oppositions are playing out on the American stage in the current era where religiously motivated antiabortion forces have succeeded in overturning *Roe v. Wade*, an action that was unthinkable for most Americans until the Supreme Court decision in *Dobbs v. Jackson* was issued on June 24, 2022.[29]

After the *Roe v. Wade* Supreme Court decision legalized abortion in 1973 there was an increase in religiously motivated antiabortion activism. The politics of abortion heated up in multiple ways. *Roe* held that abortion was protected based on a constitutional right of privacy and that states might have an interest in restricting that right under some circumstances. The right to abortion was protected during the first trimester; state intervention was allowed beginning in the second trimester to protect the pregnant woman's health. After viability (24 weeks in 1973), *Roe* held that the state's interest in protecting fetal life meant that abortion could be banned, except to protect the mother's life or health.[30] Giving women the unimpeded right to abortion for at least part of a pregnancy enraged conservative Christians, who mobilized to fight the ruling. While the United States has been steadily moving toward secularism demographically, antiabortion legislative activity spearheaded by conservative Christians has been particularly effective at imposing regulations at the state level since the 2010 elections.

One of the most significant federal regulations restricting abortion access was the 1976 Hyde Amendment prohibiting federal funding for abortion, sponsored by Illinois Republican Henry Hyde, a conservative Catholic. The Hyde Amendment put an increased burden on poor and low-income women seeking abortion care who rely on Medicaid to cover their healthcare needs. By 2021, sixteen states had passed legislation banning abortion at various stages of pregnancy—increasingly without an exception for rape or incest—and mandating various other requirements such as waiting periods, mandatory ultrasounds, and counseling that often includes medically inaccurate information.[31]

The frustration of prolife advocates over their inability to overturn *Roe* energized many in the conservative Christian base, and grassroots organizations stepped up to fight these culture war battles. One recent Public Religion Research Institute (PRRI) poll shows that half of white evangelical Christians are Republicans and only 14 percent are Democrats, while another PRRI poll found that the partisan divide between Republicans and Democrats on the issue of abortion widened from 28 percentage points to 36 between 2014 and 2018.[32] A proliferation of Catholic- and evangelical-affiliated nonprofit organizations inundate public spaces, both virtual and actual, with their prolife messages. The national March for Life, which began as a small demonstration of concerned prolife citizens in 1974, has expanded into an event of hundreds of thousands in Washington, DC, concurrent with other gatherings in state capitols throughout the nation and internationally. So-called prolife crisis pregnancy centers constitute a massive public presence where dedicated volunteers attempt to win the hearts and minds of pregnant women considering termination. These CPCs have also increased their public presence through accessing Title X monies that are intended to support family planning, despite the fact that these centers refuse to offer comprehensive family planning services. Strong intersections of abortion and religion can also be found among more shadowy activist Christian fringe groups, which emerge onto the public stage when they commit antiabortion acts of violence. Since 1991, according to the National Abortion and Reproductive Rights Action League, eleven doctors and clinic workers have been murdered, and there were twenty-six attempted murders. Clinics and abortion providers have received 600 bioterrorism threats meant to disrupt clinic services.[33]

Intersectional and Critical Feminist Approaches to Abortion Ethics

Ethical questions are of paramount importance in every society and the task of social ethics is to help people engage in considered examination of contemporary social problems in ways that contribute to deeper analysis and understanding with the goal of developing robust ways to address those problems. While ethical topics often persist over time—sexuality, war, political-economies—how we think about the morality of these questions and how we shape our ethical responses to them are deeply influenced by a wide variety of sources, including: family and tradition; socioeconomic status; scientific knowledge and understanding; historical memory; and religious teaching, beliefs, and practices. In short, morality is a reflection of culture broadly understood, which in turn is often shaped by religious belief and practice.

As religious studies scholars, we are particularly interested in helping to shape and facilitate robust and nuanced conversations about the role of religion in larger public discourse. In collecting this particular set of readings, we seek to help reframe the abortion debate in the United States by providing a different range of materials than previously gathered in other anthologies on abortion. We believe these readings will enable a more robust and ethically rich conversation about pregnancy, abortion, and childbearing. Our own scholarship is informed by intersectional feminism, a methodology that critically analyzes the impact of intersecting forces of racism, sexism, classism, and other oppressions.[34] We are interested in epistemological questions like "How do we know what we know?" and "What persons or groups are regarded as sources of authority?" To that end, this volume provides multiple sources of knowledge—experiential, historical, social-scientific, and theological—in order to help reframe the abortion debate in America.

An intersectional and feminist methodology insists that it is insufficient merely to study each religious tradition's normative position or even to compare similarities and differences among religions on abortion. Theological statements or religious legal rulings must be contextualized in light of other relevant intersecting factors that come to light from studying cultural histories of procreation, the sociology of pregnancy and birthing, the rhetoric of abortion arguments, and the testimonies of real persons who have faced an abortion decision. These factors allow one to see the workings of power in authoritative religious institutions and the persistent, if sometime suppressed, counternarratives of pregnancy-capable people attempting to manage their complex reproductive lives.

While not every religious denomination or subgroup in Islam, Judaism, Christianity is represented, the essays in this *Reader* examine a representative span of viewpoints—from evangelical Protestant to progressive Catholic, from Reformed Jewish to Haredi, from Sunni to Shiite. We have intentionally sought contributors that represent a wide variety of identities and perspectives that have often been left out of public conversations on abortion.

This volume studies not only key principles and moral teachings in these three religious traditions' normative discourses on abortion but also the ways in which believers in North America actually navigate the complexities of their reproductive lives. By looking at lived religion, one can see a diversity of positions on sexual ethics, procreation, and family life among Christian, Jewish, and Muslim adherents. In those lives, we can see that people's experiences do not always match the narrow framework within which religious authorities consider abortion to be permissible. Normative religious teachings do not always reflect how believers actually live their religiosity, especially relating to sexuality. Moreover, religions always exist in a broader societal context, and American Muslims, Jews, and Christians interact on a daily basis with institutions and cultural practices in the broader society that are, for lack of better word, secular.

While Christianity has played the dominant role in abortion debates and religious activism in the United States, the aforementioned changing demographics and the increasingly pluralistic cultural climate warrant more attention to the impact that Jewish and Muslim perspectives have had and are having on how Americans think about abortion. The United States thus serves as a kind of in-depth case study for analogous reproductive issues affecting democracies in other parts of the world. This book offers insights into the complicated interactions of religion and abortion in a range of areas, including politics, theology, the courts, grassroots activism, and medical care.

Understanding abortion in America means understanding both how many religious sectors have been and still are invested in challenging its legality, as well as how many religious individuals and communities continue to want there to be access to abortion healthcare that is safe, private, affordable, and respectful.[35] This *Reader* differs from other anthologies on religion and abortion, which have focused primarily on official denominational statements or arguments by scholars that reinforce the prochoice/prolife binary.[36] Moreover, with the exception of a few volumes of progressive-oriented religious bioethics, the existence of religious feminist positions on abortion is largely unacknowledged, and most abortion textbooks allow secular scholars to represent a singular feminist position.[37] We intentionally have chosen to frame abortion and religion differently. By presenting abortion as a situated social practice, we recognize that reproductive ethics is informed by the experience of pregnant persons, cultural and political factors, and a spectrum of religious views.

Overview of the Book's Sections

Historically and traditionally, women's voices, experiences, knowledge, and wisdom have been excluded from government, politics, philosophy, science, religious law, and dogmatics. Given that pregnancy and childbearing have, until very recently, been the exclusive domain of those designated by heteronormative society as women, their experience and their self-understanding are important and often-ignored sources of wisdom in conversations about sexuality, having children, and terminating a pregnancy. For this reason, we have chosen to begin the book with first-person accounts of abortion decisions and experiences "in their own words." This book looks behind the curtain of stigma to see how believers from these three traditions negotiate their religion's teachings on sexuality and abortion in relation to their actual daily lives. Statistically, over half of women who have abortions are Christians, with the greatest percentage of those self-identifying as Roman Catholic or evangelical. This means that the majority of American women using abortion services affiliate with denominations where opposition to abortion is the most intense.

Relatively recent medical advances and changing cultural norms mean that there is an increasing number of people who can get pregnant but who identify as non-binary, transgender, agender, or in other ways. While data are beginning to be collected about abortions of transgender and gender non-binary (TGNB) persons, an early study indicates that these abortions account for less than 1 percent of all abortions in the United States.[38] Almost no research has been done on the religious attitudes of TGNB persons and abortion, and this volume reflects that lacuna. Understanding the cultural, theological, and political history of attitudes toward pregnancy, childbearing, and abortion requires specific feminist attention to the ways in which misogyny and patriarchy have shaped attitudes, laws, social norms, and theological and religious doctrine affecting women. Thus, we see the importance of addressing the category of woman, while also being aware of how it has been used to exclude the experience of TGNB persons. The ways in which TGNB people of all experiences have been impacted by these same histories and attitudes bear further examination. We stand firmly in support of ensuring that TGNB people are able to receive culturally sensitive and appropriate medical care and urge healthcare professionals and educators to embrace and further this work, which is beyond the scope of this volume.

Part 2 of the book includes social-scientific research that is relevant to understanding the social issue of abortion. These selections offer qualitative and quantitative insight into women's experiences of abortion and demonstrate how social psychologists, sociologists of religion, and other scholars think about and study the impact of religion on moral decision-making, political-thinking, and medical practices related to abortion. These studies are vital for contextualizing pregnancy termination, which always happens in specific bodies shaped by race, nationality, ethnicity, religion, and other factors. They also demonstrate the wide range of attitudes that people of faith hold about abortion across the country, with particular attention to the diversity of attitudes within Latinx and Asian American communities.

Part 3, "History and Context," allows readers to see different perspectives and attitudes toward pregnancy, abortion, childbearing, and parenting in select historical snapshots from the ancient world to the twentieth century. These essays elucidate the ways in which social attitudes about these topics have shifted over time and in response to different cultural and religious norms and expectations, political events, legal developments, and other historical factors. This section focuses particular attention on the history and impact of white supremacy, racism, settler colonialism, and eugenics on the reproductive lives of African American and Native peoples in the United States. Recognizing the historical context within which our contemporary conversations have developed is an essential aspect of the critical social analysis that is required for authentic engagement with the complexity of ethical questions related to reproduction and reproductive politics.

The fourth part of the book, "Religious Arguments about Abortion," demonstrates that there are no monolithic positions that represent any one of these three religious traditions on abortion. We can see how different methodological starting points, different ways of interpreting normative religious texts, and different theological assumptions about God and human beings yield a range of positions from traditionalist to progressive. These essays represent thoughtful arguments from respected scholars who offer their understanding of how their particular tradition speaks to some issue related to abortion, including: why sacred scriptures do not mention abortion, whether pregnant women's suffering should be a factor in religious legal rulings, and how ancient religious teachings on fetal development should apply to pregnancy today. The editors note their own contributions in this section of the book. It is important to acknowledge that the preponderance of articles in the Christianity section are written by white authors, which reflects the nature of theological scholarship focused on this issue. We are encouraged to be able to include the work of theologian and reproductive justice activist Toni Bond, and we hope that additional conversations from scholars of color will further expand the conversation beyond the narrow focus on abortion rights.

The final section highlights a wide variety of ways that the intersection of abortion and religion has occurred in public life over the past fifty years— often in very contentious ways. Some of these essay excerpts discuss specific historical situations, and others outline ongoing struggles, including questions of racism and exclusion, ideology and politics, life and death, morality and decision-making, and justice and compassion. These essays demonstrate the concrete ways in which religion can impact real people's lives, shape public institutions, and reverberate deep into America's constitutional self-understanding. Readers will find discussions ranging from the role of religion in the *Roe v. Wade* decision, to Catholic hospital practices, to online Muslim *fatwas* (legal rulings) on sexuality.

This book's materials can be used in a wide variety of ways in the classroom or other teaching contexts and in research projects on abortion. We invite you to visit the website abortionreligionreader.com to explore additional resources that supplement this volume, including teaching outlines, modules for courses, suggestions for videos, websites, and other materials.

It is our hope that this volume will contribute to reframing discourses and debates about abortion in the United States in ways that move beyond the many narrowly focused conversations that rehash tired binaries of prolife versus prochoice, fetal versus women's rights, or women's freedom from the shackles of religion versus women's religious subjugation. While some binary terms and concepts are found throughout this book and have a place in particular contexts and arguments, these essays offer opportunities for you to complicate familiar terminology in an effort to deepen your comprehension of the complexities of socially situated persons who face unplanned or problem pregnancies and for whom religious belief may be important for their decision of what to do next. We believe these essays offer the opportunity for readers to think carefully and critically about the historical roots and contemporary ethical questions related to abortion. More needs to be said beyond the parameters of this volume, and we welcome the diverse and robust framings that hopefully will be produced in years to come that will probe even more deeply into the justice issues related to pregnant persons' moral agency and the flourishing of families that our society so desperately needs.

Notes

1. "Ancient Civilizations and Birth Control," in *The Encyclopedia of Birth Control*, ed. Vern L. Bullough (Santa Barbara, CA: ABD-CLIO, 2001), 18.
2. John M. Riddle, *Eve's Herbs: A History of Contraception and Abortion in the West* (Cambridge, MA: Harvard University Press, 1997), 68.
3. Ibid., 44–6.
4. See Monica H. Green, "Gendering the History of Women's Healthcare," *Gender & History* 20, no. 3 (2009): 498–507.
5. Elizabeth Raisanen, "Childbirth and Confinement: Mary Wollstonecraft and the Politics of Pregnancy," UCLA: Center for the Study of Women (March 2011).
6. Deirdre Cooper Owens, *Medical Bondage: Race, Gender, and the Origins of American Gynecology* (Athens, GA: University of Georgia Press, 2017).
7. Jeanne Flavin, *Our Bodies, Our Crimes: The Policing of Women's Reproduction in America* (New York: New York University Press, 2009), ch. 2.
8. Emily E. Petersen et al., "Racial/Ethnic Disparities in Pregnancy-Related Deaths—United States, 2007–2016," *Morbidity and Mortality Weekly Report* 68, no. 35 (September 6, 2019): 762–5.
9. Rachel K. Jones, "People of all Religions Use Birth Control and Have Abortions," *Guttmacher Institute* (October 2020).
10. Lawrence B. Finer and Mia R. Zolna, "Declines in Unintended Pregnancy in the United States, 2008–2011," *New England Journal of Medicine* 374, no. 9 (2016): 843–52.
11. Nick S. Macklon, Joep P. M. Geraedts, and Ban C. J. M. Fauser, "Conception to Ongoing Pregnancy: The 'Black Box' of Early Pregnancy Loss," *Human Reproduction Update* 8, no. 4 (July 1, 2002): 333–43.
12. Kendra G. Hotz, "Happily Ever After: Christians without Children," in *Encountering the Sacred: Feminist Reflections on Women's Lives*, ed. Rebecca Todd Peters and Grace Y. Kao (Boston: Beacon, 2018).

13. Laura Kurzman, "Major Complication Rate after Abortion Is Extremely Low," *UCSF News Center* (December 8, 2014).

14. Jasveer Virk, Jun Zhang, and Jø Olsen, "Medical Abortion and the Risk of Subsequent Adverse Pregnancy Outcomes," *New England Journal of Medicine* 357, no. 7 (2007): 648–53; American College of Obstetrics and Gynecology, "Induced Abortion and Breast Cancer Risk," ACOG Committee Opinion No. 434 (June 2009): 1417–8; Gail Erlick Robinson, Nada L. Stotland, Nancy Felipe Russo, Joan A. Lang, and Mallay Occhiogrosso, "Is There an 'Abortion Trauma Syndrome'? Critiquing the Evidence," *Harvard Review of Psychiatry* 17, no. 4 (2009): 268–90.

15. Anusha Ravi, *Limiting Abortion Access Contributes to Poor Maternal Health Outcomes* (Washington, DC: Center for American Progress, 2018), 1–7.

16. Rachel K. Jones and Jenna Jerman, "Population Group Abortion Rates and Lifetime Incidence of Abortion: United States, 2008–2014," *American Journal of Public Health* 107, no. 12 (2017): 1904–9.

17. Charlotte Elisheva Fonrobert, *Menstrual Purity: Rabbinic and Christian Reconstructions of Biblical Gender* (Stanford: Stanford University Press, 2002); Sara Read, *Menstruation and the Female Body in Early Modern England* (Houndmills, Basingstoke: Palgrave, 2013).

18. Kathryn M. Kueny, *Conceiving Identities: Maternity in Medieval Muslim Discourse and Practice* (Albany: SUNY Press, 2013), especially ch. 4; Anne Stensvold, *A History of Pregnancy in Christianity: From Original Sin to Contemporary Abortion Debates* (New York: Routledge, 2015), 71–3.

19. Mary Daly, *Beyond God the Father: Toward a Philosophy of Women's Liberation* (Boston: Beacon, 1973), 19.

20. Pew Research Center, May 2022, "America's Religious Quandary."

21. Rebecca Todd Peters, *Trust Women: A Progressive Christian Argument for Reproductive Justice* (Boston: Beacon, 2018), 124.

22. Since 1972, the US public has consistently supported the PRIM reasons for abortion with 87 percent support when a woman's life is endangered, 78 percent supporting in circumstances of rape (and presumably incest which is, by definition, not consensual), and 77 percent support for serious prenatal health issues. See Tom W. Smith and Jaesok Son, "Trends in Public Attitudes towards Abortion," *General Social Survey 2012 Final Report* (May 2013), 2.

23. Margaret D. Kamitsuka, *Abortion and the Christian Tradition: A Pro-choice Theological Ethic* (Louisville: Westminster John Knox, 2019), 150–4.

24. Peters, *Trust Women*, ch. 4 and 6; James C. Mohr, *Abortion in America: The Origins and Evolution of National Policy* (New York: Oxford University Press, 1978); Leslie J. Reagan, *When Abortion Was a Crime: Women, Medicine, and Law in the United States, 1867–1973* (Berkeley: University of California Press, 1996).

25. See Robert P. Jones and Daniel Cox, *America's Changing Religious Identity* (Washington, DC: Public Religion Research Institute, 2017), 1–46.
26. See Pew Research Center, "The Future of World Religions: Population Growth Projections, 2010–2050" (April 2, 2015), 1–13.
27. See Pew-Templeton Global Religious Futures Project, "Jews," Pewforum.org.
28. Jon D. Levenson, "The Idea of Abrahamic Religions: A Qualified Dissent," *Jewish Review of Books* 1, no. 1 (2010): 1–14.
29. For an interactive annotated summary of the decision, see "The Dobbs v. Jackson Decision, Annotated," *New York Times* (June 24, 2022), https://www.nytimes.com/interactive/2022/06/24/us/politics/supreme-court-dobbs-jackson-analysis-roe-wade.html.
30. "Roe v. Wade," Oyez, https://www.oyez.org/cases/1971/70-18. In a later ruling, *Planned Parenthood v. Casey*, the trimester framework was jettisoned, and states were allowed to restrict abortion as long as the laws did not impose an "undue burden" before viability. "Planned Parenthood of Southeastern Pennsylvania v. Casey," Oyez, https://www.oyez.org/cases/1991/91-744.
31. Guttmacher Institute, "An Overview of Abortion Laws" (July 1, 2021).
32. Jones and Cox, *America's Changing Religious Identity*, 9; Robert P. Jones, Natalie Jackson, Maxine Najle, Oyindamola Bola, and Daniel Greenberg, *The State of Abortion and Contraception Attitudes in All 50 States* (Washington, DC: Public Religion Research Institute, 2019), 8.
33. National Abortion Federation, "2018 Violence and Disruption Statistics," Prochoice.org, 1–10.
34. Kimberle Crenshaw, "Mapping the Margins: Intersectionality, Identity Politics, and Violence against Women of Color," *Stanford Law Review* 43 (1990): 1241–99.
35. Abortion is still legal in many states. See "Is Abortion Still Legal in My State Now that Roe v. Wade Was Overturned?" Planned Parenthood, https://www.plannedparenthoodaction.org/abortion-access-tool/US.
36. Lloyd H. Steffen, ed., *Abortion: A Reader* (Eugene, OR: Wipf and Stock, 2010); Robert M. Baird and Stuart E. Rosenbaum, eds., *The Ethics of Abortion: Pro-Life vs. Pro-Choice* (Buffalo, NY: Prometheus, 2001); Louis P. Pojman and Francis J. Beckwith, eds., *The Abortion Controversy: 25 Years After Roe v. Wade: A Reader* (Belmont, CA: Wadsworth, 1998).
37. Charles E. Curran, Margaret A. Farley, and Richard A. McCormick, eds., *Feminist Ethics and the Catholic Moral Tradition* (Mahwah, NJ: Paulist 1996); Patricia Beattie Jung and Thomas A. Shannon, eds., *Abortion and Catholicism: The American Debate* (New York: Crossroad, 1988).
38. Rachel K., Jones, Elizabeth Witwer, and Jenna Jerman, "Transgender Abortion Patients and the Provision of Transgender-Specific Care at Non-Hospital Facilities That Provide Abortions," *Contraception: X* 2 (January 1, 2020): 100019.

Part 1

In Their Own Words

Introduction to Part 1

Recognizing that the situated knowledge of people who have abortions is a critical source of wisdom and insight for thinking about pregnancy, abortion, and childbearing, and noting the historical erasure of women's experience as a source of knowledge, this volume begins with the narratives of those who alone can gestate and give birth.[1] Listening to and prioritizing women's voices, experiences, and perspectives has been a fundamental pillar of feminist scholarship and, given women's historic exclusion from official theological and legal determinations about women's reproductive health,[2] beginning with these stories is a significant step toward reframing how we think and talk about abortion.

Over the nearly fifty years since the legalization of abortion in the United States, people of many different socioeconomic, religious, racial, and other backgrounds and gender identities have exercised their constitutional right to an abortion. Nevertheless, for religious people especially, abortion is rarely a decision taken lightly. The readings in this section include contemporary first-person accounts of reproductive stories, which reveal the thought processes, emotions, and faith struggles experienced by those who have terminated a pregnancy. Listening to their stories offers the opportunity to consider the variety of circumstances and situations that accompanied various unplanned, unwanted, or problem pregnancies. These narratives also demonstrate the kinds of moral questions and considerations that shaped decision-making and illustrate the care with which these individuals engaged in moral discernment as they considered whether to terminate a pregnancy.

While these stories reflect the abortion experiences of six individuals in a context where abortion is safe and legal, that does not mean that their decision or what they went through was uncomplicated. Some believers voice a sense of feeling alienated from their conservative religious communities, as seen in "Alex's" moving account as a genderqueer teenager living in the Bible Belt of rural Iowa. While "Alex" was able to reconnect with God after their abortion, this is not always the case. Christian scholars Kate Ott and "América Gonzalez" and Muslim religious studies student "Iman" proclaim powerful theological insights affirming women's moral consciousness and God's compassion. Rachael Pass recounts how her rabbinical studies, her close support network, and Jewish rituals all factored into her thinking about her unplanned pregnancy and in carrying her through the process of a medical abortion at home. CoWanda Rusk speaks about how her Christian faith sustained her in navigating abortion access as a seventeen-year-old African American high school student. We intentionally did not include stories of "postabortion trauma"—stories that can be liberally found in prolife publications and on websites touting the myth that abortion causes, among other things, post-traumatic stress syndrome. Reputable scholars have debunked this claim as based on faulty science.[3]

Many factors influenced how these people made their decision and how they coped with it afterward, including family support or lack thereof, existing children, as well as their cultural, religious, and family background. The stories chosen for this section do not exhaustively represent abortion experiences for Muslims, Christians, and Jews, but they offer a glimpse into the diversity of abortion experiences. While the current, albeit incomplete, data show that abortions among the nonbinary and transgender population are less than 1 percent of abortions, we included Alex's account because transgender experiences are often overlooked in conversations about abortion and because increasing numbers of younger people identify as genderqueer. Some writers have courageously chosen to reveal their identity, and others have judiciously chosen to remain anonymous, and we respect both decisions. We believe the stories are compelling and hearing these voices is integral to the feminist methodology of doing scholarship rooted in lived experience, which the editors support.

As you read the essays in this section, we encourage you to consider the following:

1. In what ways are these stories different from or similar to what you expected? Where did your expectations come from? How do these stories help you think about abortion differently?

2. What different factors did people identify as important in making their decision and in terminating their pregnancy? How did they make their decisions?

3. What kind of theological and ethical reflections emerge from these accounts, not only from those with formal religious studies education but also from ordinary believers who share their evolving views of God and faith?

Notes

1. Rebecca Todd Peters, "Listening to Women," *Journal of Religious Ethics* 49, no. 2 (2021): 290–313.
2. Zahra Ayubi discusses the problem of male-only jurists deciding reproductive matters in Islam in "Authority and Epistemology in Islamic Medical Ethics of Women's Reproductive Health," *Journal of Religious Ethics* 49, no. 2 (2021): 245–69.
3. Brenda Major, Mark Appelbaum, Linda Beckman, Mary Ann Dutton, Nancy Felipe Russo, and Carolyn West, "Abortion and Mental Health: Evaluating the Evidence," *American Psychologist* 64, no. 9 (2009): 863–90.

1

So Many Lives at Stake

"América Gonzalez"

This piece by "América Gonzalez" (a pseudonym) is an original contribution to this volume. She is a Catholic scholar who teaches theology and ethics in the Northeast and has been active in mentoring and promoting greater diversity in theological education. She is one of a number of Catholic scholars who walk a precarious line between researching, writing, and teaching about abortion in ways that may deviate from official Roman Catholic positions when their livelihood is dependent on employment in a Catholic institution.

Terminating a pregnancy is about life and choice, about sex and death, about fear and condemnation. But I think, most of all, it is about loss and benefit. Who benefits when an abortion is performed? Who gets the most out of that termination? Who loses? And how do those categories shift over time and circumstances? I've had to consider these questions for myself as a woman, as a Puerto Rican Catholic feminist. I cannot look at the four children I have ushered into the world without considering the ones I did not.

When my oldest daughter was sixteen years old, our family received the horrifying news that our sixteen-year-old niece had run away from the uncle's home where she had been living, finally escaping the sexual abuse she endured by him for over a year, if not longer. We would have discovered the abuse sooner, I think, if he hadn't taken her to have an abortion. The pregnancy would have exposed his crime against this child.

In the research I've done about sexual violence in Latin America, I read so many testimonies of Latin American girls and women who, after being trafficked across international and national borders, after being forced to work in the sex trade industry, after having their bodies and their sex pummeled day after day, that abortion is as commonplace as doing the laundry, getting it clean so it can be worn again.

For these cases, abortion has served as a cover-up, a way of erasing something that cannot or refuses to be faced, to allow for lies, deceit and abuse to continue unchallenged. As a feminist, what does "choice" mean in these circumstances? The culture of feminism in this country has been so framed by the abortion debate, that to be feminist is often understood as synonymous with a pro-choice stance. Sidney Callahan's famous essay "Abortion and the Sexual Agenda" (1986) has succeeded to some degree by pushing the two terms – pro-life and feminism – together when she claims, "Pro-life feminists . . . argue on good feminist principles that women can never achieve the fulfillment of feminist goals in a society permissive toward abortion." While I agree with the latter part of this statement, I am still suspicious of the way she dismisses the very cogent socio-moral arguments made by Christian ethicists, particularly when "culture of death" language is used to serve the antiabortion stance. I would rather ask "who/what does this particular abortion benefit," a question which doesn't try to create absolutes regarding fetal life or any life for that matter. In all the stories I mentioned, male control and dominance was the beneficiary, because each served to cover-up the abuses and violence of men inflicted upon women, of male control – individual and societal – over women's bodies. But then, compulsory pregnancy can do the same exact thing.

There are very few people with whom I've shared my experience of terminating a pregnancy in 1989. I didn't want my parents to know; I couldn't let my parents know. I was recently married and in my twenties. I couldn't face the prospect of pregnancy, which was less about having a child and more about being a mother. That was my insurmountable fear based on a past of sexual assault that I wanted to erase, knowing that having my body taken over by another being would be too strong of a reminder of my body being controlled and violated by rape.

As a Catholic, sanctity of life is fundamentally connected to quality of life, achieved in community and solidarity. The notion of the common good, of all being able to flourish into the fullness of humanity, of the balance of rights and responsibility, are the pillars of my understanding of Catholic social teaching. The liberal tolerance of pro-choice feminism with its emphasis on the rights of the individual, with less consideration of the consequence of those rights on the community, feels foreign and somewhat destructive to me. At the same time, the forceful emphasis of conservative

Catholicism's equating of the sanctity of life with procreation, in such a way as to put women's bodies at the service of all humanity and of God, is nothing more than biological determinism that has paraded itself as divine natural law. I can't buy into either one. But "trusting women" still echoes with individualism to me; reproductive justice doesn't seem to address the need for communal accountability and wisdom. I think my Puerto Rican identity, and my connection to African cultural practice, has something to do with it.

My spouse is from the global south and his culture values children as a blessing by the joy they bring and the connection they maintain between the past and the future. For him, thwarting the possibility of that blessing would go against ancestral wisdom; in fact, doing so without the consent of the community (including the ancestors) could lead to being cursed. After the abortion, for many years since, he interpreted every bad turn our family experienced—illnesses, premature death, job loss, financial struggles, a cancer diagnosis—as a result of that decision made in a limited vacuum of an individualized context.

My own Puerto Rican sensibility complicates this even further because reproductive control has been used on Puerto Rican women from the 1920's up to very recently (late 20th century). But this project of reproductive control did not occur in a vacuum either; it is set within the history of U.S. colonialism in Puerto Rico, with pharmaceutical company and U.S. governmental complicity in contraceptive experimentation without consent and forced sterilization. As Iris López writes, "The reshaping of the Puerto Rican population and economy was not accomplished by emigration alone. A complementary government policy of sterilization arose simultaneously and the Puerto Rican and U.S. governments developed Puerto Rico's economy through both emigration and sterilization, especially during the industrialization phase known as Operation Bootstrap [which began in 1948]. In essence, migration was used as the temporary response to Puerto Rico's overpopulation problem, while sterilization became the permanent solution."[1]

I had no idea of this history of sterilization and reproductive control until years after I terminated that pregnancy. Historical amnesia has deadly consequences and that is precisely the goal of the colonial project. It serves to mask the truth of all that has come before us and who we are; how can we be moral agents without this deep, ancestral knowing? Puerto Rican history has been erased from the Puerto Rican collective consciousness and, as a result, many Puerto Rican women are completely ignorant of how the current debate around reproductive justice is set within a history of an intentional and systematic effort to reduce and eventually eliminate the number of Puerto Rican children born. I'm not saying that, had I known this, I would have come to a different decision. But having this knowledge about my people, my community, would have informed my decision in a much more nuanced way, that might have considered having a child as a revolutionary act of resistance against colonial erasure. And every reproductive decision made by Puerto Rican women has to be informed by this history and a heightened sense of communal accountability and wisdom. The ancestors are still speaking to us.

I don't disagree with the fundamentals of reproductive justice as a movement; yet, these communal factors of moral decision-making need to be more explicit because my culture and experience require that I make room for the ancestors (which includes our history) to speak to us; we are still accountable to them. I am accountable to them.

I am also accountable to the two angels who are with me always. One is of the child who, had I carried him/her to term, would be a 31-year-old adult with their own life, loves and dreams. That loss was experienced in the sterile technology of an abortion clinic, where the only things I recall were the blurred outline of the anesthesiologist and the uncontrollable chills I felt as I lay in the recovery room. The other is the child whose undeveloped body I held in my hands as I knelt in the pool of my own blood on the bathroom floor during the summer of 2001. He (because we knew at that point we were having a boy) would have just completed his sophomore year of college, and be considering next steps for the future. I won't forget these two, one voluntary and one involuntary but both described using the same word: abortion. The categories of liberal tolerance and conservative Catholicism are both too limited to do their lives and their deaths justice. The movement for reproductive justice, as a third way, has its own lacuna. So I'll continue to struggle, praying for grace and forgiveness that extends beyond all categories. Because so many lives are at stake, not the least of which is my own.

Note

1. Iris López, *Matters of Choice: Puerto Rican Women's Struggle for Reproductive Freedom* (New Brunswick: Rutgers University Press, 2008), 7.

2

In the Shade of Allah's Mercy

Anonymous

In this essay, a Muslim woman, married and a mother of two, grapples with becoming pregnant again when she is already struggling with existing family and graduate school obligations. She is an observant *hijabi* (she wears a *hijab*, or head covering) who follows a spiritual Sufi path. She describes her abortion decision-making, which in her case involved study of religious texts and the support of her husband and her *shaykh* (Muslim spiritual mentor). The essay reveals how understanding religious teachings about abortion is only one dimension of a believer's abortion experience.

I am a Muslim woman and I recently chose to have an abortion. I consider my religion to be one of the defining aspects of my life. I am an active member of the community in which I live, particularly in the area of women's education and empowerment. I am a wife and a mother of two little girls, both of whom I am still nursing while pursuing a post-graduate degree in Islamic Studies. My husband and I plan to have more children in the future, God Willing. . . .

Having gone through the termination of a pregnancy, I am by no means promoting abortion as a routine means of contraception, even while I uphold at the same time women's reproductive autonomy. However, with personal knowledge now that pregnancies that are unintended and unplanned do happen and that contraception can fail, I know too that under particular circumstances, Islam does and should permit abortion. It is these particular circumstances that I focus on.

. . .

Source: Anonymous, "In the Shade of Allah's Mercy: Reflections on Islam, Embodiment and Abortion," *Journal for Islamic Studies* 33 (2013): 204–15.

I became pregnant by accident at a time when another pregnancy or baby would have been very difficult; both physically and emotionally I was not ready for either. I reflected and meditated for days over the decision to terminate the pregnancy. As a student in a *madrasa* (religious seminary) for girls, I had studied the *fiqh* (Islamic law) on pregnancy and women's bodies but at the time had done so as a neutral observer, hardly imagining it had anything to do with me. I never envisaged that one day *I* would find myself agonising over the ethical and spiritual dimensions of the rulings on abortion and my reproductive body, written by men centuries earlier.

I consider myself pro-choice when it comes to the female body—to an extent. That extent is determined by the Divine Hand which guides us as human beings but all the while allows us to make choices, a faculty which we alone as children of Adam and Eve have been granted.

As a pro-choice feminist and a deeply religious Muslim, arriving at a decision to terminate the pregnancy was thus doubly difficult for me. The academic in me researched every aspect of abortion to a fine degree, from medical and health perspectives to the views of different Islamic schools of thought. In fact, I even poured over the diverse standpoints of other religions, interrogating the issue from both feminist and traditional lenses of women from diverse cultures. Wrestling with this monumental personal decision forced me to scrutinise and reflect closely on the convictions I professed to hold. I realised that despite years of study and work experience in women's rights, the effects of the early socialisation I had experienced as a girl in a conservative Muslim community, which controlled, negated and commoditised the female body and sexuality, was still deeply embedded in my unconscious.

In beginning to consider the choice of abortion, I looked first to the law. Islamic law makes allowances for abortion up to 16 weeks into the pregnancy, and beyond if the mother's life is put to risk by the pregnancy. The Prophet Muhammad (pbuh) said,

> Verily, each of you is gathered together in his mother's womb for forty days, in the form of a drop of fluid. Then it is a clinging object for a similar period. Thereafter, it is a lump looking like it has been chewed for a similar period. The angel is then sent to him [the foetus] and breathes into him the spirit.[1]

Based on this *hadith*, classical scholars theorised that ensoulment occurs between three to four months in-utero and thus built their rulings on abortion on this timeframe. The views of the different schools of thought differ considerably as regards when and why abortion is permissible, ranging from outright prohibition to neutral permissibility. I was raised and schooled in what is considered the most liberal of the legal schools on this issue, the Hanafi *madhhab*. This school allows abortion at any time before 120 days after conception, with some scholars even ruling that it can be performed without a specific reason or the permission of the pregnant woman's husband, while other jurists require a reasonable justification.

. . .

My preliminary research reassured me that at only six weeks pregnant I was clearly far from the stage of ensoulment by the standards of classical Muslim jurists. And being in a devoted monogamous marriage, having undergone a miscarriage, pregnancy and childbirth already, I was not someone capriciously choosing abortion as a means of contraception.

. . .

During the time I spent contemplating my decision, one of the Quranic verses I meditated on extensively was "Allah knows what every female carries and what the wombs lose or exceed. And everything with Him is by due balance" (Q. 13:8). I was so desperately seeking balance in my life, balance between work, spirituality, motherhood, marriage and community service, that I found comfort in this verse, which emphasised for me that true balance rests only with God. Therefore, whatever my decision, it was already known, already part of the Divine grand scheme of my life.

. . .

When my husband and I began to discuss this immensely important decision, he jolted me to self-realisation by pointing out something I had not considered. He believed that for me to choose termination was actually the more difficult decision, the struggle or the *jihād* as he put it, because ending my pregnancy would mean reversing years of social conditioning which I had so long fought against. So, together we came to the agonising decision to terminate my six-week pregnancy. I could not have made this decision without my husband's full support and compassion every step of the way.

. . .

In my reading about abortion, I became alarmed at the lack of support available to women facing the question of unplanned pregnancies both in the virtual and material Muslim communities. . . . I turned to two people for whom I have profound respect and love. The first is a professor of Islamic Studies whose work informs much of my own gender sensitivities. I presented her with my dilemma, and after a thoughtful pause, she replied, "whatever emerges as your and your husband's joint decision, [if] you have both made [it] with a sincere, prayerful and surrendered intention, [it] will be best.

Keep in your heart's eye that surrender to Allah is not always conforming to either established notions or even your own intellectual notions."

. . .

The second person whom I approached for advice was my *Shaykh*, someone for whom the title "scholar" is inadequate in describing the depth and breadth of his knowledge and spirit. . . . I confessed to him the reasons for considering a termination shortly before the procedure. I had not realized the disquietude in my soul over this decision until he comforted me and I felt the anxiety leaving my spirit.

. . .

The abortion itself was relatively painless, with only minor cramping, discomfort and bleeding. While undergoing the procedure, I found my thoughts automatically turning to women who do not have access to safe, medically sound contraception and pregnancy termination options, women who are forced to resort to untrained practitioners who use dangerous herbs, chemicals and instruments to induce abortion, risking these women's lives, health and future fertility options in the process. I realised how fortunate I am to live in a country where both my reproductive and religious rights are enshrined in its Constitution.

. . .

The process of ending a pregnancy is indeed that—a process. Post-abortion recovery is as important, particularly in coming to terms with the decision on the emotional and spiritual planes of being. I am comforted by knowing that I have a most-Compassionate, Loving God to turn to, a God whose love is described as more than a mother's love for her children. As a mother myself, I am in awe of the intensity of such love and my inner-being is replenished by it, allowing me to be at peace with myself and my decisions. I remain perpetually in the shade of Allah's mercy, accountable to Allah alone for my actions.

Note

1. Muslim ibn al-Hajjaj, *Sabi Muslim*, Vol. 6 (Darus Salaam Publications: London, 2007).

3

Reproducing Justice

Kate Ott

A professor of ethics at Drew University Theological School, Kate Ott also has extensive experience in the nonprofit sector as an educator on issues of sexual health, youth faith development, and sex education in religious communities. Ott speaks personally in this excerpt about her Roman Catholic background, her academic interests, and a devastating prenatal test result of a severe fetal abnormality that was discovered in a planned pregnancy.

For me, growing up Roman Catholic was a source of pride and confusion. In my middle and high school years, I realized we were to feed the hungry, clothe the naked, and aid the sick but never raise questions about gender or sexuality. Why was there controversy over the girl altar servers? Why were only the boys questioned about their future careers and encouraged to participate in Church leadership? Why were girls to guard themselves from sex and protect their virginity from boys? How come there were so few scripture lessons about women? Why couldn't women be ordained? The deepest and most meaningful parts of my Catholic faith experience—service to those in need, community building, and rigorous education—seemed to be in opposition to what was being promoted related to sexuality and gender. What I hadn't realized was that asking too many questions and not accepting the prescribed answers would push me further from the institutional church and deeper into theological snares.

Source: Kate Ott, "Reproducing Justice," in *Women, Religion, and Revolution*, ed. Gina Messina-Dysert and Xochitl Alvizo (Cambridge, MA: Feminist Studies in Religion), 59–65.

As I studied more and moved further to the margins of Roman Catholic communities, I found that sexuality and gender raised very volatile issues that could not be resolved. Love, it seemed, was not simple, nor were the relationships that surrounded it. My questions became more complex, mostly in response to the suffering and pain I witnessed within my family and by my friends; family structures challenged by interracial dating, a son or daughter coming out as gay, out-of-wedlock pregnancies, and abortion. I realized I had only imprecise language and categories, limited by what the Roman Catholic Church had provided, for my questions regarding sexuality, gender, relationships, and so on. It was as if sexuality was a trap and no one I knew could escape being a sinner in the eyes of the Church.

In my own faith development, I began to recognize how Church doctrines about family and marriage perpetuated exclusion, shame, and gendered double standards. In college, conversations in women and gender studies helped me uncover systemic sexism and its relationship to other oppressions like racism and classism. I learned about my own privilege as well as the damages I had suffered to my body image and self-confidence as a woman. Yet, feminism without religion felt like living free in a foreign land— exciting, eye-opening, and not quite right. Then, I found feminist theology and ethics. These writings respond to the very same issues I found myself struggling to reconcile. They uncover the intersections of religious patriarchy and systemic oppression in an effort to identify liberatory needs in our current world. They often compare the lived reality of the faithful and the power of the church hierarchy to show the diversity and struggle of living out faith values in an institutional religion while also creating new spaces for reinterpretation of harmful teachings. Some make arguments on behalf of women's ordination. Others offer feminist interpretations of the Bible, including outright condemnation of those passages that are death-dealing to women. Still others concentrate on engaging the sexual ethics of the hierarchy and making room for women's lived experiences as resources for theological reflection.

Indeed, much of my personal experience has helped me better understand the everyday sexuality and reproductive health struggles that women of faith face. Months into my marriage and the start of my theological education, I became pregnant. Twenty weeks into the pregnancy, we were given a diagnosis of abnormal development and fetal demise. After a battery of tests, we had three options: abortion by dilation and curettage, abortion by inducing early delivery, or just waiting for fetal death to occur and risking toxicity to my body. Not only was I emotionally blindsided but I was morally torn. I supported better access to health care, sexuality education, and antipoverty initiatives to help reduce teen pregnancy but didn't think mothers who intentionally became pregnant faced abortion decisions. To be handed a piece of paper that read "Sign here: I agree to have an abortion" shook me theologically.

In my soul-searching discernment, I had many conversations with my husband, friends, and Roman Catholic spiritual advisors. These advisors told me the truth about the Church's teaching. They told me that the final choice was mine and should be based on my conscience. That no priest or religious leader could know what was in my conscience and that Church teachings had developed over time and always needed to be put into pastoral context to promote the flourishing of humanity not the destruction or harm of lives and relationships. I knew what had to be done in order to bring closure, dignity, and safety. I signed the paper and consented to abortion.

I know this story can be seen as one of the medical reasons for abortion that people dismiss as "not what they are talking about" when it comes to abortion debates. Some will claim it was not actually abortion because the procedure was aiming at saving my life and preserving the dignity of the fetus. Whatever rhetorical hoops we jump through, the reality is not all abortions are the same. Regardless, we should always trust women's moral agency to make such decisions. The Roman Catholic tradition values conscience in moral decision making. Conscience is not a "gut reaction"; conscience is well formed through relationship and personal experience and informed by Church teachings and wider bodies of knowledge. The Church says that we are required to follow our conscience, first and foremost in moral decisions. Had I not learned about the Catholic tradition of conscience and had faithful guides to assist me in forming my decision, I would have thought the Church disowned me. I grieved the loss of that pregnancy, but never once have I felt that God did not support me in my decision. Loving oneself as one's neighbor often makes for very complex moral decisions. Many women face a similar decision, often without the same access to health care or relational support that I had, believing their faith communities will condemn and expel them. Women deserve to be valued equally to men in their ability to make moral decisions in the best interest of their lives and that of their current and future families.

4

Christ Was There for Me during My Abortion

CoWanda Rusk

CoWanda Rusk published the article from which this story was taken while serving as a leader with Youth Testify, a collaborative online site that supports young people who have abortions. Rusk speaks about how her Christian faith helped her through the process of obtaining legal access to abortion care as a minor by means of judicial bypass when parental involvement was not an option. She publishes on various social media platforms and continues to be active working for reproductive health, reproductive justice, and the liberation and sovereignty of Black and Indigenous peoples globally.

Christ told me that having an abortion was the right decision for me.

I know this isn't something that people hear often, but given that a majority of abortion patients are religious, I suspect it's true for a lot of those who choose the procedure. Religion and abortion have always been pitted against one another, but as a 17-year-old high-school senior when I learned I was pregnant, I was already praying about my future as I filled out college applications, asking where God was going to lead me.

Society tells women in a million small ways that mothering is our natural role, but I knew that I could not have a baby. Several of my friends were teenage mothers, so I knew they would be there for me if I continued the pregnancy; as it turned out, they were also there for me when I told them that I wanted to terminate it. But as a teen, I didn't have access to the resources

---

Source: CoWanda Rusk [Co Jackson], "Christ Was There for Me during My Abortion," *Bitchmedia*, March 25, 2019.

I needed. My school had information and resources for teen parenting, but not abortion—and I knew next to nothing about them.

I also wasn't ready to tell my family about either the pregnancy or my choice to end it. But Texas requires parental consent for people under 18 to get an abortion. *Roe v. Wade* made abortion legal, but 38 states require minors to notify or obtain consent from their parents—and for many of us this isn't possible, and poses a huge and often dangerous barrier to our Constitutional rights. One of my friends explained that I could petition for a judicial bypass, meaning I would have to go to court and get a judge to sign off on the procedure. . . .

A friend told me about Jane's Due Process, a Texas organization that helps young people go through the judicial-bypass process. (It's named for "Jane Doe," the anonymous identifier given to young people going through a judicial bypass process.) After waiting a few days, I called.

A woman named Tina made me feel safe almost as soon as she picked up the phone, asking me a series of questions to better understand my case. When had I found out I was pregnant? Was I experiencing pain? How was my relationship with my parents? How was I feeling emotionally? I appreciated her motherly compassion. Shortly after talking to Tina, I met with a lawyer who interviewed me and helped me put my case together. Part of this process involved preparing information about my medical history and my grades, and explaining why I needed an abortion and couldn't go to my parents for permission.

It's a weird feeling to try to put forth the best version of yourself for a stranger just so you can go see a doctor. Again, I turned to Christ for support: "*Hey, God: You know, if this is something you don't want me to do, don't let it happen.*" But God meets you where you are, and it did happen. From there, the doors just opened: From having my friends support me to getting the text with the phone number for Jane's Due Process, it was clear that God provided for me, offering me a way forward when I thought I had nothing. . . .

Sometimes people ask how I can be a follower of Christ and have an abortion. My response is that God is a God of love, and if you know that then you've answered your own question. God is the ultimate author of our lives, and I had an abortion as a believer of God because He planned it, so that I could stand for His people and people like me. Anything that involves people getting the love and the care they deserve is something that He would be a part of, and God was with me . . . through the entire decision.

Now that I'm back in school, I mentor other Janes going through the experience of judicial bypass, and I believe it's all according to God's plan. Recently I've had several people in my life turn to me when they were deciding to have abortions, and I was able to both support them emotionally and direct them to our local abortion fund for financial help. I believe that God has set me on this path to be a resource and support for others.

Not long ago, I was thanking Christ for my abortion. I was praising God for my abortion. Some people no doubt feel that I didn't make the right choice, but for me it was the foundation from which to start a new relationship, and strengthen the one I have with my family.

5

Lo Teivoshi, You Will Not Feel Ashamed

Rachael Pass

In this original piece Rachael Pass shares her reflections about her experience of an unplanned pregnancy while she was a rabbinical student at Hebrew Union College-Jewish Institute of Religion. Her reflections center the role that Judaism played in her experience of pregnancy, her moral decision to end the pregnancy, and how she navigated the complicated feelings she had associated with the termination. Pass went on to write her rabbinic thesis related to this experience, "*B'chesed Uv'rachamim*: How Creative Jewish Rituals Theologize Abortion," and serves as an associate rabbi at the T'Shuvah Center in Brooklyn. She has written extensively on Jewish views of abortion, creative Jewish rituals including reclaiming *mikveh*, and feminist Jewish thought and Goddess-concepts.

The story of my pregnancy and abortion happened while I was in rabbinical school. Much of my experience terminating my pregnancy intertwines with my journey towards becoming a rabbi; therefore, my experience of my abortion is a deeply Jewish one. I conceived one month into my second year of rabbinical school at Hebrew Union College-Jewish Institute of Religion. I had just moved to Manhattan after a year of living and learning in Jerusalem. I was working my first High Holy Day pulpit in a small college town, where a dear friend of mine had grown up. He flew to his hometown for Rosh Hashanah to watch me lead services for the first time as a rabbinic presence. That night, the night between days one and two of Rosh Hashanah, underneath the tiniest sliver of the new moon of Tishrei, we had sex. I conceived.

Twenty-three days later, sitting in my introductory Talmud course, I took a sip of my smoothie and felt immediately nauseated. I rushed to the bathroom and vomited. I knew why. Tuesday, in my Hebrew Grammar and Literature course, I had an intense craving for pickles on pizza. Thursday, in *shacharit* (morning services), I prayed to the sound of Dan Nichols' voice, a guest service song leader who I have known since I was a young child. And on Friday morning, Rosh Chodesh Cheshvan (the new moon), I peed on a small plastic stick. When it read positive, I uttered the blessing "*asher yatzar et ha'adam b'chochmah*, who has created the human body with wisdom." That night, I attended a required class Shabbaton (Shabbat retreat) and I prayed with my whole body, soul, being to the harmonic, dissonant sounds of our community's voices. I called the would-be father, I called my mother, and I called my rabbinic mentor, the only three people I would tell before making my decision. They all said the same wonderful, horrible thing: "I'll support you no matter what, but the decision is ultimately yours."

I spent the next two weeks researching midwives in Manhattan. I made a pros and cons list, which is still saved in my Google Drive. I scrolled through every picture of every friend's baby on Facebook. I discovered Planned Parenthood is right down the street from HUC-JIR. I read every Jewish legal and nonlegal text on abortion. I found myself focusing on the one published ritual for someone having an abortion that I could find, a *mikveh* (ritual bath) ceremony written by Rabbi Tamar Duvdevani. I didn't tell anyone else I was pregnant. I continued to vomit constantly. I basically stopped eating, because every time I ate anything, it came back up. I was very sick. I wanted a baby; I did not want a baby. I felt like my queer identity would be entirely erased in having conceived through heterosexual sex. It was the first semester of second year, and I had midterms to complete. I got A's on all of them. I turned them all in on time. I didn't skip a single class.

My friends were clearly worried about me, but I knew as soon as I told someone else I was pregnant, they would have a reaction or an opinion that might affect what I would do. I needed to make this decision on my own. It was so lonely. But it was the only way I felt I could ensure that I had autonomy over my decision. I eventually decided that I could not raise a child in Manhattan, that I could not be a mostly single mother while studying full-time to be a rabbi.

On a Thursday afternoon, at eight weeks and six days pregnant, I made the short walk from HUC-JIR to the Margaret Sanger Planned Parenthood. I listened to Debbie Friedman's "Sow in Tears," on repeat in my headphones, willing the words to be true: "those who sow, who sow in tears, will reap in joy, will reap in joy. . . ." I thought about my mother, and how she volunteered at Planned Parenthood in graduate school. I thought about my grandmother, who wrote a PhD dissertation on the language of *Roe v. Wade*, only for it to be rejected for espousing a pro-choice stance. I thought about my schooling, my work, my calling, and I chose to prioritize my own life, as we are taught to do in Mishnah Ohalot 7:6 "*chayeiha kodmin l'chayyav*, the life of the [pregnant person] takes precedence over the life of [the fetus]." When I took the Mifepristone pill, I whispered again the blessing for my body. The next night, while holding the four Misoprostol pills in the corners of my mouth, I live-streamed a Shabbat service from bed, humming along to the insistence in Lecha Dodi, "*lo teivoshi*, you will not feel ashamed." The next evening, still bleeding, I did *havdalah*, the ritual for ending Shabbat.

Two weeks later, I took a printed copy of the *mikveh* ritual that I had found with me to ImmerseNYC, a liberal *mikveh* project on the Upper West Side. I performed the ritual, singing to myself as I bathed in the healing waters. The next morning, some of my classmates and closest friends joined me in completing the ritual, by dipping a challah that I had baked into some honey to symbolize future sweetness. I repeated the words I had prayed over and over again, "*hazorim b'dimah b'rinah yoktzoru*, those who sow in tears will reap in joy."

Over the next few months, I compiled a list of verses from Tanakh which I turned into my own sort of prayer. Every day for the months leading up to what would have been my due date, I prayed these verses as a way to recognize my prolonged grief, joy, and healing. I used that ritual as a way to check in with myself, to notice the emotions I continued to feel and the changes in my beliefs about my abortion over time. These two rituals, the *mikveh* ritual and my ongoing prayer, provided a space for me to express my experience. I eventually wrote my rabbinical thesis on the subject of creative Jewish rituals for people who have had abortions, and now write and speak on the subject around the country. Each time I teach about abortion and ritual, I end with the same profound truth: my abortion was a blessing in my life, and my Judaism embraces blessing.

6

You're the Only One I've Told

"Alex" (with Meera Shah)

This narrative is co-written by "Alex" (a pseudonym) and Meera Shah, an Indian American abortion care physician, who collaborated with a number of interviewees to tell their abortion stories. In this excerpt, Alex describes their experience of navigating an unwanted high school pregnancy as a genderqueer Christian who had been raised in a prolife context.

Alex had plans, big plans. They were going to become a writer, penning screenplays for TV shows and indie movies. They were creative and loved the arts from the very beginning. "I was a marching band nerd—I played French horn in my high school's marching band," Alex told me. But most of all, they were going to get the hell out of Iowa.

As a kid, Alex had lived with their parents and two siblings in Los Angeles. But when they were nine years old, Alex and the family relocated to the land of corn dogs, cornfields, and conservatives—a six-thousand-person town where the fanciest restaurant was a Famous Dave's Barbecue and the cutest boy was the son of a Pentecostal minister.

. . .

Alex did their best to fit in, dating bland boys and echoing the rhetoric of religious conservatism that seemed to be swirling around everywhere. And back then, Alex didn't have much reason to think any differently from the people around them. Not about Jesus, or church, or abortion. "I was one of those obnoxious, pro-life vegetarians who didn't want anything to die." Still,

Source: "Alex," with Meera Shah, "Alex," in *You're the Only One I've Told: The Stories behind Abortion*, ed. Meera Shah (Chicago: Chicago Review Press, 2020), 79–90.

none of it felt right—too baggy, as Alex likes to say. A pair of pants that didn't quite fit. Alex is a genderqueer person who uses they/them pronouns.

. . .

The term *transgender*, or *trans*, means that an individual's gender identity is different from the sex they were assigned at birth. *Cisgender*, often shortened to cis, means that an individual's gender identity is the same as the sex they were assigned at birth. One's gender can also fall on a spectrum and some people identify as nonbinary, genderqueer, or gender expansive. Gender identity is not related to sexual orientation. In other words, one's gender identity does not determine who they are attracted to or have sex with.

. . .

During the fall of their junior year, Alex's parents split up for good. Alex stayed in Iowa with their dad and had a front-row seat to his slow unraveling. In the sixteen-year-old parlance of the time, there was only one way to put it: It sucked.

Luckily, there was Brandon.

Brandon was the distraction Alex needed—a warm body to collapse into when everything in their world felt like it was crashing down. Alex's boyfriend Brandon was safe, albeit a bit boring. Though the sex wasn't great, it helped to make Alex feel less alone. And though they'd been together for two years, Alex admits that there wasn't love there. "I just wanted to feel close to someone. I clung to this relationship as a lifeboat."

. . .

Their homecoming, like so many others, was in the high school cafeteria. "My friend's parents were the DJs and there were these strobe lights going." It was a warm fall night when Alex got pregnant—Brandon had just driven them home, and they had sex standing up between a pair of parked cars in the driveway . . . Sure enough, a few weeks later when their period didn't arrive as expected, a deep hollow of fear started to tunnel within Alex's gut. They needed to take a pregnancy test, fast. While on their way to Famous Dave's Barbecue, Alex asked Brandon to stop at a grocery store for a snack. A silly request in retrospect, but it worked. Not wanting to wait, Alex took the test right there in the store.

. . .

Up until now, Alex would have considered themself to be pro-life. It was conservative Iowa, right in the middle of the Bible Belt, and the thought that they'd be "killing a baby" by getting an abortion was something that passed through their mind. "I was so ashamed," Alex said. "And it felt like everything around me was dying: my grandmother was dying of cancer, my parents' marriage had just fallen apart, and I was sixteen, so everything was like, double huge." Add to that an unintended pregnancy, a seismic shift of their life in which all of the things they'd dreamt about would be pushed altogether out of reach.

. . .

Getting pregnant brought them out of that fog very rapidly.

"I felt so sad that I had to make this decision. I knew what I had to do, I just didn't want to have to do it. There was no doubt in my mind that I was going to have an abortion, even though I felt riddled with guilt about it and felt pressure from my boyfriend's parents. They would call me and tell me not to kill the baby, not to kill their grandchild." But Alex had to do what was right for them.

. . .

Alex found that having an abortion had an unintended side effect: it made them crave community and solace in the idea that there is something out there that's bigger than all of us. "I wasn't a freaky Jesus kid, but I've always been a very spiritual person. I got to a point when things were really falling apart, with the divorce and with the abortion, where I started getting like 'U2 Christian,' that God was way bigger than anything I could imagine. Bigger than gender, bigger than race, bigger than sexuality. I would go to youth group every week."

More than anything though, Alex said that feeling part of a community was what it took to make them feel like they were forgiven. "God understands my situation," Alex said. I hear echoes of similar feelings from my patients. The same religion that gave them complex feelings of guilt and shame around abortion is often the same religion that provides them with comfort after. "It was the first time that I'd ever experienced something that was truly that controversial. So the first time I experienced something like that, it really opens up your human capacity and different things that can happen to you," they said.

These days, Alex is thinking about getting pregnant with their husband, Kyle. "I'm really excited about pregnancy," they say, to know what it feels like to be pregnant with a baby they actually want. But finding the right ob-gyn who can adeptly handle genderqueer pregnancy and birth has been a challenge.

. . .

"I don't want my body to be explained to me by a man," Alex stressed. "I won't see male doctors anymore and I specifically seek out female and femme doctors who mention pronouns in their bios.

"I can always tell that someone is on my team when they're emailing and they have a pronoun in their signature. It's like a little wave that says they'll be open," Alex explained.

Part 2

Social-Scientific Studies

Introduction to Part 2

Developing a nuanced and informed public conversation about a contemporary social problem requires attention to a wide range of sources and information that can offer insight into the topic from a wide variety of perspectives. Part 1 of this volume began with the voices and stories of individual people who have terminated pregnancies. In Part 2, we turn from stories to data. Chapters in this section allow readers to see a variety of ways in which the issue of abortion is being studied by scholars and how these studies can contribute to public understanding of this social issue.

There are three key ways that the social-scientific research collected here contributes to a more robust public conversation about abortion and religion. First, social-scientific research can help correct and dispel deep-seated stereotypes and assumptions associated with abortion and can document the very real harm that results from abortion stigma. This research can also be used to shape more effective social and public policy that helps address the real problems that people face in their reproductive lives, and it can be used to improve healthcare and access to healthcare. There are several respected research centers that carefully study and collect data about abortion and contraception such as the Guttmacher Institute, Advancing New Standards in Reproductive Health (ANSIRH), and IPAS. The first three articles in this section offer information from research studies with women who have abortions—studies that complement and deepen the individual stories found in Part 1.

Two essays (Biggs et al.; Cockrill and Nack) provide significant data in the American context to show the predominance of economic stresses as an influence, the pervasiveness of concern about being a good enough mother, and the detrimental effects of abortion stigma. Contrary to misogynous myths about women who terminate a pregnancy as selfish, callous, or ignorant, these studies demonstrate that women who have an abortion seriously weigh a number of personal, social, and religious factors in deciding to terminate a pregnancy. Based on this data, most pregnant people take this process seriously, with concern for themselves, their other dependents, and the welfare of a potential child. However, most social scientists are not trained in religious studies, and attention to religion can be incidental in studies that originate from the perspective of fields like sociology or public health.

The second way that the articles in this section contribute is by educating people about religion and religious difference and demonstrating the role that religion plays in people's lives, attitudes, and decision-making. Such information can prove useful to a variety of constituencies, including healthcare workers, counselors, religious leaders, and even family and friends of people who have abortions. These studies can help us complicate stereotypical understanding of how religious authority functions and what it means to talk about lived religion or the ways in which religious people interpret, understand, and embody their faith. For example, while ultra-Orthodox Jewish women often invoke God's will as a reason not to terminate a pregnancy after an adverse prenatal diagnosis, the qualitative study by Teman et al. indicates that these women are aware that they could, if they wished, petition their rabbi for permission for an abortion—and receive it. A small but diverse study (Wiebe et al.) shows that devout Canadian Muslim women experienced feelings of guilt even while they felt that they were religiously permitted to have their abortion. The mixture of guilt and religiosity can also be found in an American study of women who reflect on which procedure to use to terminate a pregnancy because of severe fetal anomaly (Kerns et al.).

The last three articles in this section demonstrate the third way that this volume contributes to the public understanding of abortion and religion. All of the lead authors of these articles are trained in sociology or the sociology of religion, and these studies show how focused attention to the complicated combination of ethnicity, national origin, political party, and religion offers a more nuanced view of how religion and religious beliefs intersect with other identity markers and ideological frames. The work of PRRI (Jones et al.) offers a detailed and potentially surprising snapshot of religious people's attitudes toward legal access to abortion care. This information is particularly important in a cultural landscape with a dominant public perception that religions and religious people oppose abortion. The final two articles (Bartkowski et al.; Wu & Ida) illustrate the important point that diversity of opinion exists within most religious communities. Diversity of opinion exists within Latinx Catholic communities as well as Protestant. The same diversity is found among Asian American Christians.

Many people reduce the relationship of religion and abortion to the normative positions they hear in their places of worship or in discourses that dominate news cycles. However, even these religious positions are rarely developed apart from some understanding of or assumptions about the societal context in which unplanned or crisis pregnancies occur. Theologians and ethicists, however, are usually not also social scientists, and their abortion positions may not always be informed by the facts on the ground. While sociologists, anthropologists, clinical researchers, and other scientists provide crucial qualitative and quantitative analyses that can fill this knowledge gap, there is still a dearth of critically informed religious studies scholarship that thoughtfully interrogates the biases that some religious thinkers might have about the person who gets an abortion and why. The essays in this section give data and analyses about the real-life cultural factors and dynamics that affect pregnant women. Particularly given the outsized role that religion plays in shaping public attitudes about abortion, we believe that theo-ethical thinking on reproductive issues should be supported and expanded by social-scientific researchers and funders.

As you read the essays in this section, we encourage you to consider the following:

1. There are many ways to study a topic. Try to identify what kinds of questions social-scientific research helps us ask and answer. Why and how are these questions important as we consider how to reframe the public conversation about abortion in the United States?

2. What did you learn about abortion decision-making from these studies, and how does that reinforce or challenge how you think about abortion?

3. Several of these articles illustrate the breadth of diversity within religious communities and traditions. What have you learned about religious authority? How does the concept of lived religion impact how you think about abortion? How do religious attitudes and beliefs intersect with and impact other identities and experiences? Why and how are these insights important in developing a deeper understanding of abortion and religion in public life?

7

Understanding Why Women Seek Abortions in the United States

M. Antonia Biggs, Heather Gould, and

Diana Greene Foster

Biggs, Gould, and Foster are part of the collaborative research group ANSIRH (Advancing New Standards in Reproductive Health) at Bixby Center for Global Reproductive Health, University of California, San Francisco. This study draws on the qualitative and quantitative data from the Turnaway Study, a major study that documents what happened to patients who were "turned away" from clinics because they had passed the gestational age set for abortions at that facility. This paper offers a comprehensive overview of the variety and complexity of issues that factor into women's abortion decision-making and is particularly insightful due to the large sample size and the methodological decision to ask open-ended questions rather than limiting reasons by offering options for people to choose.

Background

While the topic of abortion has long been the subject of fierce public and policy debate in the United States, an understanding of why women seek abortion has been largely missing from the discussion [1]. In an effort to maintain

Source: M. Antonia Biggs, Heather Gould, and Diana Greene Foster, "Understanding Why Women Seek Abortions in the US," *BMC Women's Health* 13, no. 1 (2013): 1–13.

privacy, adhere to perceived social norms, and shield themselves from stigma, the majority of American women who have had abortions— approximately 1.21 million women per year [2]–do not publicly disclose their abortion experiences or engage in policy discussions as a represented group [3-5].

. . .

A description of study participants is presented in Table 1.

. . .

Reasons for Abortion

Women gave a wide range of responses to explain why they had chosen abortion. The reasons were comprised of 35 themes which were categorized under a final set of 11 overarching themes (Table 2). While most women gave reasons that fell under one (36%) or two (29%) themes, 13% mentioned four or more themes. Many women reported multiple reasons for seeking an abortion crossing over several themes. As one 21year-old woman describes, *"This is how I described it [my reasons for abortion] to my doctor 'social, economic', I had a whole list, I don't feel like I could raise a child right now and give the child what it deserves."* A 19-year old explains *"[There are] so many of them [reasons]. I already have one baby, money wise, my relationship with the father of my first baby, relationship with my mom, school."* A 27-year old enumerates the reasons that brought her to the decision to have an abortion *"My relationship is newer and we wanted to wait. I don't have a job, I have some debt, I want to finish school and I honestly am not in the physical shape that I would want to be to start out a pregnancy."*

Financial Reasons

A financial reason (40%) was the most frequently mentioned theme. Six percent of women mentioned this as their only reason for seeking abortion. Most women (38%) cited general financial concerns which included responses such as *"financial problems," "don't have the means," "It all boils down to money"* and *"can't afford to support a child."* As one unemployed 42-year-old woman with a monthly household income of a little over $1,000 describes *"[It was] all financial, me not having a job, living off death benefits, dealing with my 14 year old son. I didn't have money to buy a baby spoon."*

Table 1 Participant characteristics (n=954)

Participant characteristics	N	%
Race/ethnicity		
White	353	37
Black	281	29
Hispanic/Latina	199	21
Other	121	13
Age group		
15–19[a]	173	18
20–24	345	36
25–34	365	38
35–46	71	7
Marital status		
single, never married	753	79
Married	86	9
separated, divorced, widowed	115	12
More than High-School education	450	47
Enough money in past month to meet basic needs	569	60
Received public assistance in past month	428	45
Employed	507	53
Gestational age at interview		
<=13 weeks	393	41
14-19 weeks	136	14
20+ weeks	425	45
Pregnancy intentions (mean)	954	2.7
Parity (mean)	943	1.27
Nulliparous	359	38
baby under one	101	11
1+ previous births, no new baby	233	24
2+ previous births, no new baby	261	27
Has a health care provider	422	45
History of depression or anxiety diagnosis	260	27
Self-rated health good/very good	775	81

[a]This age category includes one participant aged 14 who was recruited early in the study before the minimum enrollment age was changed to 15.

Table 2 Major themes and reasons women gave for seeking abortion (n=954)

	Freq.	Percent
Not financially prepared	386	40%
General financial	365	38%
Unemployed/underemployed	41	4%
Uninsured or can't get welfare	6	0.60%
Don't want government assistance	4	0.40%
Not the right time for a baby	347	36%
Bad timing/not ready/unplanned	321	34%
Too busy/not enough time	17	2%
Too old	16	2%
Partner related reasons	298	31%
Relationship is bad, poor and/or new	89	9%
Respondent wants to be married first/not a single mom	80	8%
Partner is not supportive	77	8%
Partner is wrong guy	61	6%
Partner does not want baby	29	3%
Partner is abusive	24	3%
Need to focus on other children	275	29%
Too soon after having had a child/busy enough with current children/have enough children right now	239	25%
Concern for other children she is rearing	51	5%
Interferes with future opportunities	194	20%
Interferes with educational plans	132	14%
Interferes with vocational plans	63	7%
Want better life for self/don't want to limit future opportunities	49	5%
Not emotionally or mentally prepared	180	19%
Health related reasons	114	12%
Concern for her own health	59	6%
Concern for the health of the fetus	51	5%
Drug, tobacco, or alcohol use	46	5%
Prescription drug (not illicit) or contraceptive use	14	1.50%
Want a better life for the baby than she could provide	119	12%
Want better life for baby	67	7%
Living or housing context not suitable for baby	46	5%
Lack of childcare or help from family to care for baby	13	1.40%

(Continued)

Table 2 (Continued)

	Freq.	Percent
Don't want her children to have a childhood like hers	5	0.50%
Not independent or mature enough for a baby	64	7%
Too young or immature	47	5%
Can't take care of self	12	1.30%
Too dependent on parents or others right now	9	0.90%
Influences from family or friends	48	5%
Would have a negative impact on family or friends	22	2%
Don't want others to know/worried others would judge	19	2%
Pressure from family or friends	11	1.20%
Don't want a baby or place baby for adoption	38	4%
Don't want a baby or don't want any children	33	3%
Don't want adoption	7	0.70%
Other	11	1.20%
Total	954	100%

Note: Respondents gave reasons under multiple themes and subthemes.

A small proportion of women (4%) stated that lack of employment or underemployment was a reason for seeking an abortion. A 28-year old college educated woman, receiving $1,750 a month in government assistance, looking for work, and living alone with her two children while her husband was away in the Air Force explains "*[My husband and I] haven't had jobs in awhile and I don't want to go back to living with other people. If we had another child it would be undue burden on our financial situation.*" Six (0.6%) women stated that their lack of insurance and/or inability to get government assistance contributed to their desire to terminate their pregnancies.

. . .

Not the Right Time for a Baby

Over one third (36%) of respondents stated reasons related to timing. Many women (34%) used phrasing such as "I wasn't ready", and "wasn't the right time." A 21-year old pointed to a number of reasons why she felt the timing of her pregnancy was wrong "Mainly I didn't feel like I was ready yet - didn't feel financially, emotionally ready. Due date was at the same time as my externship at school. Entering the workforce with a newborn would be difficult - I just wasn't ready yet." A small proportion of women described not having enough time or feeling too busy to have a baby (2%). A 25-year old looking for work, already raising a child, and who reported "rarely" having enough money to meet her basic living needs explains how she has "So many things going on now physically, emotionally, financially, pretty busy and can't handle anymore right now." Similarly, a 19-year old describes how she "didn't have time to go to the doctor to make sure everything is OK like I wanted to. So busy with school and work I felt it [having an abortion] would be the right thing to do until I really have time to have one [a child]." Few women described being too old to have a baby (2%).

. . .

Partner-related Reasons

Nearly one third (31%) of respondents gave partner-related reasons for seeking an abortion. Six percent mentioned partners as their only reason for seeking abortion. Partner-related reasons included not having a "good" or stable relationship with the father of the baby (9%), wanting to be married first (8%), not having a supportive partner (8%), being with the "wrong guy" (6%), having a partner who does not want the baby (3%), and having an abusive partner (3%). For a more extensive analysis of partner-related reasons for seeking an abortion see Chibber et al. [7].

Need to Focus on Other Children

The need to focus on other children was a common theme, mentioned by 29% of women. Six percent of women mentioned only this theme. The majority of these reasons (67%) were related to feeling overextended with current children *"I already had 2 kids and it would be really overwhelming. It's kind of hard to raise 2 kids by yourself,"* that the pregnancy was too soon after a previous child *"I have a 3-month-old already. If I had had that baby, he wouldn't even be one [year old by the time the baby came]"*, or simply not wanting any more children *"I just felt inadequate-I have a teenager and 2 pre-teens and I couldn't see starting over again."* A small proportion (5%) of women felt that having a baby at this time would have an adverse impact on her other children. *"I already have 5 kids; their quality of life would go down if I had another."* A 31-year-old with three children spoke of the need to focus on her sick child as a reason for seeking abortion *"My son was diagnosed with cancer. His treatment requires driving 10 hours and now we found out we need to go to New York for some of his treatment. The stress of that and that he relies on me."*

A New Baby Would Interfere with Future Opportunities

One in five women (20%) reported that they chose abortion because they felt a baby at this time would interfere with their future goals and opportunities in general (5%) or, more specifically, with school (14%) or career plans (7%). Usually the reasons were related to the perceived difficulty of continuing to advance educational or career goals while raising a baby: *"I didn't think I'd be able to support a baby and go to college and have a job."* states an 18-year old respondent in high school. A 21-year-old woman in college with no children explains that she *"Still want[s] to be able to do things like have a good job, finish school, and be stable."* Similarly, a 26-year old desiring to go back to college explains *"I wanted to finish school. I'd been waiting a while to get into the bachelor's program and I finally got it."* . . . A 21-one-year old holding two part-time jobs and raising two children states: *"I wouldn't be able to take the time off work. My work doesn't offer maternity leave and I have to work [to afford to live] here. If I took time off I would lose my job so there's just no way."*

. . .

Not Emotionally or Mentally Prepared

Nineteen percent of respondents (19%) described feeling emotionally or mentally unprepared to raise a child at this time. Respondents in this category were characterized by a feeling of exasperation and an inability to continue the pregnancy— *"I can't go through it"*, *"I just felt inadequate"*— or feeling a lack of mental strength to have the baby— *"[I am] not mentally stable to take that on"*, *"emotionally, I couldn't take care of another baby,"* and *"I couldn't handle it."* A 19-year old mother reporting a history of depression and physical abuse describes seeking an abortion because, *"I have a lot of problems- serious problems and so I'm not prepared for another baby."*

. . .

Health-related Reasons

Twelve percent of respondents (12%) mentioned health-related reasons ranging from concern for her own health (6%), health of the fetus (5%), drug, tobacco, or alcohol use (5%), and/or non-illicit prescription drug or birth control use (1%). Maternal health concerns included physical health issues that would be exacerbated by the pregnancy or due to the pregnancy itself, "*My bad back and diabetes, I don't think the baby would have been healthy. I don't think I would have been able to carry it to term*" as well as mental health concerns. Five percent of women (5%) chose abortion because they were concerned about the effects of their drug and/or alcohol use on the health of the fetus or on their ability to raise the child.

. . .

Want a Better Life for the Baby than She Could Provide

Twelve percent of women gave reasons for choosing abortion related to their desire to give the child a better life than she could provide. Responses related to generally wanting to give the child a better life (7%) were characterized by a concern for the child "*I'm afraid my kid will be suffering in this world*" and "*wouldn't have been good for me or the child,*" or a feeling of inadequacy to parent the child: "*I can't take care of a kid because I can barely take care of myself and I don't want to bring a child into the world when I'm unmarried and not ready.*" As reflected in this previous quote, sometimes statements stemmed from a desire for the baby to have a father, or the feeling that the father of the baby was not suitable. "*I didn't want to do it by myself. I couldn't and the man was abusive and horrible . . . I didn't want my kid to grow up with a father like that (knowing his father had left).*"

. . .

Approximately 5% of respondents explained that their living or housing context was not suitable for a baby and mentioned this as one of the reasons they chose abortion. According to a 22-year old who described herself as being unable to work, on welfare, and rarely having enough money to meet basic living needs: "*My mom pays my rent for me and where I live I can't have kids. I can't get anyone to rent to me because I have had an eviction and haven't had a steady job.*"

. . .

Lack of Maturity or Independence

Less than 7% of women explained that their reliance on others or lack of maturity was a reason for choosing abortion. Some women felt they were too young (5%), unable to take care of themselves (1%), or too reliant on others to raise this baby (1%). "*I'm not grown up enough to take care of another person. I can't take care of myself yet, let alone another person. I wouldn't want to bring a baby into this world with parents who aren't ready to be parents.*"

Influences from Friends and/or Family

Around 5% of women described a concern for, or influences from family or friends as a reason for seeking abortion. Two percent feared that having a baby would negatively impact their family or friends "*It would have been a strain on my family*" and a similar proportion (2%) didn't want others to know about their pregnancy or feared judgment or reaction from others. A 19-year old explains that the reason she chose abortion was because "*I was scared to go to my parents.*" Another woman feared what the family would think about her having a biracial child. A small minority reported influences or pressure from family or friends (n=11) as a reason for seeking abortion.

. . .

Don't Want a Baby or Place Baby for Adoption

Four percent (4%) of women gave reasons falling under the theme not wanting a baby or not wanting to place a baby for adoption. Three percent (3%) explained succinctly that they do not want a baby or don't want children "*I just didn't want any kids*", "*It [a baby] is something I just didn't want.*" A small number (n=7) mentioned adoption was not an option for them. As one 25-year old describes "*We are not really sure if we ever want kids. I don't think that I would be strong enough to give it up for adoption.*" Another respondent states that "*adoption isn't an option for me-so it was kind of a no brainer decision.*"

. . .

Discussion

. . .

As indicated by the differences we observed among women's reasons by individual characteristics, women seek abortion due to their unique circumstances, including their socioeconomic status, age, health, parity and marital status. Even with changes in the climate surrounding abortion and the shifting demographics of the women having abortions, the predominant reasons women gave for seeking abortion reflected those of previous studies [6]. Reasons related to timing, partners, and concerns for the ability to support the child and other dependents financially and emotionally were the most common reasons women gave for seeking an abortion, suggesting that abortion is often a decision driven by women's concerns for current and future children, family, as well as existing commitments and responsibilities. Some women held the belief that her unborn child deserves to be raised under better circumstances than she can provide at this time; in an environment where the child is financially secure and part of a stable and loving family. This intersection between abortion and motherhood is described qualitatively in a study by Jones and colleagues where women indicate that their abortion decisions are influenced by the idea that children deserve "ideal conditions of motherhood" [8]. Some women also seem to have internalized gendered norms that value women as self-denying and always thinking in the best interest of her children, over making self-interested decisions. Experiences of stigma, fear of experiencing stigma, or internalized stigma around her abortion may have prompted women to give more socially desirable responses to make her appear or feel selfless, to justify her abortion decision. Other studies have reported abortion-seeking women's fear of being judged as having made a selfish decision [9]. At the same time, some of the women seeking abortion in this study were aiming to secure themselves a better life and future-chances for a better job and a good education. These women may be more stigmatized than the former since they don't fall into a discourse of the selfless and all-sacrificing woman. In an effort not to further contribute to the abortion stigma in our culture, we must be careful not to use women's reasons for abortion as a way to rationalize or justify their abortions, but rather to better understand their experiences [10].

References

1. Herold S: The new public face of abortion: connecting the dots between abortion stories. In *RH Reality Check*; 2012. Available at: http://rhrealitycheck. org/article/2012/07/08/new-public-face-abortion-connecting-dots-between- abortion-stories/.
2. Jones RK, Kooistra K: Abortion incidence and access to services in the United States, 2008. *Perspect Sex Reprod Health* 2011, 43(1):41–50.
3. Kumar A, Hessini L, Mitchell EM: Conceptualising abortion stigma. *Cult Health Sex* 2009, 11(6):625–639.
4. Norris A, Bessett D, Steinberg JR, Kavanaugh ML, De Zordo S, Becker D: Abortion stigma: a reconceptualization of constituents, causes, and consequences. *Women's Health Issues* 2011, 21(3 Suppl):S49–S54.
5. Shellenberg KM, Moore AM, Bankole A, Juarez F, Omideyi AK, Palomino N, Sathar Z, Singh S, Tsui AO: Social stigma and disclosure about induced abortion: results from an exploratory study. *Glob Public Health* 2011, 6(Suppl 1):S111–S125.
6. Kirkman M, Rowe H, Hardiman A, Mallett S, Rosenthal D: Reasons women give for abortion: a review of the literature. *Arch Womens Ment Health* 2009, 12(6):365–378.
7. Chibber K, Gould H, Biggs MA, Roberts S, Foster DG: *Partner reasons for seeking an abortion*. Under review.
8. Jones RK, Frohwirth LF, Moore AM: "I would want to give my child, like, everything in the world" - how issues of motherhood influence women who have abortions. *J Fam Issues* 2008, 29(1):79–99.
9. Ellison MA: Authoritative knowledge and single women's unintentional pregnancies, abortions, adoption, and single motherhood: social stigma and structural violence. *Med Anthropol Q* 2003, 17(3):322–347.
10. Cockrill K, Nack A: "I'm not that type of person": managing the stigma of having an abortion. *Deviant Behavior* 2013. In Press.

8

"I'm Not That Type of Person":

Managing the Stigma of Having an Abortion

Kate Cockrill and Adina Nack

Kate Cockrill, MPH, studied abortion stigma for over a decade and collaborated with Adina Nack on this research while Cockrill was at Advancing New Standards in Reproductive Health (ANSIRH) at the University of California, San Francisco, Bixby Center for Global Reproductive Health. Nack is a medical sociologist at California Lutheran University who has published on issues of women's sexual health, social psychology, and social inequality. Using a grounded theory approach, which allows knowledge and theory to emerge from the data (here the experiences of women who had abortions), the Cockrill and Nack qualitative study involving thirty-four women offers evidence that women simultaneously navigate three different kinds of abortion stigma: internalized stigma, felt stigma, and enacted abortion stigma (see Table 1). This piece offers insight into how stigma functions and how women manage it; of particular note is the role religion plays in both.

There is a striking disconnect between statistics about abortion in the United States and women's lived experiences. Abortion is as common a medical procedure as C-Section, with nearly one-third of women having at least one abortion during their reproductive years (Jones and Kooistra 2011). Yet,

Source: Kate Cockrill and Adina Nack, "'I'm Not That Type of Person': Managing the Stigma of Having an Abortion," *Deviant Behavior* 34, no. 12 (2013): 973–90.

Table1 Respondent Demographics

Pseudonym	Age	Ethnicity=Race	Religion	Education	Number of children	Number of abortions	Which study?
Aisha	21	white=Native American	none	Some Tech	1	2	1
Alicia	27	black	Baptist	College Grad	1	1	2
Allison	29	white	No Current/raised Catholic	Bachelor's	0	1	2
Amanda	25	white	Baptist	Some College	4	1	1
Angela	20	black	none	Some College	1	2	1
Beth	39	white	none	Some College	2	1	1
Brandy	21	black	Christian—Not Specified	Some College	0	1	2
Cassie	25	white	none	College Grad	0	1	1
Cheryl	43	white	Baptist	GED	2	1	1
Cynthia	36	white	none	Graduate School	1	2	2
Deb	41	white	No Current/raised Catholic	Graduate School	3	1	1
Jackie	unknown	black	unknown	Some College	3	2	1
Jennifer	27	white	none	College Grad	0	1	1
Jessie	18	Asian/Native American	Baptist	High School	0	1	1
Jordan	25	black	Baptist	High School	1	1	1
Joy	28	White/Native American	None	Some Graduate School	0	3	1

Name	Age	Race	Religion	Education			
Julie	40	white	Christian—Not Specified	Some Graduate School	2	1	2
Katia	25	Peruvian/British	Spiritual/raised Catholic	College Grad	0	1	2
Kelly	43	black	Christian- Not Specified	College Grad	1	2	2
Lana	28	Asian	none	College Grad	0	2	2
Laura	37	white	Christian—Not Specified	Graduate School	0	2	2
Lisa	23	white	Christian—Not Specified	Some College	2	2	1
Lyndsay	18	white	Christian—Not Specified	High School	0	1	1
Makayla	27	black	Baptist	Some Graduate School	2	1	1
Maricel	24	Latina	none	Some High School	1	2	1
Melinda	29	white	none	College Grad	0	1	2
Michelle	39	white	Christian—Not Specified	College Grad	1	2	2
Nicole	38	white	None	Graduate School	2	1	2
Sonja	25	black	Christian—Not Specified	College Grad	0	2	1
Susan	47	white	None	College Grad	8	4	2
Tamara	35	white	None	College Grad	0	1	2
Tanya	25	black	Baptist	College Grad	4	1	1
Tricia	19	white	Methodist	Some College	0	1	1
Vanessa	23	black	none	College Grad	0	1	1

many of these women report feeling silenced and isolated (Ellison 2003), and nearly 40% of Americans claim they do not know anyone who has had an abortion (Jones et al. 2011).

Women who have abortions do so in the midst of a polarizing public discourse that narrows and decontextualizes abortion (Jelen and Wilcox 2003; Joffe 2010). Prior to having an abortion, women are likely aware of negative attitudes toward abortion—in everyday discussions and through media, especially during elections. Research shows that a significant proportion of women who have abortions come from communities with anti-abortion views, and some women who have abortions are in favor of restrictions on abortion access (Cockrill and Weitz 2010; Jones et al. 2008). Given how selectively women disclose their abortion history to others and the often-negative public status of abortion, there is evidence of prevailing abortion stigma (Major and Gramzow 1999; Shellenberg and Tsui 2012).

. . .

Theoretical Framework

Herek's (2009) framework of three manifestations of sexual stigma informs our understanding of individual women's abortion experiences. First, *internalized stigma* results from a woman's acceptance of negative cultural valuations of abortion. Second, *felt stigma* encompasses her assessments of others' abortion attitudes, as well as her expectations about how attitudes might result in actions. Then, *enacted abortion stigma* is a woman's experiences of clear or subtle actions that reveal prejudice against those involved in abortion: for example, physical or emotional abuse, discrimination, hate speech, as well as verbal judgments/assumptions, avoidance, and displays of discomfort, anxiety, or even disgust (Crocker et al. 1998). These three manifestations are related but distinguishable facets of individual-level abortion stigma.

The literature on the gendered constructions of deviance helps explain how and why abortion stigma attaches to girls/women[1] who have an abortion. All stigmas stem from shared, socially constructed knowledge of the devaluing effects of particular attributes (Herek 2009). Kumar and colleagues define abortion stigma as "a negative attribute ascribed to women who seek to terminate a pregnancy that marks them, internally or externally, as *inferior to the ideals of womanhood*" (2009: 628, emphasis added). Abortion stigma is rooted in narrow, gender-specific archetypes that inform cultural meanings of pregnancy termination (Luker 1984), including archetypal constructs of the "feminine," of procreative female sexuality, and of women's innate desire to be a mother (Kumar et al. 2009).

. . .

Internalized Stigma

Many of the women in our study had learned negative stereotypes about girls/women who receive abortions (e.g., they are unintelligent, naïve, uneducated, promiscuous, irresponsible, cruel, and/or selfish). Learning these stereotypes facilitated the women's internalizations of abortion stigma, which could be expressed as prejudice or self-stigma. As evidence of such prejudices, six women used the words "irresponsible" or "careless" as general descriptions for women who have abortions.

. . .

Once pregnant and considering an abortion, the women had to reconcile their own sexual behaviors and abortion decisions with previous attitudes toward "bad" women. Some revised previous prejudices; while, others turned their prejudice inward. Thus, self-stigma manifested when a woman had (1) been exposed to negative discourses about women who have abortions, (2) believed the discourses were legitimate, and (3) believed they applied to her. Those who believed that women are responsible for preventing pregnancy judged themselves harshly: five described feeling that they were "stupid" once they were seeking an abortion. Self-stigma appeared most regularly in interviews with women who had grown up in families or communities with strong, negative attitudes toward abortion as the norm.

. . .

Eight of the women in our sample expressed having strong feelings of guilt associated with their abortion; one participant used the word "guilt" 16 times in her one-hour interview, attributing these feelings to her Catholic upbringing. Our data suggest a strong relationship between religion and self-stigma. Half of our sample identified as currently practicing Christians, Protestant or Catholic. Among these 17 women, 65% made statements revealing self-stigma. Among the 17 non-religious participants, only 35% indicated self-stigma. Self-stigma was not exclusive to religious women; it simply appeared at a lower rate among non-religious women.

Felt Stigma

Women's narratives revealed felt stigma: they imagined many unsupportive reactions to disclosing an unplanned pregnancy, an abortion decision, or an abortion history. Most respondents anticipated that certain individuals would be unsupportive or judgmental (e.g., religious family members, significant others who are anti-abortion, friends who struggled to conceive, and Ob/Gyns who had delivered their babies). These women feared that disclosing abortion would result in unwanted advice, guilt-trips, condemnation, name-calling, or ostracism.

. . .

The stigmatizing interactions women expected varied widely and depended on the values and attitudes they perceived in their communities and the people around them. Allison felt stigma related to community attitudes toward abortion but also pre-marital sex. She explained, ". . . it's a very conservative town . . . there's a lot of Catholic people that I encounter, a lot of people who just don't believe that abortion is right no matter what. . . ." Another participant, Brandy, anticipated the strongest stigma from anti-abortion friends who she feared would label her a "murderer or killer." In contrast, Julie feared her pro-choice older sister would label her "irresponsible" because the abortion showed she had failed to use contraception. Although their expectations differed, the women's most common response to felt stigma was to control information, carefully managing personal interactions.

Enacted Stigma

Confrontations between patients and protestors exemplify enacted stigma and were mentioned by 14 participants. However, participants also described many other subtle interactions which demonstrated their loss of status when seeking an abortion or disclosing an abortion experience.

Cheryl, a 43-year-old woman whose youngest child was entering college, sought healthcare for excessive vomiting and abdominal tenderness. At her appointment, she found out she was pregnant and also had a large mass on her uterus. She was consistently clear with her Ob/Gyn that she wanted to terminate the pregnancy; yet, her anti-abortion doctor refused to provide an abortion or to remove the mass for fear of harming the fetus . . . Enacted stigma from anti-abortion medical practitioners reflects the *moral surveillance* type of practitioner interaction style (Nack 2008).

. . .

Enacted stigma from one's sexual partner was also devastating. Tanya's partner told her that abortion "is the same as going out there and shooting somebody." Since they were raising four children together, he did not try to prevent her from having an abortion, but he would not help pay for the abortion and made sure she knew he thought it was a sin. Judgment or abandonment can inspire a woman's use of secrecy and information-control strategies and also reinforce negative feelings about herself.

Managing the Damaged Self

. . .

Some women managed internalized stigma by accepting the legitimacy of stigma, while simultaneously challenging its application to their particular experiences. They rationalized why the abortion happened and why it was a legitimate behavior, despite its taboo. Two ways of rationalizing included *excuses* and *justifications* (Scott and Lyman 1981 [1968]). Excuses allow women to avoid the label of "irresponsibility"; whereas, justifications serve women who accept responsibility for their abortions but deny the wrongfulness of the act, therefore denying any negative devaluations of moral character.

Excuses and justifications appeared with high frequency in the abortion narratives. Lyndsay, introduced above, described her own rationale:

> I had a baby, and I gave her up for adoption, and then . . . I got pregnant . . . it was more like of a date rape kind of thing . . . adoption is hard . . . but I'm okay with my [abortion] decision. Especially, like already going through having a baby and all that.

Lyndsay defends her abortion with two excuses: (1) she was not expecting to get pregnant so soon after the birth of a child and (2) the sex that resulted in the need for abortion was not consensual. Her justification for the abortion is that she has already gone through with one adoption, an emotionally difficult experience, and cannot go through with another.

. . .

Maintaining a Good Reputation

For women who have abortions, the knowledge of the abortion carries a great risk to their reputation. After her second-trimester abortion, Deb described the following conversation with her doctor:

> He called me the next day . . . and he said, "You are a high profile person in this area. Everybody knows you. You need to tell people that you had a miscarriage. Do not tell anybody that you had an abortion. . . . Do not tell your closest friend. . . . Anybody that you tell there's a risk of it getting out."

Women who anticipated stigmatizing interactions because of abortion often tried to reduce the likelihood of negative outcomes by withholding their experience from others. For example, some used deceptive *cover stories:* at least three of the women created fictional explanations for why they needed childcare on their abortion appointment dates.

After the abortion, women may also try to *pass* as having not had an abortion when the topic comes up in conversation. . . . Brandy discussed how she felt when someone who does not know her abortion status talks about their own abortion, "I feel uncomfortable because it's like, 'Okay, I've had one [too] but they don't know it.'"

. . .

The consequences of passing, covering, and telling outright lies about abortion can be negative for the individual. Major and Gramzow (1999) found that women who kept their abortion secret were more likely to need to suppress thoughts of their abortion and to experience intrusive thoughts about their abortion, which increased their risk of abortion-related distress.

. . .

Managing the Damaged Reputation

Stigma experiences led some women to begin to name and critique the stigma they were experiencing. . . . Additionally, enacted stigma motivated some women to try to *normalize* (Elliot et al. 1990) the abortion experience for those who might judge not only them but also other women like them. Unlike the other types of stigma management behaviors, these types of management may take place in varying scopes, one-on-one, with small groups, online through social media, or through broader advocacy efforts. Through *condemning the condemners*, a woman can assign the greater sin to those who have judged abortion to be wrong and who work to limit women's access to abortion. This neutralizes the act of abortion by socially constructing the anti-abortion value system as more unjust and immoral than having an abortion.

Cassie described a level of hypocrisy among Christians in her community:

What gets me with that whole argument is they want to talk about how it's murder and . . . you know, the child should be born, but they don't talk about all the children that are born that are unloved, that are abused, that are psychologically . . . damaged, because instead of having an abortion the parents kept the child. . . . you don't see them trying to support . . . single mothers. You, you don't see the churches getting out to . . . help children.

Cassie's critique of anti-abortion individuals was not her only strategy for resisting stigma. She also sought to *normalize* the experience for herself and other women: "Abortion is abortion. People want to specify it only should be for rape victims, or abuse victims. No, it should be available for everybody."

. . .

Discussion and Conclusion

In the United States, women have abortions in an environment fraught with controversy and judgment, shaping painful stigma that may have ongoing ramifications throughout a woman's life. We find evidence that abortion stigma is deeply entangled with social constructions of feminine "goodness," such that it disproportionately impacts women and incentivizes concealment of a woman's abortion status.

. . .

All of the women who called the talkline verbalized a need for social and emotional support beyond what was available to them in their social networks. Even so, as time passes even these women may perceive their abortion as less salient and need less support, decreasing the likelihood of disclosure.

. . .

Given the inter- and intrapersonal consequences of stigma for women who have abortions, our analysis also helps to inform potential destigmatization strategies. . . . Abortion secrecy promotes invisibility of the abortion experience and can hinder opportunities for such collective stigma management. Clinics, talklines, and counseling services help women who have abortions to connect with individuals who can listen nonjudgmentally and may share their stigma. However, one-on-one interactions cannot create the kind of collective stigma management that is necessary for changing sociocultural norms.

. . .

It is common for advocates, policymakers, and researchers to highlight women's justifications and excuses for abortion. While these efforts produce short-term successes, they fail to disrupt the narrow gender constructs that fuel individual experiences of stigma. Excuses and justifications may ease the burden of internalized stigma or stigmatizing encounters, but they will not reduce stigma in the long term. A longer-term strategy will seek to problematize the expectations placed on women and deconstruct stigmatizing labels such as "good mother" and "irresponsible."

Note

1. Hereafter we will use the word "women" to refer to women and girls together.

References

Cockrill, Kate and Tracy Ann Weitz. 2010. "'Abortion Patients' Perceptions of Abortion Regulation." *Women's Health Issues* 20:12–19.

Crocker, Jennifer, Brenda Major, and Claude Steele. 1998. "Social Stigma." Pp. 504–553 in *The Handbook of Social Psychology*, edited by D. Gilbert, S. Fiske and G. Lindzey. Boston: Oxford University Press.

Elliot, Gregory, Herbert Ziegler, Barbara Altman, and Deborah Scott. 1990. "Understanding Stigma: Dimensions of Deviance and Coping." Pp. 423–443 in *Deviant Behavior*, edited by C. Bryant. New York: Hemisphere.

Ellison, Marcia A. 2003. "Authoritative Knowledge and Single Women's Unintentional Pregnancies, Abortions, Adoption, and Single Motherhood: Social Stigma and Structural Violence." *Medical Anthropology Quarterly* 17:322–347.

Herek, Gregory. 2009. "Sexual Stigma and Sexual Prejudice in the United States: A Conceptual Framework." Pp. 65–112 in *Contemporary Perspectives on Lesbian, Gay, and Bisexual Identities*, edited by D. Hope. New York: Springer.

Jelen, Ted G. and Clyde Wilcox. 2003. "Causes and Consequences of Public Attitudes toward Abortion: A Review and Research Agenda." *Political Research Quarterly* 56:489–500.

Joffe, Carole. 2010. *Dispatches from the Abortion Wars: The Costs of Fanaticism to Doctors, Patients, and the Rest of Us*. Boston: Beacon Press.

Jones, Rachel K. and Kathryn Kooistra. 2011. "Abortion Incidence and Access to Services in the United States, 2008." Perspectives on Sexual and Reproductive Health 43:41–50.

Jones, Rachel K, Lori F. Frohwirth, and Ann M. Moore. 2008. "'I Would Want to Give My Child, Like, Everything in the World': How Issues of Motherhood Influence Women Who Have Abortions." Journal of Family Issues 29:79–99.

Jones, Robert P, Daniel Cox, and Rachel Laser. 2011. "Committed to Availability, Conflicted About Morality." Public Religion Research Institute. Retrieved March 26, 2013. (http://publicreligion.org/site/wp-content/uploads/2011/06/Millenials-Abortion-and-Religion-Survey-Report.pdf)

Kumar, Anuradha, Leila Hessini, and Ellen M. H. Mitchell. 2009. "Conceptualising Abortion Stigma." Culture Health & Sexuality 11:625–639.

Luker, Kristin. 1984. Abortion and the Politics of Motherhood. Berkeley: University of California Press.

Major, Brenda and Richard H. Gramzow. 1999. "Abortion as Stigma: Cognitive and Emotional Implications of Concealment." Journal of Personality & Social Psychology 77:735–745.

Nack, Adina. 2008. "From the Patient's Point of View: Practitioner Interaction Styles in the Treatment of Women with Chronic STD." Research in the Sociology of Health Care 26:95–122.

Scott, Marvin B., and Stanford Lyman. 1981 [1968]. "Accounts." Pp. 343–361 in Social Psychology through Symbolic Interaction, edited by G. P. Stone and H. A. Farberman. New York: Wiley.

Shellenberg, Kristen M. and Amy O. Tsui. 2012. "Correlates of Perceived and Internalized Stigma among Abortion Patients in the USA: An Exploration by Race and Hispanic Ethnicity." International Journal of Gynecology & Obstetrics 118, Supplement 2:S152–S159.

9

Women's Decision Making Regarding Choice of Second Trimester Termination Method for Pregnancy Complications

Jennifer Kerns, Rachna Vanjani,

Lori Freedman, Karen Meckstroth,

Eleanor A. Drey, and Jody Steinauer

Jennifer Kerns, a physician and clinical researcher with a focus on patient decision-making in complicated pregnancies, notes that patients rely heavily on advice from healthcare providers when making abortion decisions after diagnosis of a fetal anomaly. Patients must choose between a D&E and an induced labor-and-delivery. While women were not asked about their religious affiliation, references to baptism and church indicate that for at least some of the study's participants religion was a factor in why they opted for one abortion procedure over the other. This qualitative research highlights the importance of developing a better understanding of the role of religion in abortion decision-making, particularly when serious problems arise in wanted pregnancies, and of educating healthcare workers in ways that increase sensitivity and support for patients.

Source: Jennifer Kerns, Rachna Vanjani, Lori Freedman, Karen Meckstroth, Eleanor A. Drey, and Jody Steinauer, "Women's Decision Making Regarding Choice of Second Trimester Termination Method for Pregnancy Complications," *International Journal of Gynecology & Obstetrics* 116, no. 3 (2012): 244–8.

Termination of pregnancy for fetal anomalies or pregnancy complications is common. Approximately 150,000 women in the USA per year are faced with the diagnosis of a fetal anomaly [1,2], and most women will terminate for that reason [3–6]. The 2 methods of second trimester termination, dilation and evacuation (D&E) and medical abortion, are similar in safety and efficacy [7], but are very different experiences for women [8]. D&E is shorter and typically done as an outpatient with deeper anesthesia [9]. Medical abortion, also referred to as labor induction, is most often done on labor and delivery, takes longer, more consistently allows for an intact autopsy specimen and offers the chance for contact with the fetus.

Women rely heavily on advice from providers when terminating for a fetal anomaly [10], but with little data to direct patient counseling regarding method, providers often recommend a method based on personal beliefs and practices [11]. In fact, there may be a bias toward recommending medical abortion with the belief that viewing the fetus helps women grieve and recover [12]. Grief and posttraumatic stress symptoms are not uncommon after termination for fetal anomaly [10,13–15] and undergoing a procedure that is contrary to a woman's emotional needs may potentially complicate her grief and delay recovery.

. . .

Between July 2009 and February 2010, women terminating pregnancies for fetal anomalies, pregnancy complications, or those undergoing treatments for fetal demise were recruited to the study and interviewed about their decision to undergo D&E or medical abortion.

. . .

Of the 37 eligible women, 31 were enrolled: 20 (65%) who underwent D&E and 11 who (35%) underwent medical abortion.

. . .

Nearly all women expressed strong feelings about abortion with negative attitudes expressed among those who chose medical abortion and positive attitudes among those who chose D&E. One woman who underwent a medical abortion for preterm premature rupture of membranes illustrated this point (Table 3, quote 1). Some women directly linked their attitudes about abortion to their decision regarding the method. Specifically, half of the women who chose medical abortion did so because it represented something other than an abortion (Table 3, quotes 2, 3). Many of these women equated a D&E to an abortion, often using the words "D&E" and "abortion" interchangeably. Women who chose to have a D&E expressed much more positive attitudes about abortion (Table 3, quote 4).

Table 3 Theme 2: Abortion attitudes

Subthemes	Quotes
Choosing induction because it is not an abortion	1 "When I was a teenager . . . I was very active in church . . . they just gave us the information, and let us choose what, what we thought about it . . . which has helped me form my opinion against abortion, personally." (Patient 17, 31 years)
	2 "I believe that [D&E] was more like an abortion because . . . the baby would be taken out in parts and . . . we wouldn't be able to see the baby." (Patient 1, 45 years)
	3 "I could either go about having her through the abortion or I could go with labor and I immediately picked the labor." (Patient 20, 23 years)
Positive abortion attitudes and D&E	4 "I have been a pro-choice person my entire life and so there wasn't ever that wavering, you know, ever. I actually will probably become an even more stronger advocate for pro-choice."
Right and wrong reasons for abortion	5 "If it [the pregnancy] was something that was unplanned . . . it wouldn't have bothered me [continuing the pregnancy], but I didn't want to bring a child sick into the world." (Patient 2, 37 years)
	6 "I believe it's a woman's right to choose. I don't think that it should be used as a form of birth control, like a lot of women use it for. I think if you're going to have unprotected sex, then you need to be prepared for the consequences." (Patient 8, 25 years)
Abortion as unexpected but necessary	7 "I believe it has to be an option available to women because, you know, there are circumstances when it's necessary." (Patient 16, 41 years)
	8 "I've heard a lot of criticism about late-term abortion and I've always thought now that's a strange thing to do, you know, to make that choice so late. And now I see you can really get boxed in as a pregnant person and, by the time you get all this testing done it's like it's really late." (Patient 16, 41 years)

Women with negative abortion views, regardless of method chosen, sought to separate themselves from women terminating a pregnancy for other reasons (Table 3, quotes 5, 6). These women drew distinctions between terminating an anomalous pregnancy versus terminating an unplanned pregnancy, thus describing what they considered right and wrong reasons for abortion.

. . .

Women's attitudes about religion played important roles in the decision to terminate, as well as the decision to undergo a particular procedure. For

Table 4 Theme 3: Religious attitudes

Subthemes	Quotes
Pregnancy termination as an act of compassion	1 "I felt like my faith was being tested and I prayed and I prayed for a good outcome because this was a situation where we didn't know every step of the way what we were going to do . . . And my husband and I really had to stop and think about that and, you know, and I think it's so personal for everybody but we didn't want a disabled child. And my husband and I talked about it and quality of life was just so, it was exactly what we want to give our kids, is to have a quality of life." (Patient 15, 39 years) 2 "Yeah, it was [about living a] meaningful life, that and the way they explained it to us, the doctor's office, what was wrong with the baby. There was no way that the baby was even going to survive the night . . ." (Patient 1, 45 years)
Choosing induction for religious reasons	3 "So the baby could be baptized and . . . it was important for me to be able to see the baby and baptize it and be able to go about it that way." (Patient 1, 45 years) 4 ". . .because we don't, we really don't believe in abortion, and we wanted to meet our child and be able to baptize him. So, it kind of played a role, 'cause he had to be baptized, and . . . we were able to get him baptized, instead of just having the other procedure done and not seeing him at all." (Patient 18, 20 years)

many women who identified themselves as religious, terminating the pregnancy was an act of compassion whereby they were sparing their child from living a poor quality life (Table 4, quotes 1, 2). For some women, choosing medical abortion was directly related to religious beliefs such as baptism (Table 4, quotes 3, 4) For 1 woman who underwent medical abortion, religious beliefs and abortion attitudes were inextricably linked and formed the basis of her decision.

. . .

Some clinicians believe that medical abortion is the best way for women to cope with pregnancy termination [11,12]. The findings of the present study indicate that while this is true for some women, other women find the prospect of a medical abortion traumatizing. Choosing D&E as a way to avoid compounding an already traumatic experience was not reflective of ambivalence about the pregnancy or an avoidance of coping. Instead, it was a nuanced expression of an individual woman's attempt to place herself on an emotionally concordant coping path.

. . .

The findings from this study add to and complement existing data on how women cope after termination for fetal anomaly. A study of parental coping after pregnancy loss found no association between religious beliefs and coping, but found an association between negative religious coping practices such as guilt and persistent grief [16]. Although the present study found that women who identified as religious were more likely to choose induction, emotional coping style more consistently predicted method choice than did religiosity. Another study showed no difference in grief resolution or depression between women undergoing D&E or medical abortion [17]. A possible reason for these findings might be that women self-selected the method that was most congruent with their emotional needs.

References

1. ACOG Committee on Practice Bulletins. ACOG Practice Bulletin No. 77: screening for fetal chromosomal abnormalities. Obstet Gynecol 2007;109(1):217–27.
2. Crane JP, LeFevre ML, Winborn RC, Evans JK, Ewigman BC, Bain RP, et al. A randomized trial of prenatal ultrasonographic screening: impact on the detection, management and outcome of anomalous fetuses. The RADIUS Study Group. Am J Obstet Gynecol 1994;171(2):392–9.
3. Anderson N, Boswell O, Duff G. Prenatal sonography for the detection of fetal anomalies: results of a prospective study and comparison with prior series. AJR Am J Roentgenol 1995;165(4):943–50.
4. Boyd PA, Devigan C, Khoshnood B, Loane M, Garne E, Dolk H. Survey of prenatal screening policies in Europe for structural malformations and chromosome anomalies, and their impact on detection and termination rates for neural tube defects and Down's syndrome. BJOG 2008;115(6):689–96.
5. Pryde PG, Drugan A, Johnson M, Isada NB, Evans MI. Prenatal diagnosis: choices women make about pursuing testing and acting on abnormal results. Clin Obstet Gynecol 1993;36(3):496–509.
6. Shaffer BL, Caughey AB, Norton ME. Variation in the decision to terminate pregnancy in the setting of fetal aneuploidy. Prenat Diagn 2006;26(8):667–71.
7. Lohr PA, Hayes JL, Gemzell-Danielsson K. Surgical versus medical methods for second trimester induced abortion. Cochrane Database Syst Rev 2008(1):CD006714.

8. Kaltreider NB, Goldsmith S, Margolis AJ. The impact of midtrimester abortion techniques on patients and staff. Am J Obstet Gynecol 1979;135(2):235-8.

9. O'Connell K, Jones HE, Lichtenberg ES, Paul M. Second-trimester surgical abortion practices: a survey of National Abortion Federation members. Contraception 2008;78(6):492-9.

10. Korenromp MJ, Page-Christiaens GC, van den Bout J, Mulder EJ, Visser GH. Maternal decision to terminate pregnancy in case of Down syndrome. Am J Obstet Gynecol 2007;196(2):149.e1-149.e11.

11. Freedman LR. Willing and Unable: Doctors' Constraints in Abortion Care. Nashville, TN: Vanderbilt University Press; 2010.

12. Sloan EP, Kirsh S, Mowbray M. Viewing the fetus following termination of pregnancy for fetal anomaly. J Obstet Gynecol Neonatal Nurs 2008;37(4):395-404.

13. Kersting A, Kroker K, Steinhard J, Hoernig-Franz I, Wesselmann U, Luedorff K, et al. Psychological impact on women after second and third trimester termination of pregnancy due to fetal anomalies versus women after preterm birth-a 14-month follow up study. Arch Womens Ment Health 2009;12(4):193-201.

14. Korenromp MJ, Page-Christiaens GC, van den Bout J, Mulder EJ, Hunfeld JA, Potters CM, et al. A prospective study on parental coping 4 months after termination of pregnancy for fetal anomalies. Prenat Diagn 2007;27(8):709-16.

15. Korenromp MJ, Page-Christiaens GC, van den Bout J, Mulder EJ, Visser GH. Adjustment to termination of pregnancy for fetal anomaly: a longitudinal study in women at 4, 8, and 16 months. Am J Obstet Gynecol 2009;201(2):160.e161-7.

16. Cowchock FS, Lasker JN, Toedter LJ, Skumanich SA, Koenig HG. Religious beliefs affect grieving after pregnancy loss. J Relig Health 2010;49(4):485-97.

17. Burgoine G, Van Kirk SD, Romm J, Edelman AB, Jacobson SL, Jensen JT. Comparison of perinatal grief after dilation and evacuation or labor induction in second trimester terminations for fetal anomalies. Am J Obstet Gynecol 2005;192(6): 1928-32.

Muslim Women Having Abortions in Canada:
Attitudes, Beliefs, and Experiences

Ellen Wiebe, Roya Najafi, Naghma Soheil,

and Alya Kamani

Ellen Wiebe is a physician and clinical professor in British Columbia, whose research focuses on women's health. In this study, she and her research team conducted a quantitative study about Muslim women's experience of abortion in Canada, where Islam is the largest non-Christian religion. Published in a medical journal, this article documents the role that religion and religious authorities play in the decision-making of some Muslim patients, and it also offers rudimentary explanations about Islam to educate physicians and other healthcare workers about some basic beliefs and the wide diversity of practices within Islam. To provide high-quality care for religious patients, it is critical for providers to understand the diversity of beliefs and practices that exist within all religious traditions.

Islam is the largest non-Christian religion in Canada, with 579,640 Canadians identifying themselves as Muslim (or Moslem) in the 2001 census.[1] The

Source: Ellen Wiebe, Roya Najafi, Naghma Soheil, and Alya Kamani, "Muslim Women Having Abortions in Canada: Attitudes, Beliefs, and Experiences," *Canadian Family Physician* 57, no. 4 (2011): e134–8.

proportion of Canadian Muslims is growing considerably: from 0.9% of the population in 1991 to 2.0% in 2001. In 2001, 0.6% of nonimmigrants and 7.6% of immigrants identified themselves as Muslim. The estimate for 2009 was that 2.5% of the population—approximately 850,000 Canadians—would be self-identified Muslims.[2] Unlike the Muslim population of European nations,[3] this group is ethnically diverse; 36.7% are South Asian, 21.1% are Arab, 14.0% are West Asian, and 14.2% are part of other minority groups including Chinese, African, Filipino, Latin American, Korean, and Japanese. In the 2001 census, 14.2% of the Canadian Muslim population said they did not consider themselves to be visible minorities. This group could partially reflect the number of converts to Islam.

In order to best care for our Muslim patients, it is useful to understand something about Islamic concepts of abortion. There are 2 main branches of Islam, Sunni and Shia, with many subdivisions, including Hanafi, Shafi, Hanbali, Salafi, Maliki, Twelver, Ismaili, Kharijites, Sufis, Ahmedis, and many more. The primary source of Islam is the Quran (or Koran) and the oral statements of the prophet Mohammad and his practices (Sunna). In addition, Muslims all over the world might follow different Imams (Islamic religious leaders).

Some Muslims oppose all abortions based on the following passage from the Quran: "Do not kill your children for fear of poverty, for it is we who shall provide sustenance for you as well as for them."[4] Some Muslims believe abortion is permitted if the mother's health is endangered, based on another passage, which states that, "A mother should not be made to suffer because of her child."[5]

Most of the schools of Islam that permit abortion insist that there must be a serious reason for it, such as a threat to the mother's life or the probability of giving birth to a deformed or defective child. The gestational age is important; for example, the Hanafi (Turkey, the Middle East, and Central Asia) and Shafi (Southeast Asia, southern Arabia, and parts of East Africa) schools allow abortions to take place until day 120, while in the Maliki (North and Black Africa) and Hanbali (Saudi Arabia and United Arab Emirates) schools, an abortion is permissible only up to day 40.[6-9]

Muslim jurists have agreed that abortion is prohibited after the fetus is completely formed and has been given a soul, unless it is reliably shown that the continuation of the pregnancy would necessarily result in the death of the mother. Then, in accordance with the general principle of the Shari'ah, that of choosing the lesser of 2 evils, abortion is not only permissible, but *must* be performed.[6] The effects of religious convictions and culture on a woman's decision to have an abortion and her experience of guilt are important for health practitioners to consider. The purpose of this study was to discover what our Muslim patients actually believed about the permissibility of abortion and to examine how this might affect their experiences. We also wanted to assess the anxiety level of our Muslim patients to see how it compared with previously published levels of anxiety in abortion patients.

We received 53 completed questionnaires. It is not clear what percentage of our Muslim patients agreed to complete questionnaires, as we do not routinely ask women to identify their religion.

Demographics

Participants had been born in 17 different countries, including Iran (n= 22, 41.5%), other West Asian countries (n=7, 13.2%), Canada (n= 5, 9.4%), Pakistan (n= 5, 9.4%), and African countries (n= 4, 7.5%). Most women identified their race as Persian (n= 17, 32.1%) or Asian-Indian (n= 15, 28.3%). They varied in age from 17 to 47 years, with a mean of 29 years. Twenty-six (49.1%) were married; 26 (49.1%) had no children. Participants had lived in Canada for between 1 and 31 years, with a mean of 10 years.

. . .

Attitudes

When asked about their Muslim beliefs and practices, 51 participants (96.2%) agreed with the statement "Any Muslim woman has the right to have an abortion," 17 (32.1%) "agreed with Islamic principles," 14 (26.4%) agreed (always or sometimes) that "Islam prevented a woman from having another child after an abortion," 26 (49.1%) said they felt guilty because of Islam, 24 (45.3%) said they prayed every week, and 21 (39.6%) said that they used prayer and meditation to deal with their guilt. A third of the women (n= 16, 30.2%) were completely pro-choice and said all the reasons a woman should be allowed to have an abortion listed in the questionnaire were acceptable, while the others had reservations and 11 (20.8%) identified only one acceptable reason.

Experience

Women who indicated that some reasons to have abortions would not be acceptable (Table 2) and women who said they agreed that abortion went against Islamic principles (Table 3) had higher anxiety and guilt scores than those who did not: 6.9 versus 4.9 ($P=.01$) and 6.9 versus 3.6 ($P=.004$), respectively. Depression scores were not significantly different for these women. Women who said they prayed more than once per week had similar scores to women who prayed less often ($P=.54$). Twenty-one women said they used prayer and meditation to deal with their guilt about having the abortion.

Table 2 Mean anxiety, depression, and guilt scores by attitude toward abortion: *Scores are rated on a scale of 0 to 10 (N= 50).*

SCORE	MORE PRO-CHOICE (LISTED ACCEPTABLE REASONS) N = 16	LESS PRO-CHOICE (SOME REASONS NOT ACCEPTABLE) N = 34	PVALUE
Anxiety	4.9	6.9	.01*
Depression	4.2	5.4	.17
Guilt	3.6	6.9	.004*

*Statistically significant using *t* test.

Table 3 Mean anxiety, depression, and guilt scores by attitude toward Islamic principles: *Scores are rated on a scale of 0 to 10 (N= 48).*

SCORE	STRONGLY AGREE THAT ABORTION IS AGAINST ISLAMIC PRINCIPLES N = 3	DO NOT STRONGLY AGREE THAT ABORTION IS AGAINST ISLAMIC PRINCIPLES N = 45	PVALUE
Anxiety	9.3	5.9	.03*
Depression	5.0	4.9	.98
Guilt score	9.5	5.3	.03*

*Statistically significant using *t* test.

Women's Comments

At the end of the questionnaire, women were given space to provide comments; 14 women wrote about how they felt about their religion and abortion, representing various views. One woman noted: "I feel guilty; it is against Islamic law." Others explained: "In Islam you can have an abortion up to 3 months—I don't feel guilty" and "Islamic beliefs don't influence sad feelings." Other women talked about the lack of support they felt in their community: "It is hardest for unmarried woman to face family [when pregnant]."

Discussion

The group of Muslim women that we surveyed was so diverse that no generalizations can be made about them. Their attitudes toward abortion ranged from being completely pro-choice to believing abortion was wrong unless done to save a woman's life. Many reportedly found their religion to be a source of comfort as well as a source of guilt, turning to prayer and meditation to cope with their feelings about the abortion.

In a previous study of anxiety and attitudes toward abortion, women who held more anti-choice views had greater anxiety related to their abortion experiences.[10] In our study, although we had a smaller number of subjects, the women who were less pro-choice were also more anxious and reported feeling more guilt. Our Muslim patients in this study had a higher mean anxiety score (6.1) than women in the previous study (5.2).[10] Specifically, the women who most strongly believed that abortion was against Islamic principles were most likely to report high levels of both guilt and anxiety.

Most women in the study (96.2%) agreed that Muslims have the right to have abortions. As only 30.2% were fully pro-choice and agreed that women should be able to have an abortion for any reason, for the rest of the women, the right to have an abortion might simply mean that they believe Muslims should not be discriminated against on the basis of their religion in terms of having the freedom to access abortion care.

Conclusion

Canadian Muslim women presenting for abortion come from many different countries and schools of Islam. It is important that physicians caring for Muslim women understand that their patients come from a variety of backgrounds and can have widely differing beliefs. It might be helpful to be aware that patients who hold more anti-choice beliefs are likely to experience more anxiety and guilt related to their abortion than pro-choice patients do.

References

1. Statistics Canada. *Major religious dominations, Canada, 1991 and 2001*. Ottawa, ON: Statistics Canada.
2. Wikipedia. *Islam in Canada*. San Francisco, CA: Wikimedia Foundation Inc; 2011.
3. Hessini L. Abortion and Islam: policies and practice in the Middle East and North Africa. *Reprod Health Matters* 2007;15(29):75–84.
4. *The Holy Quran*, Surah Al-An'am, 6:151
5. *The Holy Quran*, Surah Al-Baqara, 2:233.
6. Al-Qaradawi Y. *Lawful and the prohibited in Islam*. Baltimore, MD: Islamic Book Service, American Trust Publications; 1982.
7. Hedayat KM, Shooshtarizadeh P, Raza M. Therapeutic abortion in Islam: contemporary views of Muslim Shiite scholars and effect of recent Iranian legislation. *J Med Ethics* 2006;32(11):652–7.
8. Serour GI. Islamic perspectives in human reproduction. *Reprod Biomed Online* 2008;17(Suppl 3):34–8.
9. Schirrmacher C, Syed IB. *Abortion*. Article no. 112. Louisville, KY: Islamic Research Foundation International Inc; 2009.
10. Wiebe ER, Trouton KJ, Fielding SL, Grant H, Henderson A. Anxieties and attitudes towards abortion in women presenting for medical and surgical abortions. *J Obstet Gynaecol Can* 2004;26(10):881–5.

11

Ultra-Orthodox Jewish Women Navigating the Uncertainty of Pregnancy and Prenatal Diagnosis

Elly Teman, Tsipy Ivry, and

Barbara A. Bernhardt

Elly Teman has her PhD in social anthropology from Hebrew University, Jerusalem. Tsipy Ivry is a senior lecturer on reproduction and biotechnology at the University of Haifa. Barbara Bernhardt has her MS in epidemiology and works as a researcher and genetics counselor at the University of Pennsylvania. This ethnographic study investigates how Ultra-Orthodox Jewish women in the northeast United States negotiate their religious beliefs with practices of prenatal testing and abortion. The authors capture a range of opinions among the women interviewed, who live in tight-knit Haredi and Hassidic communities that encourage strict religious observance, arranged marriages, large families, minimal use of contraception, and opposition to abortion.

This study looked at a particular religious group that has primarily been referred to as "ultra-Orthodox" or "Orthodox" Jews and are now customarily referred to with the term Haredi (meaning God-fearing)

Source: Elly Teman, Tsipy Ivry, and Barbara A. Bernhardt, "Pregnancy as a Proclamation of Faith: Ultra-Orthodox Jewish Women Navigating the Uncertainty of Pregnancy and Prenatal Diagnosis," *American Journal of Medical Genetics* Part A 155, no. 1 (2011): 69–80.

Jews. This population follows a deeply religious lifestyle in accordance with the five books of Moses (the [T]orah) as well as a broad spectrum of rabbinic literature, commentary, and rulings. Distinguished from the larger and more liberally oriented Reform and Conservative branches of the US Jewish population by their more strict interpretation of Jewish Law, Haredi Jews also distinguish themselves from the modern orthodox, who are typically more open to Israel's statehood, secular knowledge, and modern society [Friedman, 1991]. Haredi society actually refers to a plurality of communities each with its own religious leaders or rabbis and style of religious observance [Comenetz, 2006]. In each of these groups, a particular rabbi or group of rabbis serve as "community gatekeeper" [Mittman et al., 2007]. Rabbis are consulted on all matters related to the interpretation and application of Jewish Law in everyday life, including medical issues. . . . Haredi communities may be visually distinguished by their dress code of black hats and dark suits for men and long skirts and covered hair for women. . . . The case of Haredi women is particularly interesting to consider in terms of prenatal diagnosis because of the high number of pregnancies among the women of this population and their tendency to continue bearing children up until the time of menopause when the risk for having a child with a chromosome anomaly increases significantly. All Haredi communities practice arranged marriages, usually within their specific sect, which results in a high rate of consanguinity. Having children is believed to be a divine commandment, so birth control is not encouraged and women tend to begin reproducing shortly after marriage. Women normally continue having children at short intervals up until menopause, often reaching a family size of 10 or more children by their 40s [Birenbaum-Carmeli, 2008]. Consanguineous marriages, the possibility of being a carrier for the genetic diseases that have been traced among Ashkenazi Jews, and advanced maternal age increase the risk that babies will be born with congenital anomalies or genetic disorders.

   . . .

The Discourse of Faith

The women in this study ascribe to a worldview in which they believe in a concept of divine providence [*hashgacha pratis*], which imparts the understanding that God oversees the universe and humans are not in control of their fate. The concept of divine providence includes the belief that God has an overarching plan and has envisioned a unique mission [*tafkid*] in life for every soul [*neshama*]. Each being on this Earth has the obligation to carry out the tailor-made role that God has envisioned for him or her.

In everyday life, the practice of conceding control to God is expressed in having faith [*emunah*]. As Shainy, age 27 and a mother of four explained: "We're not God. God chooses to make things happen. Who knows what he chooses? Who knows why he chooses?" The challenge for individuals who hold this worldview is not only to have faith in God but also to have trust and certainty (*bitachon*) that God will take them on the right path, even if that path is not what they would have envisioned for themselves.

Pregnancy, as a "way of life" for these women [Teman, N.D.], is a situation that is rife with possible uncertainties; the women often referred in the interviews to the many stories of miscarriages, stillbirths, and health-impaired babies being born. One younger woman noted: "Every other block in Brooklyn has another Down syndrome child." Yet in all of these stories, whether speaking about themselves or a sister, cousin, or friend, they always ended the story with the affirmation that these are events that are beyond human control. Batya, age 23, mother of two, relayed that because her sister and sister-in-law had each had miscarriages in their first pregnancies, she had "sort of assumed that I'd have a miscarriage." This feeling accompanied her throughout pregnancy: "Even up till the end I was still really nervous something would happen. [. . .] It's scary but you don't really have that much control over it." When probed how she deals with the uncertainty, Batya answered: "You just pray a lot and don't do stomach crunches."

Batya's situation illustrates that of many of the women in this study. She has been surrounded by the multiple pregnancies of her mother, aunts, sisters, and other relatives from childhood. She feels a certain amount of anxiety and uncertainty during her pregnancy because of her knowledge of what might possibly go wrong, but at the same time she believes that God is in control and trusts with certainty that He will do what He sees as right. Nevertheless, she still makes an effort to be careful in her physical behavior (not to do stomach crunches) and she prays to God to ask for health and safety in pregnancy for herself and for her baby. The idea that a person can take action to help their situation even as they understand that ultimately these actions may not alter God's plan is encapsulated in the mediating concept of "obligatory effort" [*hishtadlus*]. When applied to health, obligatory effort means that one has an obligation to seek out medical care while at the same time praying to God to affect a cure as if your own efforts are meaningless [Parkoff and Linas, 2002; Kahn, 2006; Fertig, 2007].

. . .

Pregnancy and the Ideal Woman of Faith

A discourse about the ideal way of practicing faith and certainty was common amongst the women in the study and formed a basic model of religious devotion to aspire to. Stories circulated about women who proved the strength of their faith and certainty through their unwavering commitment to carrying out any task God had envisioned for them. These women achieved an almost mythological status—they faced the uncertainty of their predicament with a steadfast belief that anything God had planned for them was for the best. These stories about the "ideal woman of faith" were relayed in nearly every interview conducted, relating to someone the interviewee knew or had heard about in the community who exemplified this type of ultimate faith and certainty in the midst of a pregnancy-related crisis. Such women represented the gold standard that women tried to live up to and in telling these stories women expressed admiration for these displays of unwavering righteousness.

Shterna, age 23, mother of three, worked as an ultrasound technician in a clinic with a Haredi clientele. As a strictly observant mother herself, she recounted stories of women she had met in the clinic who had "remembered God" while experiencing moments of crisis related to pregnancy:

I remember one particular woman, she had just had her fourth miscarriage in a row and she was obviously devastated and she said like, "Okay, God's giving me another blow—I'll deal with it and we'll go on. He'll give me a healthy child." She remembered God in the moment of such despair. She saw that the heart was not beating and she said, "Okay." She was so strong in her faith [emunah]. . . .

As an ultrasound technician, Shterna had also participated in situations in which women had been told their baby had a fetal anomaly. These situations, in which the women had chosen to continue to carry the pregnancy to term and had accepted this as a God-sent ordeal made a particularly strong impression on her:

I saw also one lady whose baby had a heart defect and she also, she was just so positive. "Okay, so we'll do whatever we need to do. We'll find the best care that we could. And so she went, she spent a couple months of her pregnancy in [a hospital far from home]. She had to leave behind her four other children at home and her husband was back and forth, back and forth, taking care of the kids and running to her. It was not an easy situation . . . they did not say, 'I wish we could just abort this baby.'" No, they were just so good, like they were just, I don't know, very accepting. "Okay, this is what God gave us and we are just gonna go on. This is what He knows we can handle."

Shterna's words convey that mothers of disabled children in these communities are more likely to be valorized for caring for any child sent by God than criticized for not having used all the technologies available to "select" a "perfect baby" [Landsman, 2008; Ivry, 2009]. While giving to charity, doing good deeds (mitzvoth), and being a good wife and mother are all measures that are honored in this society, true religious commitment is measured in times of crisis. To become pregnant again and again is to face the many uncertainties of this period head on; in this way, pregnancy as a "way of life" is in itself a proclamation of faith. These times of crisis were viewed through the concept of the *nisayon*, or test of faith, as explored below.

The Test of Faith

While the discourse of the ideal woman of faith was circulated as a model of religious devotion, there was a gap between this ideology and the reality of raising a disabled child. Baila, age 56, mother of eight, exemplifies this. On the one hand, she refers to special needs children as "gifted" and their mothers as "chosen":

[My friend] told me that these children are considered gifted, they are highly evolved souls [*neshamas*]. It is considered by people that you are on a spiritual [*ruchniyus*] basis enough to accept it [*mekabel*]. It's considered really a divine privilege [*zchut*]. You have to be on a very high level to embrace it that way.

On the other hand, Baila spoke with ambivalence about her personal ability to live up to that ideal. As she relayed the story of a friend who had two special needs children, Baila inserted a plea to God mid-sentence, changing her voice as if addressing God directly and saying, "Don't give me such a task.

I mean I don't feel I could handle it." She then continued to tell about other families she had heard about in her community with multiple children who had given up a special needs child to adoption because they "just couldn't handle it," adding, "If I was in that situation I'm telling you . . . God did not give me that test. He didn't give me that."

Like Baila, other women spoke of large families they knew who had been unable to "handle" caring for a special needs child. The child was either given up for adoption or institutionalized. Decisions such as these were never made by the couple on their own; such decisions were always made by rabbis, whose rulings were formed on a case by case basis in consideration of the particular circumstances of the family seeking counsel. The women spoke of consulting a particular rabbi by phone on a regular basis regarding assorted issues even if that rabbi was in another state or in Israel; they also noted stories of women they knew who had been referred to specific rabbis who specialized in genetic and reproductive issues. Some spoke of rabbis who were known for more lenient or more strict rulings, and some knew of women who had received rabbinical permission to terminate their pregnancies after serious fetal anomalies were diagnosed, such as anencephaly or Tay-Sachs disease.

. . .

Discussion

Our interviews revealed that there were a wide range of positions related to certainty and uncertainty that Haredi women expressed in the context of pregnancy and prenatal diagnosis. The elements of fatalism and inevitability in their way of thinking, as well as the aspiration to be guided by faith and certainty, were not singular to pregnancy. Pregnancy, however, with its specific discourse of risk and uncertainty, brings their navigations of certainty–uncertainty in their faith-based worldview into focus.

There were many reasons for the women to experience uncertainty during pregnancy, as pregnancy was not a one-time event in their lives. Pregnant or caring for a small infant continuously throughout their childbearing years, these women faced continuous uncertainties with regard to the outcome of pregnancy and the health of their children. The women were highly aware of the chance that in one of their pregnancies they might give birth to a baby with physical and developmental disabilities. Dor Yeshorim screening had made them aware of the increased risk of being a carrier of Jewish genetic diseases, and many of the women were aware of Down syndrome babies being born to younger women in the community and not only to women of "advanced maternal age." The women were also regular consumers of prenatal care, so they were aware of the existence of prenatal tests that could screen for fetal anomalies because they had been offered the tests during routine prenatal care. These potential reasons for uncertainty were offset by the women's understanding that pregnancy termination was prohibited unless rabbinical permission was given in extreme cases.

The women's articulations of uncertainty were shaped in conversation with two mutually exclusive trajectories of certainty. Although they longed for reassurance of a healthy outcome to their pregnancies, they devalued the type of "secular certainty" that prenatal testing offered them—a calculated certainty based on technological predictions and probabilities. Conversely, they valued the type of "religious certainty" that could be measured by a woman's faith in God's plan, her knowledge that He is in control, and her acceptance of the idea that God may test her faith in any given situation. In this sense, to pursue secular certainty to ease their qualms about fetal health signified a problem of faith. The "ideal woman of faith" was expected to overcome the temptation to do prenatal tests, accept the challenge of raising a disabled child if God willed it and continue to bear more children. Alternately, accepting the offer of prenatal tests was understood as allowing uncertainty to direct one's actions and thus represented spiritual weakness. Seeking out an abortion when a fetal anomaly was diagnosed because you "could not handle it" was understood as a failure to live up to the gendered ideal of righteousness. Facing the unknown head-on by repeatedly becoming pregnant and overcoming the temptation of prenatal tests was thus a *proclamation of faith.*

. . .

However, faith did little in these circumstances to relieve the uncertainty of the women, many of whom remained scared throughout their pregnancies. In fact, the women's faith seemed to add an additional layer of pressure to the already existent burdens of commitment and responsibility that pregnant women tend to carry [see Rapp, 1999; Landsman, 2008; Ivry, 2009]. The orthodox women may not have struggled with the moral quandaries that have been described in the scholarship on women's experiences of prenatal diagnosis [Rothman, 1986; Rapp, 1999]; for most, refusing prenatal tests was a choice they accepted, and the option of termination—the "burden of choice"—was not perceived to be an option because of religious law, despite rabbinic exceptions. However, the women did struggle with spiritual ideals—with the principles of faith and certainty—and the tensions they experienced in trying to rise to the challenge of having full certainty to match their faith were performed not only in the private and social sphere but also in the spiritual sphere between themselves and God. Faith serves as a tool for coping with uncertainty but simultaneously contributes to additional pressures on pregnant women who are trying to fulfill the ideal gendered model of faith in their community.

References

Birenbaum-Carmeli D. 2008. Your faith or mine: A pregnancy spacing intervention in an ultra-Orthodox Jewish community in Israel. Reprod Health Matters 16:185–191.

Comenetz J. 2006. Census-based estimation of the Hasidic Jewish population. Contemp Jewry 26:35–74.

Fertig A. 2007. Bridging the Gap: Clarifying the Eternal Foundations of Mussar and Emunah for Today. Jerusalem: Feldheim Publishers.

Friedman M. 1991. The Haredi Ultra-Orthodox Society: Sources Trends and Processes. Jerusalem: The Jerusalem Institute for Israel Studies.

Ivry T. 2009. Embodying Culture: Pregnancy in Japan and Israel. New Brunswick, NJ: Rutgers University Press.

Kahn S. 2006. Making technology familiar: Orthodox Jews and infertility support, advice, and inspiration. Cult Med Psychiatry 30:467–480.

Landsman G. 2008. Reconstructing Motherhood and Disability in the Age Of "Perfect" Babies. New York: Routledge.

Mittman IS, Bowie JV, Manan S. 2007. Exploring the discourse between genetic counselors and Orthodox Jewish community members related to reproductive genetic technology. Patient Educ Couns 65:230–236.

Parkoff RE, Linas E. 2002. Trust Me: An Anthology of Emunah and Bitachon. Jerusalem: Feldheim Publishers.

Rapp R. 1999. Testing Women, Testing the Fetus: The Social Impact of Amniocentesis in America. New York: Routledge.

Rothman BK. 1986. The Tentative Pregnancy: Prenatal Diagnosis and the Future of Motherhood. New York: Viking.

Teman E. N.D. Pregnancy as a Way of Life Among Ultra-Orthodox Jewish Women. Unpublished manuscript in preparation. Philadelphia.

12

The State of Abortion and Contraception Attitudes in All 50 States

Robert P. Jones, Natalie Jackson, Maxine Najle, Oyindamola Bola, and Daniel Greenberg

Public Religion Research Institute (PRRI) is a nonprofit organization that studies the intersection of religion, culture, and public policy in the United States. For this piece, scholar of religion Robert P. Jones and his team gathered polling data on abortion attitudes in relation to religious denomination and political party affiliation. Though exact numbers shift over time, longitudinal polling data in the United States has consistently demonstrated majority support for legal access to abortion. This study confirms that wide majorities of most religiously identified people also favor legal access to abortion in all or most cases.

The Legality of Abortion

A majority (54%) of Americans believe that abortion should be legal in most (31%) or all (23%) cases, while four in ten (40%) believe that abortion should be illegal in most (25%) or all (15%) cases. These numbers are essentially

Source: Robert P. Jones, Natalie Jackson, Maxine Najle, Oyindamola Bola, and Daniel Greenberg, "The State of Abortion and Contraception Attitudes in All 50 States," *Public Religion Research Institute* (March 26, 2019): 1–32.

unchanged since 2014 when a similar majority (55%) of Americans said abortion should be legal in most (34%) or all (21%) cases, and about four in ten (41%) believed that abortion should be illegal in most (25%) or all (16%) cases.

Although a few states such as Alabama and Missouri have recently passed laws that—should they survive court challenges—would make abortion illegal with virtually no exceptions, there is no state in which more than one quarter of residents say abortion should be illegal in all cases. . . . States with the largest proportion of residents who say abortion should be illegal in all cases include: Louisiana (23%), Mississippi (22%), Arkansas (21%), Nebraska (21%), Tennessee (21%), Kentucky (20%), and North Dakota (20%). In all other states, including Alabama (16%) and Missouri (19%), fewer than one in five think abortion should be illegal in all cases. Fewer than one in ten residents say abortion should be illegal in all cases in Vermont (5%), the District of Columbia (7%), and New Hampshire (8%).

Party Affiliation

Attitudes about the legality of abortion are highly stratified by partisan affiliation. Democrats (70%) are twice as likely as Republicans (34%) to favor the legality of abortion; six in ten (60%) Republicans are opposed to the legality of abortion, although notably only 22% of Republicans say abortion should be illegal in all cases.

The partisan gap has widened from 28 percentage points in 2014 to 36 points today. Democrats have become three percentage points more supportive of the legality of abortion (up from 67%), while Republicans have become five percentage points less supportive (down from 39%) over the last four years. Notably, this increase in support among Democrats is accompanied by a shift in intensity. The percentage of Democrats who say abortion should be legal in *all* cases has increased by six percentage points, from 29% in 2014 to 35% today. There is no corresponding shift in intensity among Republicans.

Party by Ideology

Across party lines, a majority of liberals and moderates support abortion. The biggest intra-party divide is among Democrats: 82% of liberal

Democrats think abortion should be legal in most or all cases, compared to 63% of moderate Democrats and 46% of conservative Democrats. Among Republicans, majorities of liberal (54%) and moderate (53%) Republicans think abortion should be legal in most or all cases, compared to only 28% of conservative Republicans.

Interestingly, liberal Republicans (54%) are more supportive of abortion legality than conservative Democrats (46%). Liberal Democrats (82%) are more supportive of legality than conservative Republicans (68%) are opposed to it. Conservative independents (37%) resemble Republicans overall, but both moderate (61%) and liberal (70%) independents show strong support for abortion legality.

. . .

Religious Affiliation

Among religious groups, opposition to the legality of abortion is largely confined to white evangelical Protestants and other smaller conservative Christian groups [Figure 4]. Strong majorities of Hispanic Protestants (58%), white evangelical Protestants (65%), Mormons (66%), and Jehovah's Witnesses (68%) say abortion should be illegal in most or all cases. Notably, even among white evangelical Protestants, only one quarter (25%) say abortion should be illegal in all cases.

Majorities of other large Protestant groups, such as white mainline Protestants (59%) and black Protestants (56%), say abortion should be legal in most or all cases.

Catholics are divided (48% support legality in most or all cases vs. 46% oppose legality in most or all cases), but there are significant differences by race and ethnicity. A majority (52%) of white Catholics, compared to 41% of Hispanic Catholics, support the legality of abortion.

Majorities of all non-Christian religious groups support legal abortion in most or all cases. Notably, some of these groups, such as Jews (70%) and Unitarian Universalists (83%), support the legality of abortion by wide margins. Muslims (51%) have the narrowest majority, but all other groups have more than six in ten in favor of abortion legality. More than seven in ten (72%) religiously unaffiliated Americans support the legality of abortion, including more than one-third (36%) who say it should be legal in *all* cases.

. . .

Figure 4 The Legality of Abortion, by Religious Affiliation.

Percent who say abortion should be:

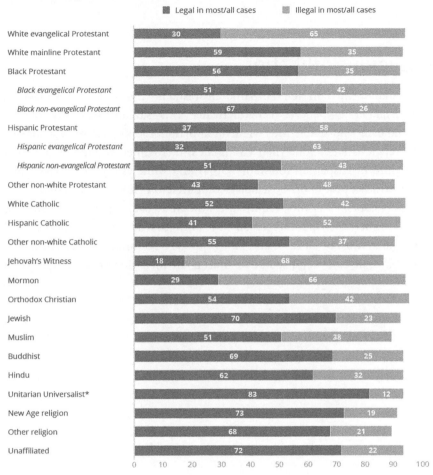

■ Legal in most/all cases   ■ Illegal in most/all cases

	Legal	Illegal
White evangelical Protestant	30	65
White mainline Protestant	59	35
Black Protestant	56	35
Black evangelical Protestant	51	42
Black non-evangelical Protestant	67	26
Hispanic Protestant	37	58
Hispanic evangelical Protestant	32	63
Hispanic non-evangelical Protestant	51	43
Other non-white Protestant	43	48
White Catholic	52	42
Hispanic Catholic	41	52
Other non-white Catholic	55	37
Jehovah's Witness	18	68
Mormon	29	66
Orthodox Christian	54	42
Jewish	70	23
Muslim	51	38
Buddhist	69	25
Hindu	62	32
Unitarian Universalist*	83	12
New Age religion	73	19
Other religion	68	21
Unaffiliated	72	22

*Sample size is less than 100 (N=97).

Source: PRRI 2018 American Values Atlas.

How Abortion Opinion Impacts Vote Choices

About one in five (21%) Americans consider a political candidate's view on abortion a deal-breaker and say they would only vote for a candidate who shares their opinion on abortion. Americans who oppose the legality of abortion (27%) are significantly more likely than those who support the legality of abortion (18%) to say they will only vote for a candidate who shares their views on the issue.

. . .

Religious Affiliation

Just under three in ten Hispanic Protestants (29%), white evangelical Protestants (28%), and Jewish Americans (27%) say they will only vote for a candidate who shares their view on abortion, the highest proportions of any religious affiliation. Their candidates likely differ, though: More than one-third of Hispanic Protestants (36%) and white evangelical Protestants (35%) who oppose abortion legality, compared to 19% and 15% of those who support abortion legality, require a candidate to share their views. Among Jewish Americans, that is reversed: 31% of those who think abortion should be legal in most or all cases and 22% of those who think it should be illegal in most or all cases say a candidate must share their views to earn their vote.

13

Faith, Race-Ethnicity, and Public Policy Preferences:

Religious Schemas and Abortion Attitudes among US Latinos

John P. Bartkowski, Aida I. Ramos-Wada,

Chris G. Ellison and Gabriel A. Acevedo

Studies examining the relationship between religion and abortion attitudes have historically focused on white Christians and have documented the role that increased religiosity plays in those attitudes. Here, sociologist John Bartkowski leads a team of researchers in a study that represents more diverse communities. This quantitative bilingual research project about the lived religious experience of those in the Latinx community in the United States offers insight into the differences in abortion attitudes of those affiliated with traditional Latin American Roman Catholicism and those Latino/as who attend one of the many fast-growing conservative Protestant churches. Understanding the variation of perspectives within a given religious tradition is an important aspect of the study of religion.

Source: John P. Bartkowski, Aida I. Ramos-Wada, Chris G. Ellison, and Gabriel A. Acevedo, "Faith, Race-Ethnicity, and Public Policy Preferences: Religious Schemas and Abortion Attitudes among US Latinos," *Journal for the Scientific Study of Religion* 51, no. 2 (2012): 343–58.

Scholars have long studied the links between religion and abortion, and have found that people who are highly religious tend to be more opposed to abortion (see, e.g., Gay and Lynxwiler 1999; Guth et al. 1993; Jelen and Wilcox 2003; Steensland et al. 2000). Moreover, conservative religious adherents who are highly active in their faith tradition evince the greatest opposition to abortion (e.g., Guth et al. 1993; Hoffmann and Johnson 2005; Hoffmann and Miller 1997; Steensland et al. 2000). Conservative Protestants[1] are now considerably more likely to oppose abortion than are Catholics, and there is little attitudinal variability among conservative Protestants on this issue when compared with those from other faith traditions (Hoffmann and Johnson 2005; Hoffmann and Miller 1997, 1998). Despite the consistency of these observations across studies conducted in different years with various data sources, the literature on religion and abortion could benefit from additional consideration of the pathways through which opposition to this practice is formed. For the most part, scholars have argued that religious communities, particularly theologically orthodox faith traditions, create a moral ethos that lends itself to political conservatism. While this interpretation is plausible, it fails to examine the social mechanisms associated with religious involvement that might underlay the connections between religiosity and public policy views.

Moreover, relatively little attention has been given to the linkages between religion, race ethnicity, and abortion attitudes. Non-Hispanic white Americans have received the lion's share of attention in the religion and abortion attitudes literature (Jelen and Wilcox 2003). And, where race ethnicity has been explored, African Americans have most often been the subject of investigations (e.g., Gay and Lynxwiler 1999; Lynxwiler and Gay 1994), with Latinos[2] receiving scarce attention on this score. This oversight is lamentable, given the rapid growth of Latinos as a proportion of the American population and the increasing religious diversity observed among American Latinos. Decennial U.S. Census data reveal that there were 35.3 million Latinos in the United States in the year 2000, up significantly from 22.4 million in 1990 (U.S. Census Bureau 2010). In 2000, Latinos were estimated to make up 12.5 percent of the American population, and this figure registered at 16.3 percent in 2010. Long-term growth projections estimate that 20 percent of Americans will be of Latino origin by 2030, with additional increases to just under a quarter of the overall U.S. population expected two decades thereafter.

This fast-growing racial-ethnic group is also experiencing significant religious diversification (Barton 2006; De La Torre 2008; Diaz-Stevens and Stevens-Arroyo 1998; Dolan and Deck 1994; Espinosa, Elizondo, and

Miranda 2005; Hunt 1999; Maldonado 1999, 2002). While the Catholic Church had enjoyed a longstanding monopoly on Latino religious affiliation, recent years have witnessed increasing inroads that Protestant faiths have made into the Latino religious market. Some have argued that Hispanic Protestants are "doubly marginalized" by being situated outside the Latino Catholic mainstream and at the edges of predominantly non-Hispanic white American Protestantism (De La Torre 2008; Maldonado 1999). A review of multiple national studies has revealed that Latinos are still quite likely to be born and raised Catholic (about 70 percent), even as a significant minority of Latinos now identifies as non-Catholic Christian (about 20 percent) (Perl, Greely, and Gray 2006). Most of the remainder (about 8 percent) claims no faith at all (Pew Hispanic Center and Pew Forum on Religion & Public Life 2007). Conservative Protestant denominations have been especially successful at attracting Latino adherents, with over 15 percent of Latinos now claiming such an affiliation (Pew Hispanic Center and Pew Forum on Religion & Public Life 2007). The "evangelicalization" of American Latinos raises important questions not only about the contours of religious diversity among America's largest, fastest-growing racial minority. It also prompts questions about the cultural and political sensibilities of conservative Protestant Latinos when compared with their Catholic counterparts.

This study is designed to examine the influence of religion among Latinos on a key public policy issue, namely, abortion. In undertaking this study, we explore how a combination of racial-ethnic homology (shared Latino heritage) and religious diversity (Catholic vs. conservative Protestant affiliation) is associated with abortion attitudes. We use nationally representative data with a rich repository of religion measures to do so. In addition, we seek to advance theoretical understandings of the linkages between race-ethnicity, religion, and abortion. We identify religious schemas (cognitive frameworks) as a key mechanism through which abortion attitudes are formed, and compare the efficacy of religious schemas across denominational contexts. While we recognize that both Catholic and conservative Protestant schemas are linked to antiabortion attitudes, our comparison of these two religious groups within the broader Latino population permits us to consider how religious schemas influence public policy attitudes differently across faith traditions. We anticipate that the greatest opposition to abortion will be expressed by devout Latino conservative Protestants given (1) the especially robust antiabortion attitudes among conservative Protestants at large, (2) the market niche status and voluntaristic nature of religious affiliation among conservative Protestant

Latinos, and (3) the degree of network integration and cultural exposure of highly churched Latino conservative Protestants. Where public policy preferences are concerned, Latino conservative Protestantism is expected to contrast markedly with the near-monopolistic and more institutionalized nature of religious affiliation within Latino Catholicism.

. . .

Discussion

Given the rapid growth and religious diversification of U.S. Hispanics, this study examined abortion attitudes expressed by Latino Americans of different religious affiliations, with particular attention to Catholic and conservative Protestant preferences toward legalized abortion. We defined schemas as cognitive frameworks that at once enable social actors to interpret the worlds they inhabit and provide recipes for appropriate action. Using recent data collected from a nationally representative sample of American Hispanics, we found that regularly attending conservative Protestant Latinos were decidedly more opposed to abortion than their regularly attending Catholic counterparts. We explained this finding in two ways.

First, Latino conservative Protestants may have transposed religious schemas from the broader evangelical subculture within which they are situated. These schemas yield robustly antiabortion social attitudes not only among white religious conservatives, as demonstrated in previous research (reviewed above), but also among Latino conservative Protestants (as shown here). Although leaders in the Catholic Church have condemned abortion, sometimes likening it to murder, American Catholics and their Latino co-religionists have been inclined to appropriate Vatican pronouncements about sexual morality quite selectively. Thus, the disjuncture between official Church doctrine and laypersons' views that has long been observed in non-Hispanic white Catholicism (D' Antonio et al. 2007) also seems evident among Latino Catholics. Within conservative Protestantism, abortion is seen as an affront to motherhood, pronatalism, traditional family values, and, even more fundamentally, scriptural edicts about "God's handiwork" in creating life at conception, thereby producing little variability among conservative Protestants on this hot-button social issue (Hoffmann and Johnson 2005; Hoffmann and Miller 1997, 1998). Thus, for both Latino and white conservative Protestants, religious schemas yield strong opposition to abortion.

Second, it is reasonable to interpret greater opposition to abortion among Latino conservative Protestants as an amplification of pro-life schemas that have become diluted in Latino Catholicism. Latino conservative Protestants are affiliated with a niche, highly voluntaristic faith tradition, one strikingly at odds with Catholicism. Scholars of Hispanic religion have called attention to the "double marginality" of Latino Protestantism, which is religiously distinct from Latino Catholicism and ethnically distinct from non-Hispanic white American Protestantism (De La Torre 2008; Maldonado 1999). Abortion attitudes may be one means through which Latino conservative Protestants negotiate this numerical and cultural marginality. Strong opposition to abortion situates evangelical Latinos squarely within the broader universe of conservative Protestantism. At the same time, these convictions distinguish them from the "lukewarm" commitment to core Christian principles exhibited by their Catholic peers. Thus, even though Hispanic Catholics may far outnumber Latino conservative Protestants, the demonstration of a more aggressive commitment to a pro-life position by Latino conservative Protestants can be viewed as evidence of taking one's (evangelical) faith "more seriously" than one's Catholic counterparts. This is not to say that stronger antiabortion attitudes among Latino conservative Protestants may be reduced to political maneuvering. However, an interethnic alliance among conservative Protestants on the issue of abortion is one possible outcome of such shared pro-life convictions.

For both Latino conservative Protestants and Catholics, we found that worship service attendance was associated with stronger antiabortion attitudes. This finding was consistent with our expectation that network integration would be vital to the reinforcement of religious schemas and, consequently, would strengthen antiabortion attitudes. Interestingly, infrequently attending Catholics were about as supportive of legalized abortion as the religiously unaffiliated, whereas infrequently attending conservative Protestants evinced abortion views not terribly different than those of regularly attending Catholics. This finding suggests that Latinos who claim only a nominal Catholic affiliation have largely dis-identified with Catholic teachings on abortion, and perhaps other issues as well. By contrast, nominal conservative Protestant Latinos hold antiabortion sentiments similar to those of highly churched Catholics. So, while attendance significantly enhances antiabortion attitudes in both traditions, a lack of attendance undermines opposition to abortion quite profoundly for Catholics. The odds of observing Latino conservative Protestant opposition to legalized abortion were reduced slightly by biblical literalism and antiabortion preaching from the pulpit. However, significant effects persisted for regularly attending Latino evangelicals despite controlling for these other religious factors. This finding suggests that robust integration within conservative Protestant religious networks—that is, the confluence of affiliation and regular attendance—is a key mechanism through which Latino evangelicals' antiabortion attitudes are maintained.

These findings have a number of important implications. First, our study underscores the importance of moving beyond monolithic bloc arguments about Latino religiosity and public policy preferences. This rapidly growing sector of the American population is clearly undergoing religious diversification, and this process has important consequences for public policy attitudes. We conceived of religious diversification in multifaceted terms, focusing not only on denominational pluralism but also differences in worship service attendance, biblical literalism, and the political salience of religious beliefs. Our investigation revealed that an expansive approach to studying religious diversity among Latinos yields more holistic and robust empirical explanations of political differentiation among Latinos.

Second, our study sheds light on the nexus of race-ethnicity and American religion. While scholars have long investigated the relationship between race-ethnicity and religion in the United States (see Bartkowski and Matthews 2006 for review), our study reveals how politically oriented religious schemas are a product not only of one's faith tradition, but are influenced by racial ethnic heritage. The case of Latino abortion attitudes illustrates how religious schemas linked to antiabortion attitudes are amplified in faith traditions that could be seen as upstart religions in the Hispanic context. We have argued that the relatively weaker opposition to abortion exhibited by Latino Catholics, even those who are actively churchgoing, is a product of structural dynamics in the Hispanic religious marketplace. A near-monopolistic, highly institutionalized faith such as Latino Catholicism faces more difficulty achieving "buy-in" to its core doctrinal precepts among adherents whose faith was conferred upon them rather than intentionally chosen by them. Latino conservative Protestantism is a more "costly" faith because it places stricter, more rigorous demands on its adherents than does Catholicism, particularly where tightly cohesive evangelical opposition to abortion is concerned. And, as members of a minority faith tradition that is more likely to be chosen rather than conferred by default across generations, conservative Protestant Latinos may find themselves religiously at odds with a large segment of the Hispanic population, including their (ostensibly Catholic) family, friends, and neighbors. It seems reasonable to surmise that these factors could bolster the religious commitments and religiously based social attitudes of evangelical Latinos when compared with their Catholic counterparts.

Third, over the past three decades, some activists within the Republican Party have reached out to racial and ethnic minorities, especially Latinos and African Americans, on the basis of shared conservative religious and social values. To date, these appeals have enjoyed only limited success (McDaniel and Ellison 2008). Much of the outreach to Hispanics has been guided by the assumption that Latino cultural conservatism stems from strong Catholic roots. However, this study, along with other recent work (e.g., Ellison, Echevarria, and Smith 2005; Ellison, Acevedo, and Ramos-Wada 2011), reveals that: (a) Latino Catholic opinion is sharply divided on many hot-button social issues, and (b) the growth of conservative Protestant and sectarian (e.g., Mormon, Jehovah's Witness) groups may increase the prominence of socially conservative views within the Latino population.

Notes

1. Recognizing that many sociologists of religion use the term "conservative Protestant" as a broad category composed predominantly of evangelicals in addition to some other conservative Christian groups (e.g., fundamentalists, Pentecostals), we generally opt for this term throughout the article. In a few instances, we use the term "evangelical" interchangeably for stylistic convenience.
2. We use the terms "Latino" and "Hispanic" interchangeably for stylistic convenience.

References

Bartkowski, John P. and Todd L. Matthews. 2006. Race/ethnicity. In *Handbook on religion and social institutions*, edited by Helen Rose Ebaugh, pp. 163–83. New York: Springer.

Barton, Paul. 2006. *Hispanic Methodists, Presbyterians, and Baptists in Texas*. Austin, TX: University of Texas Press.

D'Antonio, William V., James D. Davidson, Dean R. Hoge, and Mary L. Gautier. 2007. *American Catholics today: New realities of their faith and their church.* Lanham, MD: Rowman and Littlefield Publishers.

De La Torre, Miguel A. 2008. Religion and religiosity. In *Latinas/os in the United States: Changing the face of America,* edited by Havidan Rodriguez, Rogelio Saenz, and Cecilia Menjivar, pp. 225–40. New York: Springer

Díaz-Stevens, Ana Maria and Anthony M. Stevens-Arroyo. 1998. *Recognizing the Latino resurgence in US religion: The Emmaus paradigm.* Boulder, CO: Westview Press.

Dolan, Jay P. and Allan Figueroa Deck (eds.). 1994. *Hispanic Catholic culture in the US: Issues and concerns.* Notre Dame, IN.: University of Notre Dame Press.

Ellison, Christopher G., Gabriel A. Acevedo, and Aida I. Ramos-Wada. 2011. Religion and attitudes toward same-sex marriage among US Latinos. *Social Science Quarterly* 92(1):35–56.

Ellison, Christopher G., Samuel Echevarria, and Brad Smith. 2005. Religion and abortion attitudes among US Hispanics: Findings from the 1990 Latino National Political Survey. *Social Science Quarterly* 86(1):192–208.

Espinosa, Gastón, Virgilio Elizondo, and Jesse Miranda (eds.). 2005. *Latino religions and civic activism in the United States.* New York: Oxford University Press.

Gay, David and John Lynxwiler. 1999. The impact of religiosity on race variations in abortion attitudes. *Sociological Spectrum* 19(3):359–77.

Guth, James L., Corwin E. Schmidt, Lyman A. Kellsdelt, and John C. Green. 1993. The sources of antiabortion attitudes: The case of religious political activists. *American Politics Research* 21(1):65–80.

Hoffmann, John P. and Sherrie Mills Johnson. 2005. Attitudes toward abortion among religious traditions in the United States: Change or continuity? *Sociology of Religion* 66(2):161–82.

Hoffmann, John P. and Alan S. Miller. 1997. Social and political attitudes among religious groups: Convergence and divergence over time. *Journal for the Scientific Study of Religion* 36(1):52–70.

Hoffmann, John P. and Alan S. Miller. 1998. Denominational influences on socially divisive issues: Polarization or continuity? *Journal for the Scientific Study of Religion* 37(3):528–46.

Hunt, Larry L. 1999. Hispanic Protestantism in the United States: Trends by decade and generation. *Social Forces* 77(4):1601–24.

Jelen, Ted G. and Clyde Wilcox. 2003. Causes and consequences of public attitudes toward abortion: A review and research agenda. *Political Research Quarterly* 56(4):489–500.

Lynxwiler, John and David Gay. 1994. Reconsidering race differences in abortion attitudes. *Social Science Quarterly* 75(1):67–84.

Maldonado, David, Jr. (ed.). 1999. *Protestantes/Protestants: Hispanic Christianity within mainline traditions.* Nashville, TN: Abingdon Press.

Maldonado, David, Jr. 2002. The changing religious practice of Hispanics. In *Hispanics in the United States,* edited by Pastor San Juan Cafferty and David W. Engstrom, pp. 97–121. New Brunswick, NJ: Transaction Publishers.

McDaniel, Eric L. and Christopher G. Ellison 2008. God's party? Religion, race/ethnicity, and partisanship over time. *Political Research Quarterly* 61(2):180–91.

Perl, Paul, Jennifer Z. Greely, and Mark M. Gray. 2006. What proportion of adult Hispanics are Catholic? A review of survey data and methodology. *Journal for the Scientific Study of Religion* 45(3):419–36.

Pew Hispanic Center and Pew Forum on Religion and Public Life. 2007. *Changing faiths: Latinos and the transformation of American religion.* Available athttp://pewforum.org/uploadedfiles/Topics/Demographics/hispanics-religion-07- final-mar08.pdf, accessed March 22, 2010.

Steensland, Brian, Lynn D. Robinson, W. Bradford Wilcox, Jerry Z. Park, Mark D. Regnerus, and Robert D. Woodberry. 2000. The measure of American religion: Toward improving the state of the art. *Social Forces* 79(1):291–318.

U.S. Census Bureau. 2010. *Facts on the Hispanic or Latino population.* Available at http://www.census.gov/ pubinfo/www/NEWhispMLl.htrnl/, accessed March 15, 2010.

14

Ethnic Diversity, Religion, and Opinions toward Legalizing Abortion:

The Case of Asian Americans

Bohsiu Wu and Aya Kimura Ida

In this piece, sociologists Bohsiu Wu and Aya Kimura Ida examine the diversity of attitudes about abortion across six major groups that have traditionally been designated as Asian American. While religiosity has been identified as a significant factor that shapes abortion attitudes, this quantitative research demonstrates the need to disaggregate data sets in order to examine potentially significant differences among and between groups. It also highlights the importance of more detailed analysis of the religious and ethnic diversity within groups that are often categorized together in order to examine the effect of various factors (degree of religious devotion, abortion practices in the country of origin, English proficiency, etc.) on abortion attitudes.

Despite the contentious nature of the abortion debate, public opinion toward legalizing abortion in the past decades has been stable according to several major opinion surveys. For example, Gallup Polls show that the percentage of American adults in 2014 who were pro-choice was 47% and the percentage

Source: Bohsiu Wu and Aya Kimura Ida, "Ethnic Diversity, Religion, and Opinions Toward Legalizing Abortion: The Case of Asian Americans," *Journal of Ethnic and Cultural Studies* 5, no. 1 (2018): 94–109.

prolife was 46% (Gallup, 2014). Similarly, in the studies from 1995 to 2016, the percentage of American adults who favor legalization of abortion hovers around 50% whereas those who oppose is 45% (Pew Research Center, 2016). General Social Survey (GSS) also shows a similar pattern (Smith & Son, 2013). Previous studies on opinions toward legalizing abortion show that several factors hold consistent impact on Americans' attitudes toward this controversial issue (Aydin, 2012; Lafer & Aydin, 2012; Tolba, 2018). These factors include age, education, income, religiosity, region of residence, and political ideology. Gender was found not to be a significant factor and the lack of a gender difference was attributed to a suppression effect of religiosity in a recent study using GSS data (Barkan, 2014).

. . .

Background Religion and Abortion

There is a very clear pattern from various opinion surveys regarding the role of religion in the abortion debate. American Catholics and conservative Christians including fundamentalists and evangelicals are much more likely to oppose legal abortion compared to their counterparts belonging to different faiths (Cook, Jelen, & Wilcox, 1992). The evidence from previous opinion surveys is clear (Pew Research Center, 2017). In general, frequency of church attendance is positively correlated with a prohibitive view of abortion. That is, regardless of denomination, people who attend church service more frequently are more likely to oppose abortion. Church-goers who strongly believe that the sanctity of life should prevail over the right to choose are more likely to have their faiths and attitudes reinforced by other members in the same religious institutions. These findings suggest the importance of analyzing the effects of religious affiliation and religiosity separately as they may exert differential impact on one's attitudes.

The impact of religion on people's views toward abortion is apparently strong but not absolute. Petersen (2001) found that an interactive effect exists between religion and education in a way that the impact of religion can be neutralized by education. While education has a modest liberating effect on the view of abortion among religious conservatives (Brooks, 1999), the effect of education among religious liberals is strong. That is, unlike their conservative counterparts, educated and religious liberals are less likely to oppose abortion. There is also an interactive effect between education and church attendance in that a weaker liberating effect from education is found among frequent church goers than among their infrequent counterparts regarding anti-abortion opinions. Further, among infrequent church attenders, there is little interaction effect between education and religion regarding opinions toward abortion. This is because ". . . infrequent attenders . . . generally lack significant integration into religious communities that support the conservative stance" (Petersen 2001, p.200). The effect of religion on opinion toward abortion can be moderated by other critical factors that shape people's moral universe.

. . .

Religion, Abortion, and Asian Americans

In a recent study, Min and Jang (2015) confirm that there is a high level of religious diversity among Asian Americans. In the survey included in the study, five major Asian American groups (Chinese, Filipino, Indian, Korean, and Vietnamese) are asked about their affiliation with a religious institution and church attendance. More than 80 percent of Filipino/a Americans identify themselves as Catholics. Close to 80 percent of Indian Americans report either Hinduism or Sikhism as their religions (69% and 11%, respectively). Nearly 60% of Korean Americans are Protestants. Over one in five Vietnamese choose Catholicism and close to half identify Buddhism as their current religion. Surprisingly, nearly three out of four Chinese American respondents choose "no religion" when asked about their current religion. The authors attribute this particular response to the fact that most Chinese Americans, especially new immigrants, practice folk religions which is not one of the choices in the survey. Regarding church attendance, pious Asian Americans who are Christians tend to attend church services more frequently than their American counterparts. Of all five groups, Korean Americans who are Protestants have the highest degree of church attendance in that more than half of Korean American respondents report going to church more than once a week. This contrasts with a very low level of attendance on the part of Chinese Americans who are Buddhists; more than half of them seldom or never attend services in temples. Compared to their less devout counterparts, Asian Americans who are more involved in religions, especially ethnic churches, tend to forge a stronger ethnic identity and receive a wide range of services from their respective churches.

. . .

According to the 2010 Census, Asian Americans account for about 6% of the population in the US, a rapid increase compared with data from the previous census. Census data also show that Asian Americans are made up of a great multitude of ethnicities, languages and dialects, religious preferences, socioeconomic statuses, and different immigration patterns (. . . U.S. Bureau of the Census, 2012). Whether such diverse backgrounds may affect how Asian Americans view the abortion issue is yet to be tested. Given the centrality of religion that fundamentally influences how abortion is viewed, it stands to reason that different Asian Americans' views on abortion should also be influenced by their respective religious affiliations and varying degree of religiosity.

. . .

Discussion and Conclusion

Findings from this study indicate that a distinctive difference in opinions exists among ostensibly homogeneous Asian Americans regarding legalized abortion. Asian Americans, as a group, differ sharply in this controversial domestic issue. An almost identical percentage of Asian Americans (42% disagree vs. 44% agree) hold opposing views of legal abortion. Regarding the abortion controversy, Asian Americans are a microcosm of the mainstream American society that has been sharply divided over the past decades. Among six different Asian American subgroups, opinions also evidently differ from one group to another: Japanese American are the most favorable to legalized abortion, whereas Vietnamese Americans hold the least favorable attitudes.

. . .

First, with the exception of Japanese Americans, gender appears to be a non-factor for most Asians after controlling for religiosity and other factors . . . In other words, only among Japanese Americans does a suppression effect exist which is consistent with a recent study that shows that the impact of gender is suppressed by religiosity (Barkan, 2014). That is, the reason why gender may appear not to affect opinions toward legalized abortion is because women are more religious than men and people with a high degree of religiosity and a stronger religious identity are more likely to oppose legal abortion. Further studies are warranted to examine why only among Japanese Americans is gender suppressed by religiosity. One possible explanation is that Japanese Americans are more likely to be native-born Americans compared to other Asian American subgroups. Therefore, as a result of a higher degree of acculturation in mainstream society, Japanese Americans are more likely to exhibit similar traits as their counterparts of other races and ethnicities in the mainstream American society.

Second, comparing all six Asian American groups, it appears that the most consistent and impactful factor is political self-identification with the exception of Asian Americans of Indian and Korean descent.

. . .

Third, religion, especially church attendance, is significant in shaping Asian Americans' views of abortion in an expected fashion. However, not all Asian Americans are affected by religion the same way. Religious attendance is significant for only three groups: less so Chinese, but more importantly for Filipino/a and Vietnamese Americans. As a recent phenomenon, the introduction of evangelical Christianity to Chinese immigrant communities may align some Chinese Americans with conservative Christians in holding a prohibitive view toward abortion (Kim, 2004; Yang, 1998). In contrast, the influence of Catholicism remains salient for Filipino/a and Vietnamese in forming their views of abortion.

Among Chinese Americans who hold a Buddhist view of death and rebirth as a cycle, it is possible that abortion is not considered as a life ethic issue as compared to Catholic and Christian conservatives. In the same vein, Chinese Americans who practice folk religions and ancestor worship, may also hold a cyclical view of life and death, thus forgoing a moralistic view of abortion. Evidence from previous studies also suggest that abortion was officially promoted and implemented as a pragmatic solution to population control in both mainland China and Taiwan, two main origins of emigration to the US (Smolin, 2010); therefore, immigrants from these two countries may not see abortion strictly as a moral and religious issue. Regarding the abortion issue, a moral universe that centers around religion for other ethnic Asian groups may not be the same for Chinese Americans. The void then, for Chinese Americans, is filled by a more mundane orientation such as political self-identification.

Results from this study clearly indicate that Asian Americans, as a group, differ significantly in their views toward legalized abortion, one of the most contentious social issues in the US. It is thus reasonable to speculate that such a divergence of opinions may also exist among Asian Americans in their attitudes toward other controversial social issues (CARE, 2011; Campaign for College Opportunity, 2015). The rich diversity among Asian Americans is rooted in the unique immigration history and cultural heritage of each ethnic group, which subsequently shapes each group's experience in collectively becoming the fastest growing racial minority in the US. The variation among six major Asian American groups concerning legalized abortion reflects not only such diversity but also a potential realignment in the abortion debate along racial and ethnic lines.

With globalization aided by technological advancement, the degree of ethnic and racial heterogeneity is increasing not only in the United States, but also in other [countries] (Ahmed, 2016; Corona et al., 2017; Inceli, 2015; Kaya, 2015; Ozfidan & Burlbaw, 2016). Racial and ethnic diversity can engender both cultural and economic revival as currently witnessed in many parts of the world. Unfortunately, it can also become the fault line that sharply divide a society. A better appreciation of the benefits and complications of racial and ethnic diversity will enhance the degree of mutual appreciation from all sectors in a society. Future public opinion research capable of addressing the issue of ethnic diversity will produce nuanced insights into how the public views and deal with controversial social issues including abortion.

References

Ahmed, M. (2016). Ethnicity, identity and group vitality: A study of Burushos of Srinagar. *Journal of Ethnic and Cultural Studies, 3*(1), 1–10.

Aydin, H. (2012). First-Generation Turkish Immigrants' Perceptions on Cultural Integration in Multicultural Societies: A Qualitative Case Study. *US-China Educational Review B, 2*(3), 326–337.

Barkan, S. E. (2014). Gender and abortion attitudes: Religiosity as a suppressor variable. *Public Opinion Quarterly, 78*(4), 940–950.

Brooks, J. G. (1999, December 30). *In search of understanding: The case for constructivist classrooms.* [Review of the book, by C. Halpern]. *American Journal of Qualitative Research, 1*(1), 32–36.

Campaign for College Opportunity. (2015). *The state of higher education in California: Asian American, Native Hawaiian, Pacific Islanders.* Retrieved from https://www.collegecampaign.org/wp-content/uploads/2015/09/2015 -State-of-Higher-Education_AANHPI2.pdf

[Cook, E. A., Jelen, T. G., & Wilcox, C. (1992). Between two absolutes: Public opinion and the politics of abortion. Boulder: Westview Press.]

Corona, R., Velazquez, E., McDonald, S. E., Avila, M., Neff, M., Iglesias, A., & Halfond, R. (2017). Ethnic labels, pride, and challenges: A qualitative study of Latinx youth living in a new Latinx destination community. *Journal of Ethnic and Cultural Studies*, 4(1), 1–13.

Gallup. (2014). *US still split on abortion: 47% pro-choice, 46% pro-life*. Retrieved from http://www.gallup.com/poll/1576/Abortion.aspx

Inceli, O. (2015). The Perceptions of English Teachers to the SIOP® Model and Its Impact on Limited English Proficiency. *Journal of Ethnic and Cultural Studies*, 2(1), 15–28.

Kaya, Y. (2015). The opinions of primary school, Turkish language and social science teachers regarding education in the mother tongue (Kurdish). *Journal of Ethnic and Cultural Studies*, 2(2), 33–46.

Kim, K. C. (2004). Chinatown or uptown? Second-generation Chinese American protestants in New York City. In P. Kasnitz & J. H Mollenkopf (Eds.), *Becoming New Yorkers: Ethnographies of the new second generation* (pp. 257–279). New York, NY: Russell Sage Foundation.

Lafer, S. & Aydin, H. (2012). Educating for Democratic Societies: Impediments. *Journal of Social Studies Education Research*, 3(2), 45–70.

Min, P. G., & Jang, S. H. (2015). The diversity of Asian immigrants' participation in religious institutions in the United States. *Sociology of Religion*, 76(3), 253–274.

National Commission on Asian American and Pacific Islander Research on Education [CARE report]. (2011). *The relevance of Asian Americans & Pacific Islanders in the college completion agenda*. Retrieved from http://www .apiasf.org/research/2011_CARE_Report.pdf

Ozfidan, B., & Burlbaw, L. (2016). Perceptions of bilingual education model in Spain: How to implement a bilingual education model in Turkey. *Journal of Ethnic and Cultural Studies*, 3(1), 49–58.

Petersen, L. R. (2001). Religion, plausibility structures, and education's effect on attitudes toward elective abortion. *Journal for the Scientific Study of Religion*, 40(2), 187–203.

Pew Research Center. (2016). *Public opinion on abortion: Views on abortion, 1995–2016*. Retrieved from http://www.pewforum.org/2016/04/08/public -opinion-on-abortion-2/

Pew Research Center. (2017). *Public opinion on abortion: Views on abortion, 1995–2016*. Retrieved from http://www.pewforum.org/fact-sheet/public -opinion-on-abortion/

Smith, T. W., & Son, J. (2013). *Trends in public attitudes towards abortion*. Chicago: National Opinion Research Center. Retrieved from http://www

.norc.org/PDFs/GSS%20Reports/Trends%20in%20Attitudes%20About%20
Abortion_Final.pdf

Smolin, D. M. (2010). The missing girls of China: Population, policy, culture,
gender, abortion, abandonment, and adoption in East-Asian perspective.
Cumberland Law Review, 41(1), 1–65.

Tolba, N. (2018). From Rebellion to Riots. *Research In Social Sciences And
Technology, 3*(2), 93–114.

U.S. Bureau of the Census. (2012). *The Asian population: 2010.* Washington,
DC: U.S. Government Printing Office. Retrieved from https://www.census
.gov/prod/cen2010/briefs/c2010br-11.pdf

Yang, F. (1998). Chinese conversion to evangelical Christianity: The
importance of social and cultural contexts. *Sociology of Religion, 59*(3),
237–57.

Part 3

History and Context

Introduction to Part 3

Ideas and constructs that frame how we think and talk about a variety of issues are shaped by a wide range of factors, including our personal social context (also referred to as our social location), our religious beliefs and practices, our training and education, and our experience. In turn, each of these factors has developed over a long period of time and has been influenced by historical events, movements, ideologies, and belief systems in sometimes-difficult-to-detect ways. The essays in this part address abortion in times past in two ways: in terms of the historical development of ideas known as intellectual history; and in terms of cultural, political, and economic context known as social history. Thus, some material in this chapter addresses the intellectual history of the idea of abortion. We refer here to the "idea of abortion" because one thing you will discover in these chapters is that the very understandings of what is and is not abortion and when it is a significant moral event have changed over time. Other discussions focus on social and cultural context and material practices. For example, for most of human history a pregnancy could not be confirmed until a woman felt the prenate move in her uterus (an action known as "quickening" that usually happens between the fifteenth and twentieth week of pregnancy). Women "bringing on the menses" by the use of herbal remedies was not necessarily considered an abortive act—especially if the fetus was mostly undeveloped. In this way, we can see that our very understanding of the idea of abortion and material practices related to reproductive management has changed over time. A final theme you can find in some of these excerpts is the history of how people who hold a minority status in society are othered, denigrated, and oppressed by those who hold some power over them.

This section examines both the intellectual history of pregnancy and abortion and the sociocultural context of those conversations from the ancient Greco-Roman world up through the early twentieth century. A. James Murphy suggests that there was a chasm between Judeo-Christian and Gentile attitudes and practices regarding contraception and abortion. Beverly Harrison, Zubin Mistry, and Mohammed Ghaly address the complicated mix of religious, philosophical, and medical discourses that intersected in the late antique period and early Middle Ages—discourses that still have salience in ethical and theological debates. Ignacio Castuera discusses the significant medieval Catholic development that reverberates into the present day—namely, the transition from abortion seen as a moral failing related to illicit sex to abortion categorized as a crime subject to prosecution in the courts. The Protestant Reformation inaugurated a new focus on procreative heterosexual married life. Kate Blanchard analyzes sixteenth-century reformer John Calvin's views as a backdrop to how family planning is seen as problematic in some conservative Protestant discourses today.

Christianity was brought by explorers-turned-conquerors to the Americas, and D. Marie Ralstin-Lewis recounts how this settler colonialism denigrated and decimated Native peoples. She also reveals how the US government wielded its power in supporting the development of devastating sterilization campaigns against Native women. Reproductive justice advocate Loretta Ross discusses how racist eugenic ideas and policies also impacted women of color into the twentieth century highlighting their organized resistance and noting Margaret Sanger's troubled history with eugenics as well as Sanger's partnership with some Black leaders. While Christianity's involvement in both supporting and challenging slavery is widely known, Dorothy Roberts relates the less well-known history of how chattel slavery forced African American women to find ways to wrest some reproductive control over their enslaved and sexually exploited bodies. Paul Saurette and Kelly Gordon describe how the newly founded American Medical Association in the mid-nineteenth century brought opposition to abortion for medical, religious, economic, and patriarchal reasons into the public eye. The physicians' campaign to criminalize abortion is a frightening example of the power of an elite group of white men imposing their medical and ethical values and biases on their female patients and changing public opinion in the process. This historical example of how a conservative minority shaped and controlled public mores about abortion is relevant to today. The late twentieth century similarly saw a conservative prolife Christian minority in the US slowly transform public conversations and attitudes on abortion, which has culminated in a radical reversal of reproductive rights by the Supreme Court and state legislatures in 2022.

The chapters in this part provide snapshots from the history of abortion that contribute to thinking carefully and critically about abortion and religion in contemporary life. The ways in which many people think about abortion today have been influenced accurately and inaccurately by claims that are made especially about the history of Christianity and about the ideas and pronouncements of church fathers, theologians, councils, and ecclesiastical jurists throughout history. Many of the selections in this part demonstrate the clarity that comes with seeking to understand what past thinkers meant within their own sociohistorical contexts, before we try to ascertain what, if any, their influence should be on contemporary theo-ethical discussions. Similarly, understanding the ways in which the control of women's reproductive lives is rooted in the history of patriarchy and white supremacy is essential background to unpacking the ongoing sexism, heterosexism, and racism found in some antiabortion discourses.

As you read the essays in this section, we encourage you to consider the following:

1. How is abortion defined and understood in different historical periods and cultures? What impact do these definitions have on women in different times and contexts?
2. Try to identify how the particular and interconnected factors in different times and places shaped perceptions of women, procreation, pregnancy, and children and how those perceptions in turn affected religious stances on abortion.
3. What does bringing a modern intersectional perspective on gender and race to bear on reproductive realities in the past reveal about the relationship between power and pregnant bodies at different points in history?

15

Undesired Offspring and Child Endangerment in Jewish Antiquity

A. James Murphy

A. James Murphy is a biblical scholar who specializes in the area of children in antiquity and the Greco-Roman period. This essay contests popular scholarly opinion that Judaism (and the Christian religion that emerged from it) had a protective stance toward born and unborn children in contrast to Gentile culture. In this excerpt, Murphy analyzes references and allusions to ancient practices of pregnancy termination, which indicate not only a familiarity with abortion but also a lack of an explicit condemnation of it into the rabbinic period.

Within a number of publications in recent years, some scholars have assumed or asserted without much nuance that ancient Jews, Jewish tradition, and/ or the god of Israel valued children more than did their Greco-Roman contemporaries. . . . Often, scholars have highlighted Jesus' treatment of children as unique in the ancient world of the Bible,[1] and, since Jesus was Jewish, his cultural milieu must have influenced his openness toward children. Therefore, Jewish attitudes toward children must have been distinctly more progressive than the attitudes of their Gentile contemporaries. As a result, some scholars have begun to emphasize the distinctiveness of the Jewish regard for children as well, closer to that of Jesus and Christianity, while accentuating the chasm between Judaism and broader Gentile cultures.

. . .

A. James Murphy, "Undesired Offspring and Child Endangerment in Jewish Antiquity," *Journal of Childhood and Religion* 5, no. 3 (2014): 1–36.

[I]s there evidence to suggest efforts to limit the raising of offspring or of child endangerment in the Jewish world of antiquity? . . . Is there evidence within Jewish contexts of unwanted pregnancies, or that infants' or children's lives were put at risk by parents, caregivers, Jewish society or the god of Israel? A number of texts demonstrate the situation was much more complex than we often seem willing to admit.

Undesired Offspring?—Abortion

. . .

Abortion is mentioned in Jewish sources somewhat more than contraception,[2] but nothing comparable to the amount of discussion it garners in Greco-Roman literature. Evidence shows that some of Israel's neighbors were familiar with substances thought in antiquity to have contraceptive qualities, some of which reportedly possessed abortive qualities. For example, ancient Egyptians listed certain substances including acacia gum to end pregnancy.[3] Acacia figures prominently in the building of the tabernacle in Exodus, so some ancient Jews were familiar with its use in construction. They knew of several such substances that surrounding cultures used, in part, for their abortive qualities. Yet Jewish sources never discuss them in medicinal or contraceptive terms. Possibly, the Israelites did not recognize the abortive qualities of such substances. Admittedly speculative, I think it more likely ancient Jews occasionally used such substances, even if in limited circumstances.

Some Jews clearly knew about abortion as a procedure that terminates a fetus at least by the late seventh century B.C.E., which merited attention well into the rabbinic period. Within this period, we find the entire range of what I call prescriptions, descriptions, and commentary. Our earliest reference is of Judean provenance, the prophet Jeremiah. Jeremiah 20:14-18 provides *descriptive* attestation that at least some ancient Jews near Jerusalem were familiar with abortive practices prior to the Hellenistic period: "Cursed be the day that I was born . . . Cursed be the man who brought word to my father, 'A son is born to you' . . . because he did not kill me in the womb, that my mother would be my tomb."[4] There is no way to prove that his knowledge must derive from familiarity with non-Jewish abortive practices; nor does the passage prove its practice by Jews in Jerusalem at that time. The context is a moment of rejection and anguish specific to Jeremiah and his experience.

Yet its utterance is *descriptive* evidence that abortion may have been a plausible alternative to pregnancy, that abortion was possible in his day and location.

The next indication of familiarity with abortive practices emerges from the Hellenistic Diaspora community that produced the Septuagint in Alexandria, Egypt ca. 250 B.C.E. Exodus 21:22-25 provided the source text, which is part of the ancient Covenant Code.[5] The context is that two men are fighting and injure a pregnant woman causing "her children to come out" (i.e., an unnatural expulsion of the fetus, or miscarriage). If no "harm" occurs, then the perpetrator must pay a fine to the woman's husband (v.22). If "harm" does occur, then the principle of *lex talionis* applies, an eye for an eye . . . a life for a life. As it stands this passage is vague concerning to whom the term "harm" applies. Does it apply to the woman or to the fetus? Nevertheless, the law implies an outcome that is undesirable on the part of the husband and perhaps the woman implicitly, a miscarriage. There is no prescription concerning elective abortion before the Hellenistic period. However, as Greek displaced Aramaic (and Hebrew) as the language of Diaspora Judaism, the vagueness of this passage, and its (mis)translation into Greek provided the fodder for much discussion from at least the first century C.E. into the Rabbinic period and beyond.

Hellenistic schools of thought and debate were already pervasive in the eastern Mediterranean by the mid-200s B.C.E., and the Alexandrian translators of the Septuagint were likely very knowledgeable and influenced by contemporary Greek debates over the nature of a fetus among Platonists, Stoics, and Aristotelians.[6] As a result, a tremendous change in meaning occurred when they rendered the Hebrew "harm" (אסון) into Greek as "fully formed" (ἐξεικονισμένον). This change lends to reading the verse: "When men fight and strike a pregnant woman, so that her children come out, but there is no *full form*, the perpetrator shall be fined . . . but if there is *full form*, then you shall take life for life . . ." (21:22-23).[7] In effect, this created a *prescription* against a form of abortion where there had previously been none. Any reader or audience who was henceforth dependent upon the Septuagint could understand this as a divine injunction against killing the fetus. In their appropriation of the Septuagint, early Christian authorities understood the Greek translation of Exodus 21:22-25 to relate to the developing embryo or fetus; killing either should be understood as murder. Subsequently, these different translations, the Hebrew and the Greek, contributed to differences of opinion within Rabbinic Judaism over the nature of the unborn.

Scholars generally see at least two perspectives concerning the developing fetus that emerged in the wake of the Septuagint translation of the Hellenistic period. One, referred to as the Alexandrian school, derived its interpretation from this Greek translation and reflected views that emerged from within the Jewish community of Alexandria. The other, which has been referred to as the Palestinian school of thought, remained dependent on the Hebrew tradition and eventually resulted in the Talmudic view that emerged from early halakhic midrash on the Exodus passage. Significantly, both schools viewed abortion only in terms of necessity in their day, yet they disagreed over whether or not the fetus, at a given stage of development, acquired human form according to Exodus 21:22-25, in the event of an unintended mishap leading to miscarriage.[8] Greek philosophical ideas about ensoulment, the point when the fetus was thought to first experience sensation, likely influenced both of these debates and positions.[9] The writings of Philo and Josephus demonstrate that both positions became the topic of some extended commentary by the first century C.E.

Some scholars believe the comments by Philo on the law in Exodus 21:22-25 best represent the perspective of the Alexandrian school. For him, it is imperative to convey to his audience that this passage implies that causing a miscarriage or abortion is a capital offense against a physically formed fetus.

> If a man comes to blows with a pregnant woman and strikes her on the belly and she miscarries, then, if the result of the miscarriage is unshaped and undeveloped, he must be fined both for the outrage and for obstructing the artist Nature in her creative work of bringing into life the fairest of living creatures, man. But, if the offspring is already shaped and all the limbs have their proper qualities and places in the system, he must die. . . .(*Spec.* 3.108-109)[10]

. . .

Philo seems aware of abortive practices, even if his *descriptions* consist more of accusation than reality. It remains a probability, not a certainty, that his polemic was directed to a segment of the Jewish population. Furthermore, there is no indication as to the common or uncommon nature of the practice among his intended audience, whoever they may be. Philo's writings were not authoritative for Judaism or the Diaspora community of his day, but they do represent the strong *commentary* of an elite voice against abortion from within his particular community as well as probable *descriptive* evidence for the practice.

The first-century writer Josephus also provides both *descriptive* attestations to abortive practices as well as assertive *commentary* against them, although it is unclear whether we should attribute his references to his earlier experience in Palestine or to his later experiences in Rome. In the process he also becomes an early witness to the Palestinian position rooted in the Hebrew tradition and eventually upheld in the Talmud. *Antiquities* IV, 8, 33 reads as follows:

> He that kicketh a woman with child, if the woman miscarry, shall be fined by the judges for having, by the destruction of the fruit of her womb, diminished the population, and a further sum shall be presented by him to the woman's husband. If she die of the blow, he shall also die, the law claiming as its due the sacrifices of life for life.[11]

Like its Hebrew Bible precursor and the Talmud that would follow, Josephus' Greek translation takes the capital offense to be death of the mother, not the fetus. He regards the death of the fetus as a blow to "the multitude," yet considers its death to be of lesser offense than that of one fully born.

. . .

The point is that simple statements that claim ancient Jews rejected "harsh practices toward children, including abortion"[12] obscure the complex nature of the limited references. . . . It is unclear whether they are merely responses to a Gentile practice, or to practices known or surmised within their own communities. Philo's accusation probably represents the latter. The prophet Jeremiah attests familiarity with the practice in Judah before the Hellenistic age, and there is no hint of condemnation of the practice, while the Rabbinic period demonstrates that, while limited, there was no absolute rejection of the practice.

. . .

Conclusion

This perusal through ancient Jewish literature suggests that just as with Greco-Roman sources there is also a complexity to child history within Jewish sources.

. . .

In terms of abortion, our earliest secure description is that of Jeremiah, who makes no prescription regarding the practice. Beyond this reference, Jewish tradition appears silent on the issue prior to translation of the LXX. Most references to abortive practices occur from the late Hellenistic period forward. Geographical references to abortion occur in Alexandria, and suggest Judah and Asia Minor as well.

In conclusion, although Jewish sources are much less explicit about abortion and infanticide among their own than are Greco-Roman sources, such practices were known among various Jewish populations in antiquity. Given the data in the sources at our disposal, it is probable that they occurred to varying degrees between locales and times, which led to prescriptive stories, proclamations, or polemical commentary by some who took exception to such practices. Above all, contrasting commentary, prescriptions, and descriptions of these practices should caution us against absolute claims that ancient Jews did not engage in such practices or that they valued children more than their neighbors.

Notes

1. Such studies, of course, actually serve further to reassure the uniqueness of Jesus, and perhaps Christianity, for many readers. For examples, see Anthony O. Nkwoka, "Mark 10:13-16: Jesus' Attitude to Children and its Modern Challenges," *Africa Theological Journal* 14, no. 2 (1985): 100-110; William A. Strange, *Children in the Early Church* (Carlisle: Paternoster Press, 1996); Judith Gundry-Volf, "'To Such as These Belongs the Reign of God': Jesus and Children," *Theology Today* 56, no. 4 (January 2000): 469-480. Compare her wording here with the slightly altered wording in the anthology on children and religion edited by Marcia Bunge: Gundry-Volf, "The Least and the Greatest: Children in the New Testament," in *The Child in Christian Thought* (Grand Rapids: Eerdmans, 2001), 29-60.
2. For contraception, see Gen 38 for a *descriptive* instance of *coitus interruptus*, and T. B. *Yevamot* 12b for a description of an acceptable woolen contraceptive device called a *mokh*.
3. See John M. Riddle, J. Worth Estes, and Josiah C. Russell, "Birth Control in the Ancient World," *Archaeology* 47, no. 2 (March/April 1994), 31.
4. Compare the similar lament by Job (3:16) and of Qohelet (6:3), where "stillborn" is probably the better rendering of נֵפֶל, but the consonantal root also could convey the notion of a violent death by falling.
5. The Covenant Code is considered by many scholars to have been an early independent legal code consisting of Exodus 20:22—23:19 (some 21:1—23:19).
6. [Michael J. Gorman, *Abortion and the Early Church: Christian, Jewish and Pagan Attitudes in the Greco-Roman* (Downers Grove, Ill.: Intervarsity

Press, 1982)], 35. See also the earlier work by Victor Aptowitzer who says the emerging Alexandrian view was "not genuinely Jewish but must have originated in Alexandria under Egyptian-Greek influence," a compromise between Platonists and Stoics. See Victor Aptowitzer, "Observations on the Criminal Law of the Jews," *Jewish Quarterly Review* 15 (1924), 87, 114; also quoted in [David M. Feldman, *Birth Control in Jewish Law* (New York: New York University Press), 1968], 259.

7. See Feldman, *Birth Control*, 255-262; Gorman, *Abortion and the Early Church*, 35.

8. Feldman, *Birth Control*, 251-254, 257-258; [Odd Magne Bakke, *When Children Became People: The Birth of Childhood in Early Christianity* (trans. Brian McNeil; Minneapolis: Fortress Press, 2005)], 111; Gorman, *Abortion and the Early Church*, 34. This concern over the value of the fetus is not unique to Jewish law, but fits within the general milieu of ancient Near Eastern law codes; e.g., see the *Laws of Lipit-Ishtar* P. rev. iii 2-13; *Sumerian Laws Exercise Tablet* iv 1-10; *Middle Assyrian Laws* ii 93-97; vii 63-108; translated by Martha T. Roth, *Law Collections from Mesopotamia and Asia Minor* 2nd ed. (SBL Writings From the Ancient World Series; Atlanta: Scholars Press, 1997).

9. Aristotle, *History of Animals* VII.3; Gorman, *Abortion and the Early Church*, 22.

10. All citations and quotations from the work of Philo are taken from *Philo in Ten Volumes.* (trans. F. H. Colson; LCL; Cambridge, Mass.: Harvard University Press, 1968-1985) unless stated otherwise. Philo has also taken liberty to change the passage from a fight between two men, to a deliberate attack by a man upon a pregnant woman.

11. All citations and quotations from the work of Josephus are from *Josephus in Nine Volumes* (ed. H. St. J. Thackeray et al., LCL; Cambridge, Mass.: Harvard University Press, 1926-65).

12. E.g., [Judith Gundry-Volf, "'To Such as These Belongs the Reign of God': Jesus and Children," *Theology Today* 56, no. 4 (January 2000)]: 470.

16

Selected Early Catholic Teaching on Abortion

Beverly Wildung Harrison

Beverly Wildung Harrison (d. 2012), professor at Union Theological Seminary for over thirty years, was the first woman president of the Society of Christian Ethics. She pioneered the field of feminist social ethics with critical work on power, sexual ethics, and economics and social class. Her groundbreaking book on reproductive ethics, from which this excerpt was taken, was widely regarded for decades as the definitive Christian ethical argument supporting the position that the capacity to shape their procreative lives is a social good that women require. In this excerpt, Harrison turns to the texts of the early church in order to launch a strong critique of historians and theologians claiming a consistent antiabortion tradition in Christianity. Harrison exposes a history of the church's fixation on sexual sin and inconsistency on the question of when life begins.

Our knowledge about post-New Testament Christian teaching on abortion is fragmentary at best. The earliest Christian post-canonical test invariably cited condemning abortion is *The Didache* (The Teaching) . . . [which] receives some attention in the history of Christian ethics because it is one of the few early examples of Christian morals extant from the second century. The writer of *The Didache* addresses his treatise to a young man, one who, if he would aspire to the Christian way of life, must follow the commandments. The text instructs the faithful one:

Beverly Wildung Harrison, *Our Right to Choose: Toward a New Ethic of Abortion* (Boston: Beacon, 1983).

> You shall not commit murder. You shall not commit adultery. You shall not
> corrupt boys. You shall not commit fornication. . . . You shall not kill an
> unborn child or murder a newborn infant.[1]

Precisely what context or act is implied in murdering an unborn child is not
specified. We now know, however, that *The Didache* represents the teaching
of an early Jewish-Christian writer or group. A number of historians believe
that overall proscriptions in *The Didache* in fact are related to the intense
conflict between Jewish Christians and their unconverted coreligionists.
There was considerable rivalry, especially regarding moral rigorism,
between some groups of early Jewish Christians and their non-Christian
Jewish counterparts, and it is now recognized that the author of *The Didache*
took over his moral formula from a rigorist Jewish sect. There were many
such groups in the second century vying among themselves and with the
newer Christian groups. The text tells us nothing about when in the course
of pregnancy the writer may have assumed a "child" to be present or how this
teaching relates to traditional rabbinic positions about the preeminence of a
pregnant woman's well-being in childbearing.

Apart from this code, explicit denunciations of abortion, separate from
views on the irreducible responsibility to procreation, are rare in early
Christianity. [Canon lawyer John] Noonan's claim, typical of mainstream
theological pronouncement, that "by 450 [C.E.] the teaching on abortion
East and West had been set out for four centuries with clarity and
consistency"[2] is doubtful at best, though the fragmentary evidence on the
question makes dogmatism either way impossible. The silence in canonical
New Testament writings and in most extant theology of the period is
noteworthy. . . .

Ironically, after *The Didache*, the first elaborated denunciation of abortion
in Christian theological writings appears to have been advanced to defend
Christians from the pervasive charge that they were antisocial and immoral.
In the first several centuries after Jesus, Christians composed, after all, a tiny
social minority—looked upon as a band of people espousing a religious
viewpoint, at best eccentric, at worst offensive to many "respectable"
contemporaries in the Roman Empire. Christian religious practice was often
belittled and caricatured. In fact, several early theologians defended Christians
from rumors circulating to the effect that Christian rites were cannibalistic.
No doubt the origin of such allegations lay in Christian liturgical practice.
Christians were accused of "eating" the body and blood of their leader.
Perhaps that is why Christians also met with charges of infanticide. In any

case, Christians were frequently faulted for moral laxity, and many of them responded with rigorist defenses of Christian ethical conduct.

Tertullian, a strict, even moralistic, early-third-century theologian, protested such charges of immorality, citing Christian attitudes toward abortion as an example of the extent of Christian scrupulousness about killing. In this connection, he enunciated the opinion, later influential, that "the seed" is, because of its potential, already "man." "He is a human being [*homo*] who will be one; the whole fruit is actually in the seed."[3] His comments reflect assumptions current in the time that "the seed"—that is, the sperm— was the male's contribution to procreation. In this androcentric view, a woman contributed only a place for "the seed" to germinate. As is often pointed out, this portrayal ideologically correlates with the assumption that children are really the fruit, even the possession, of men. Furthermore, any "waste" of semen or seed was considered a homicidal act in some Christian tradition, though not by Tertullian.

For Tertullian personally, as for many later rigorist theologians, abortion may have been appropriate to save a woman's life;[4] as such it was a necessary evil. . . . Tertullian elaborated a position, called in technical theological language *traducianism*—the teaching that "body" and "soul" coexist from the moment of conception.[5] It cannot be stressed too strongly that Tertullian did not formulate this doctrine in answer to the modern question "When does human life begin?" Rather, he accepted the widespread dualistic religious assumption of his day that spirit merged with matter to form human life. He attempted to clarify how body/ spirit unity was accomplished in order to interpret what Christians believed about salvation. While traducianism influenced some later Christian thinking on abortion, Tertullian himself never related it to his fragmentary comments on abortion. Nor did traducianism, as a theory of body/ spirit unity at conception, have much influence among early Christian theologians. At the time of the Reformation, debates about how body/ soul unity occurred were still under way.

Some other early Christian theologians, all celibates—namely, Justin Martyr, Origen, and Clement of Alexandria[6]—were vitriolic toward women. By contrast, Tertullian's views on women were "moderate," but, particularly in his later years, he was markedly, even phobically, antisexual. In light of this, his attitude toward abortion was less harsh than might be expected. Yet he is invariably cited as an early author of an ardent Christian anti-abortionist tradition.

Speculations about the relation between matter and spirit were standard in the writings of all learned men during the first four centuries of the

Christian era. Intellectuals already held considerably divergent views, which in turn were reformulated by various Christian theologians. The Stoics, among the most sophisticated of the philosophical elites who were to influence Christianity, believed that human life truly began only at birth. Their view was shared by many ancient groups, including several strands of Jewish culture that did not envision reality in terms of a body/ spirit or matter/ spirit dualism characteristic of wider late Hellenistic culture. It is clear, however, that most early Christian thinkers were influenced less by the Stoics or by Hebraic traditions than by the sharp dualisms of other late Hellenistic religion.

. . .

Much subsequent speculation among Christian theologians about when the full animation of body by spirit transpired was no more aimed at clarifying the meaning of abortion than were Tertullian's reflections. Rather, the discussion was carried on to determine when and how human responsibility for sin and evil emerged and to grapple with the disparity between divine ensoulment and "the fall of man." For the great fourth-century polemicist Augustine, these theological speculations took on great urgency, not because abortion posed the need for a clear-cut answer but because, by then, the Christian community was fractured with controversy over how human sinfulness related to divine salvation. Augustine adamantly opposed Tertullian's traducianist view, because he thought it unspiritual.[7] For Augustine, the infusion of rational soul, which was truly spiritual, could not be coterminous with the mere biological process of conception. At the same time, he was firmly opposed to the abortion of a "formed" fetus. Examination of his moral justifications for condemning abortion makes it clear that Augustine, who, especially in his later years, must stand fairly high on any list of antisexual phobists in Christian history, opposed it collaterally, not only with contraception but with any absence of procreative intent in sexuality. His was a litany growing more common in fourth- and fifth-century Christian theology—that sex, except for the purpose of procreation within marriage, was murderous.

. . .

Augustine, like Tertullian and most other men of the educated classes, continued to perpetuate what historian George Williams rather quaintly coined the "sire-centered" view of embryology referred to earlier[8]—that in procreation the male provided "the seed," the woman merely the generative space for fetal development. A variant understanding was that a woman supplied some of her menstrual blood as "matter" for fetal development.[9] In this theory, the spirit, or rational soul, was the male contribution. In any case, Augustine employed the distinction between formed and unformed fetal life applying a prohibition of abortion only to a "formed" fetus. In fact: several times he opined that the death of an unformed fetus was *not* homicide. Furthermore, on at least one occasion, this rigorist bishop subscribed to what may have been an uncharacteristic sympathy for the life of the pregnant woman, insisting that an embryotomy to save the life of the mother would not impair a fetus's prospects for participating in the resurrection of the dead. The absolute prohibition against abortion at the risk of killing a pregnant woman has never been the dominant Christian view. Such a position would have seemed heartless even to some of the more militant misogynists of early Christendom.

. . .

If the "evils" of abortion were as universally recognized among Christians as anti-abortion proponents suggest, it is difficult to understand the minor part given to discussion of abortion not only in theological writings but also in the developing church discipline spelled out in deliberations of church councils adjudicating controverted issues of faith. Invariably, in the attempt to demonstrate the unanimity and intensity of Christian anti-abortion teaching, anti-abortion scholars point to the teaching of two fourth-century councils, but always without full notation of what those councils specifically addressed in terms of abortion. Around the year 309 C.E., a small gathering of priests and bishops at the Council of Elvira held in Granada, a remote province of what is now Spain, attempted to codify disciplinary canons for their churches. The Council of Elvira is important precisely because it provides evidence for the early development of a specific penitential system within Christianity. The canons of Elvira introduced penances for numerous offenses, clarifying the severity of the various sins of Christians. More recently, however, this council has been identified as problematic in Christian theological development because it represents the first attempt by Christian bishops to regulate sexual offenses. . . .

It is startling, given claims in mainstream anti-abortion interpretations of Christian teaching, that the Council of Elvira, far from "proving" that early Christianity deemed abortion a heinous sin, demonstrates the intimate connection between abortion and the condemnation of "sexual sin." It is not abortion per se that is condemned, but abortion undertaken by a baptized Christian woman to conceal adultery.[10] Infanticide was a lesser crime if performed by a catechumen,[11] who could be baptized "in the end."

. . .

Just as the Council of Elvira is cited as evidence of the triumph of anti-abortion teaching in the then western church, the Council of Ancrya in 314 C.E. is cited as confirmation of the victory of anti-abortion teaching in early eastern Christianity. A council of eighteen bishops of the eastern church, more than attended at Elvira, convened to establish penances for those who had lapsed from Christianity during the Roman imperial persecutions of Christians under Maximus. Many church historians have reported on the significance of this council or summarized its actions on penance without mentioning abortion.[12] The textual evidence is oblique as to whether the council's actions referred to abortion at all. If, however, abortion was deliberated, it was treated under the rubrics of adultery, use of soothsaying, and resort to "customs of the Gentiles." The penances prescribed for adultery and abortion to conceal adultery were more moderate than those established at Elvira.[13]

Anti-abortion historians of Christianity explain the discrepancy between the supposed massive and unanimous theological condemnation of abortion and the erratic penitential treatment of abortion by church councils and, much later, in canon law, by making a sharp distinction between Christianity's "normative" moral position condemning abortion and its penitential tradition. They claim that the latter was necessarily less rigorist because of pastoral compassion and the more flexible requirements necessary to cope with the actual moral weakness of people.[14] By contrast, I believe that the early penitential treatments of abortion and the later canonical penalties established for those who performed or sought abortions reflect both the extension of control of sexual conduct by an emerging hierarchy and the disinterestedness of the church in the question of abortion—except as sexual sin.

Notes

1. *The Didache*, in *Christian Ethics: Sources of the Living Tradition*, ed. Waldo Beach and H. Richard Niebuhr (New York: Ronald Press, 1955), pp. 58-59. Many translators, believing that the reference to "child in the womb" is not an accurate rendering of the original, translate it simply as "child." See [Cyril Richardson, ed., *Early Christian Fathers*, vol. 1 (Philadelphia: Westminster Press, 1957)], pp. 111-179.
2. [John T. Noonan, Jr., "An Almost Absolute Value in History," in John T. Noonan, ed., *The Morality of Abortion: Legal and Historical Perspectives* (Cambridge: Harvard University Press, 1970)], p. 18.

3. It should be emphasized that Tertullian's teaching is always the first elaborated, not merely cited, as anti-abortionist, because, given his "traducian" theory (as explained later in the text), he penned the only extended literary example of reasoning about the *origins* of "full humanity." That his reasoning was not aimed at assessing fetal life, but at speculating about soul/body unity, is ignored. See Tertullian, *Apologetical Works and Minueus Felix Octavius*, 9:8 (New York: Fathers of the Church, 1950), p. 32. . . .

4. I say "may" because the authenticity of the relevant text is disputed. See Tertullian, *De Anima*, 25.4 (Amsterdam: Meulenhoff, 1947), pp. 35-36 and also pp. 324-326. Along with Justin, Clement, Augustine, and Jerome, Tertullian believed that sexual activity was only for procreation; otherwise, it was sensuous, and therefore violated God's spirit. See his *Treatises On Marriage and Remarriage* (Westminster, Md.: Newman Press, 1951), pp. 70- 71 and passim.

5. Tertullian, *De Anima*.

6. On Justin, see [St. Justin Martyr, *First Apology*, in Cyril Richardson, ed., *Early Christian Fathers*, vol. 1 (Philadelphia: Westminster Press, 1957), pp. 258-260]. Clement believed that abortion was an unspeakable evil, evidently for two reasons: (1) it wasted "the seed" God meant to come to fruition and (2) it was practiced invariably by women to hide sexual infidelity. See Clement of Alexandria, *Le Pedagogue*, Livre 4, 10:84 and 91 (Paris: Les Edition des Cerf, 1965), pp. 162-168 and 176. . . .

7. Augustine, *Letters*, 4: 165-203, trans. Sister W. Parsons (New York: Fathers of the Church, 1955), p. 279.

8. George Hunston Williams, "Religious Residues and Presuppositions, in the American Debate on Abortion," *Theological Studies*, vol. 31, (1970), p. 33.

9. There were, of course, a number of variants of the "sire-centered" view, on which women contributed something to the process of pregnancy, but all views presupposed the male role as the primary generative one. . . .

10. Canon 63, as translated by Samuel Laeuchli [*Power and Sexuality: The Emergence of Canon Law at the Synod of Elvira* (Philadelphia: Temple University Press, 1972)], Appendix, p. 133:

    If a woman, while her husband is away, conceives by adultery and after that crime commits abortion, she shall not be given communion even at the end, since she has doubled her crime.

11. Ibid., canon 68, p. 134:

    A catechumen, if she has conceived a child in adultery and then suffocated it, shall be baptized at the end.

12. See a Standard English reference work widely used in the early decades of the twentieth century, such as the Rev. Edward II. Landon, ed., *A Manual of Councils of the Holy Catholic Church* (Edinburgh: John Grant, 1909), pp 23ff. . . .

13. Connery correctly summarizes Ancrya's "more lenient" attitude to abortion as compared to Elvira's in [John R. Connery, "Abortion: Roman Catholic Perspectives," *Encyclopedia of Bioethics*, vol. 1 (New York: Free Press, 1978)], pp. 48ff. . . .

14. Even Connery adopts this logic—the distinction between the "normative" theological ethical tradition and the more morally "permissive" canonical tradition. I hold an alternative view, namely, that Church canons if they are less "rigorist" than the anathemas of individual theologians should be viewed as evidence of lack of moral consensus among Christians, not as lesser morality. Samuel Laeuchli's thesis about the use of hierarchical power to enforce sexual conformity at Elvira also implies that, at least with respect to sexuality, rigorist councils should be read as *imposing* homogenous practice where diversity prevailed. The use of external power to impose sexual morality suggests lack of agreement from those affected. See Connery, "Abortion: Roman Catholic Perspectives," in *Encyclopedia of Bioethics*, vol. 1 (New York: Free Press, 1978) pp. 9-13.

17

Imagining *Abortivi* in the Early Middle Ages

Zubin Mistry

A medieval historian at the University of Edinburgh, Zubin Mistry has written the definitive book on abortion in the Middle Ages. From the historical richness of this research, we have excerpted a section focusing on the towering late-fourth-/mid-fifth-century bishop, Augustine of Hippo. Mistry shows how Augustine was perplexed by the conundrum of whether *abortivi* (fetuses that die by miscarriage or abortion) might be resurrected, given the lack of the church's theological clarity regarding when a fetus becomes an ensouled person.

From late antiquity right through to the end of the Middle Ages, countless authors and artists cultivated and communicated complex meanings of fetal existence within theological tracts, sacred narratives, devotional practices and, even, iconography. It is likely that certain theological ideas about the fetus informed moral ideas about abortion (and infanticide).[1] But automatically reading the varieties of early medieval discourse on the fetus as encrypted moral arguments about abortion is more revealing of modern, rather than medieval, mental associations. We cannot simply assume that when theologians like Maximus the Confessor traced the union of body and soul to the moment of conception when reflecting on the nature of Christ, their ideas were either intended or understood to have implications for abortion.[2]

. . .

The *abortivus* was the stillborn infant, the fetus dead in the womb, the premature newborn, the product of abortion (deliberate or otherwise).

Source: Zubin Mistry, *Abortion in the Early Middle Ages, C.500–900* (Woodbridge, Suffolk: York Medieval, 2015).

Discussion of *abortivi* was not the same thing as discussion of abortion. 'Only death is certain,' Augustine once said in a sermon. 'A boy is conceived, perhaps he is born, perhaps he becomes an *aborsus*.' In societies where pregnancy loss was commonplace, unintended abortion encapsulated the contingency of mortality. Deliberately aborted fetuses were only a minority among *abortivi*.[3]

The flesh-and-blood contingencies of pregnancy loss were a social reality, imaginations of the *abortivus* haunted the margins of thought. Abortion has a long but neglected history as a symbol. In the Early Middle Ages this symbolism sometimes appeared in unexpected places. . . . In early medieval thought, the *abortivus* came to symbolize wayward sinners, defiant Jews and obdurate heretics. But if the *abortivus* was an expressive symbol, it was also an elusive reality, a fleeting presence, which created conceptual problems for theologians. How did *abortivi* fit into God's salvific plan? Would they have a share in the world to come?

    . . .

Dead or alive: Augustine and his readers on the resurrection of *abortivi*

We begin at the end, or beyond the end, at the resurrection. From early Christianity the resurrection of the body was 'always connected to divine power . . . [to] the extraordinary power necessary to create and recreate, to reward and punish, to bring life from death'.[4] In the vision of heaven sketched out by the fourth-century Syrian theologian Ephrem, whoever 'dies in the womb of his mother and never comes to life, will be quickened at the moment [of resurrection] by [Christ] who quickens the dead; he will then be brought forth as an adult'. For Ephrem, the resurrection would transfigure the calamity of death before birth into a celestial reunion between mother and child. 'If a woman dies while pregnant, and the child in her womb dies with her,' Ephrem continued, 'that child will at the resurrection grow up and know its mother; and she will know her child'.[5]

But the resurrection also threw up difficult conceptual tensions about identity and change, about the nature of bodies and souls, because at the resurrection we will be both the same as and different from our former bodily selves. Eschatology forced theologians to confront awkward metaphysical questions.[6] The residue of such intellectual challenges can be detected in an eighth-century catechetical creed. It emphasized that everyone, 'whether a small child, an old man, or after coming alive and dying in a mother's womb', would be resurrected.[7] Like Ephrem, the creed used the resurrected fetus to illustrate the all-embracing power of the resurrection. Unlike Ephrem, its author had inherited a more complicated tradition of thought. The resurrected fetus had come alive in the womb. This precise detail was a trace of vexed questions which Augustine had once confronted. What made the resurrection of *abortivi* a hard case in eschatology makes the thought of Augustine and his early medieval readers of particular interest to us. Reflection on the resurrection of *abortivi* necessitated reflection on the beginning of bodies and souls in the womb.

. . .

Augustine was confident that young infants would attain perfected bodies at the resurrection. Dead infants lacked the bodily size with which they would one day be resurrected. But 'just as all body parts are already latently in seed, even though some of them are lacking in the born', the possibility of bodily perfection was inherent in everyone at least in principle (*in ratione*). At the resurrection *parvuli* [infants] would be resurrected in the bodies, tall or short, big or small, they would otherwise have attained.[8] Augustine's confidence quickly evaporated, however, when he turned to *abortivi*:

> I dare neither to affirm nor to deny that aborted fetuses, which, when they had already lived in the womb, died there, will be resurrected; although I do not see how, if they are not discounted from the number of the dead, the resurrection of the dead should not extend to them. For either not all the dead will rise up and there will be some human souls, which had human bodies albeit within the maternal organs, without bodies in eternity; or if all human souls will receive their risen bodies, which they had wherever they left them in life and death, I do not understand how I can say that those who died in the wombs of mothers do not partake of the resurrection of the dead. But whichever of these someone thinks, what we will say about born infants ought to be understood about them too, if they will rise up.[9]

Augustine's hesitation gravitated around whether or not bodily resurrection embraced all of the dead. If bodily resurrection did not apply to all of the dead, the disembodied souls of *abortivi* would float around for eternity. Alternatively, if it did apply to all of the dead, *abortivi* who died in their mothers' wombs would be resurrected in perfected bodies just as infants would be.

In *De civitate Dei* Augustine referred to *abortivi* who numbered among the dead—or, to put it differently, to *abortivi* who had once been alive, if only fleetingly. The *Enchiridion*, which also had a wide readership in the Early Middle Ages, makes clear that the beginnings of life troubled Augustine more deeply.[10] Here Augustine's speculation was more intricate, more intensely personal and more openly riven with doubts. He introduced his section on the resurrection with one confident proposition: no Christian should doubt that all those who had been born and who would be born, who had died and would die in the future, would be resurrected. But 'I have not worked out,' he confessed, 'how I can briefly discuss [resurrection] and satisfy all the questions which are typically raised about this subject'.[11]

The first question concerned aborted fetuses, 'who have been born as it were in the wombs of the mothers, but not yet in such a way that they can be reborn'.[12] Effectively this was about very young, undeveloped fetuses. If *they* would be resurrected, then formed fetuses (*formati*) certainly would be. Augustine initially leaned towards excluding unformed abortions (*informes abortus*) from the resurrection: 'But who is not more inclined to think that unformed abortions perish, just like seeds which were not conceived?'[13] Yet he immediately began to vacillate. 'But does anyone dare to deny, though would he dare to affirm either,' Augustine equivocated, 'that the resurrection will bring it about that whatever lacked form will be filled, and in such a way that the perfection which would have come about in time is not lacking?'[14] Augustine felt the intuitive pull of the assumption that *informes abortus* would not be resurrected, but he also wondered whether this misconstrued the dramatic power of the resurrection, through which 'what is not yet whole will be made whole, just as what was deficient will be repaired'.[15] Since anyone who had died would be resurrected, the real question concerned when life—and the possibility of numbering among the dead—began in the womb:

> And through this [the question] can be asked and discussed very carefully among the most learned—I do not know whether it can be ascertained by man—namely when does a person begin to live in the womb, whether there is some kind of hidden life which does not yet appear with the movements of something living? For it seems overly rash to deny that infants, who are cut out limb by limb and thrown out of the wombs of pregnant women so that they do not kill their mothers too if they remained dead there, had ever lived. But once a person begins to live, he is then certainly able to die: and dead, wherever death managed to befall him, I cannot understand how he cannot pertain to the resurrection of the dead.[16]

Augustine knew the answer to the question of the resurrection of *abortivi* in theory. If they had been alive, and thus had been able to die, *abortivi* would also be resurrected in perfected bodies. His allusion to embryotomy—in this case, referring to the excision of dead fetuses dangerously retained in their mothers' wombs, fetuses which were presumably *formati* if they could be cut out limb by limb—illustrated the theory. But Augustine was by his own admission unsure whether the status of *informes abortus* could be ascertained.[17]

. . .

Augustine's intricacy and self-conscious uncertainty have been the most significant casualties in later interpretations and appropriations of his thinking. To reconstruct Augustine's position on abortion modern interpreters have filled the silences of his moral treatises on marriage, in which he addressed the morality of abortion or otherwise avoiding offspring without explicitly addressing when life begins, with his eschatology. The various Augustines resurrected as interlocutors in modern debate have been shorn of imperfections; after all, the resurrection perfects whatever lacked form. The assurance of these resurrected Augustines contrasts with the vacillating Augustine of the *Enchiridion*. . . . Thus, one modern Augustine does not regard the undeveloped fetus as a 'human person'.[18] Another modern Augustine, by contrast, embraces the 'value of all life, actual or potential' in the face of uncertainty over when life begins.[19]

Notes

1. Cf. [E. Koskenniemi, *The Exposure of Infants among Jews and Christians in Antiquity* (Sheffield, 2009)], pp. 23–4.
2. On Maximus, see M.-H. Congourdeau, 'L'animation de l'embryon humain chez Maxime le Confesseur', *Nouvelle revue théologique* 111 (1984), 693–709; J. Saward, *Redeemer in the Womb: [Christ Living in Mary* (San Francisco, 1993)], pp. 8–13. On the theological concerns which underlay early and late antique Christian thought on the embryo, see M.-H. Congourdeau, 'Genèse d'un regard Chrétien sur l'embryon', in V. Dasen, ed., *Naissance et petite enfance [dans l'antiquité*, ed. V Dasen (Fribourg, 2004)], pp. 349–62.
3. 'Sola mors est certa . . . Conceptus est puer, forte nascitur, forte aborsum facit', *Sermo* 97.3, PL 38, col. 590. For an attempt to generate a quantitative picture of fetal mortality from the seventeenth century onward, see

R. Woods, *Death before Birth: Fetal Health and Mortality in Historical Perspective* (Oxford, 2009).

4. C. W. Bynum, *The Resurrection of the Body in Western Christianity, 200–1336* (New York, 1995), p. 2.

5. Quoted ibid., p. 77.

6. In addition to Bynum, *Resurrection of the Body*, on later scholastic responses to such questions, see P. L. Reynolds, *Food and the Body: Some Peculiar Questions in High Medieval Theology* (Leiden, 1999); A. Fitzpatrick, 'Bodily Identity in Scholastic Theology' (unpublished PhD thesis, University College London, 2013).

7. . . . Pirminius, *Scarapsus* 28a, p. 113.

8. . . . *De civitate Dei*, 22.13 [ed. B. Dombart and A. Kalb, *Augustinus, De civitate dei*, CCSL [Corpus Christianorum Series Latina] 48 (Turnhout, 1955)], pp. 833–4.

9. . . . [Ibid], p. 833.

10. See the list of manuscripts in *Augustinus, De fide rerum invisibilium; Enchiridion ad Laurentium de fide et spe et caritate* [etc], CCSL 46 (Turnhout, 1969), pp. viii–xiv, including around twenty from the ninth/tenth century or earlier.

11. . . . *Enchiridion* 23.84, ed. M. Evans, CCSL 46, p. 95.

12. . . . *Enchiridion* 23.85, p. 95. This appears to be Augustine's paraphrase of a question, not his answer.

13. . . . Enchiridion 23.85, p. 95.

14. . . . Enchiridion 23.85, pp. 95–6.

15. . . . Enchiridion 23.85, p. 96.

16. . . . *Enchiridion* 23.86, p. 96.

17. [D. Shanzer, "Voices and Bodies: The Afterlife of the Unborn," *Numen* 56 (2009)], 348–9, referring to Augustine's 'bolder treatment' in the *Enchiridion*, interprets Augustine's position as the 'unformed *foetus* cannot be said to have lived, because it had never been born' (at 348, italics in original).

18. [D. A. Dombrowski and R. Deltete, *A Brief, Liberal, Catholic Defense of Abortion* (Urbana IL, 2000)], p. 23.

19. [M. J. Gorman, *Abortion and the Early Church: Christian, Jewish and Pagan Attitudes in the Greco-Roman World* (Downers Grove IL, 1982)], pp. 71–2. [D.A. Jones, *The Soul of the Embryo: An Inquiry into the Status of the Human Embryo in the Christian Tradition* (London, 2004)], p. 228, appears to assume that Augustine was attempting to imagine the bodies of resurrected fetuses in heaven.

18

Pre-modern Islamic Medical Ethics and Graeco-Islamic-Jewish Embryology

Mohammed Ghaly

In this excerpt, Mohammed Ghaly, scholar of biomedical Islamic ethics, critically examines two pre-modern Islamic writers who grapple with tensions between the medieval knowledge of embryology (much of which was inherited from scientific texts translated between the eighth and tenth centuries from Greek into Arabic) and the religious interpretations of prenatal development. Al-Qarāfī demonstrated a hermeneutical strategy of metaphorical interpretation of scripture. Al-Qayyim focused on the variability of medical evidence, which he argued is susceptible to error. As a biomedical ethicist, Ghaly is interested in how a study of ancient sources parallels contemporary biomedical ethical inquiry and thus might help illuminate these discussions.

[T]his microstudy aims to show that a close analysis of issues pertinent to embryology in Islamic Law can reveal new nuances in, and add to a better understanding of, the relation between Islam and science.[1] Furthermore, studying these medieval discussions will give us an idea about what pre-modern Islamic medical ethics looked like and how it might have affected the contemporary discussions on similar issues. . . . The main questions to be raised in this respect are: Were Muslim jurists aware of the embryological views recorded in the medical sources? If so, how did Muslim jurists respond to these medical sources when their embryological views seemingly contradict specific Qur'anic verses or prophetic traditions?

Source: Mohammed Ghaly, "Pre-modern Islamic Medical Ethics and Graeco-Islamic-Jewish Embryology," *Bioethics* 28, no. 2 (2014): 49–58.

This article studies the contributions of two Muslim jurists, namely the Mālikī Shihāb al-Dīn al-Qarāfī (d. 1285)[2] and the Ḥanbalī Ibn al-Qayyim (d. 1350).[3]

. . .

Graeco-Islamic-Jewish Medical Views on Human Embryology

Nutriment is one of the books attributed to the Greek physician Hippocrates (ca. 375 BC), known in Arabic literature as Būqrāṭ, Ibuqrāṭ or Abuqrāṭ.[4] This book, whose attribution to Hippocrates seems to be accepted without hesitation in the Islamic tradition,[5] was translated into Arabic under the title *Kitāb al-ghidhā'*, probably in the 8th century, by a certain al-Biṭrīq.[6] Information on the development of the embryo and fetus inside the uterus, as recorded in the translation of al-Biṭrīq, reads:

> The formation of the embryo is completed in 35 days, it moves in 70 and is perfected in 210. Others say that the formation of the embryo is completed in 45 days, that it moves in 90 and that it emerges in 270. Others say that its formation is completed in 50 days, that it moves in 100 and that it is perfected in 300. Others say that the form of the embryo is completed in 40 days, that it moves in 80 and that it emerges in 240.[7]

This text speaks of four main possibilities for the duration of pregnancy, respectively 210 days (seven months), 270 days (nine months), 240 days (eight months) and 300 days (10 months).

. . .

These Hippocratic views started to circulate later among physicians in the Muslim world. . . . The well-known Muslim physician Avicenna (d. 1037) also made reference to these medical views in his *Kitāb al-ḥayawān* (The book of animals). However, Avicenna was sceptical about the accuracy of these views and argued that they can hardly be supported with solid evidence. Furthermore, Avicenna shortened the list of pregnancy possibilities to two, namely seven- and ten-month pregnancies instead of the four possibilities mentioned in *Kitāb al-ghidhā'*. He held that seven and nine months are the common average (*al-zamān al-wasaṭ al-ʿadl*) during which the cycle of pregnancy comes to perfection.[8]

Also the two Jewish physicians who lived in Egypt; Ibn Jumayʿ (d. ca. 1198)[9] and Moses Maimonides (d. 1204)[10] commented on the same embryological views without, however, casting doubts upon their veracity from a medical point of view. In his encyclopedic medical work, which is extant in manuscript form only, *Al-irshād li maṣālīḥ al-anfus wa al-ajsād* (Guidance to the welfare of souls and bodies), Ibn Jumayʿ elaborated on the embryonic and fetal development inside the uterus. The manuscript of this work, available in the Syrian al-Ẓāhiriyya library, shows that Ibn Jumayʿ dedicated a distinct chapter for explaining these embryological views. In this chapter, Ibn Jumayʿ argued that the unborn goes through three main stages, namely formation (*takhalluq*), moving (*taḥarruk*) and finally the stage birth (*wilāda*) by the end of which a baby is born. . . .

Kitāb al-fuṣūl fī al-ṭibb (Book on Medical Aphorisms) is Maimonides' most voluminous medical work and was mainly based on Graeco-Latin and Islamic medical works. Guidelines drawn from Greek medical authorities such as Hippocrates and Galen occupied a significant position in the book.[11] In this book, Maimonides recorded his embryological views, which corresponded in broad lines with those of his contemporary Ibn Jumayʿ. Like Ibn Jumayʿ, Maimonides spoke of two possibilities for the total period of pregnancy, namely seven and nine months. Also the cycle of pregnancy was divided into the same three stages.

. . .

Medieval Islamic Law on Human Embryology

. . .

(A) Shihāb al-Dīn al-Qarāfī: Islamic scriptures reconciled with Graeco-Jewish medical views

In his book *Al-furūq* (Subtle distinctions), al-Qarāfī dedicated a distinct chapter to the Graeco-Jewish medical ideas on human embryology and their relevance to Islamic Law. . . .The chapter can be divided into four sections . . .

In the third section, al-Qarāfī focused on the religious sources, especially the tradition of Ibn Mas'ūd* and how its purport can be reconciled with the medical views already expounded in the second section. Al-Qarāfī signalled two possible conflicting points between the tradition and these medical views. The first point related to the first passage in the tradition, namely 'The creation of each one of you is put together in his mother's womb in forty days'. However, the medical views held that an embryo gets formed within 30, 35 or 45 days. Al-Qarāfī proposed that the number 'forty' in the tradition should not be taken literally. . . .[12] The second conflicting point had to do with ensouling the unborn which, according to the tradition, happens after four months of pregnancy. Medical views, however, indicated that the unborn passes the phase of moving, which is usually seen as an indication of life, much earlier. Applying the aforementioned medical views on the literal understanding of the tradition, al-Qarāfī argued, means that birth will take place after one-year of pregnancy.

. . .

According to al-Qarāfī giving birth after a twelve-month pregnancy might happen but it remains uncommon. On the other hand, the opening phrase of the prophetic tradition 'the creation of each one of you (aḥadakum)' implies that this is what happens in the normal pregnancies rather the exceptional or uncommon ones. In order to solve this conflict, al-Qarāfī proposed a metaphorical interpretation for this phrase according to which it will be read as 'any one of you' instead of 'each one of you'. According to this reading, the tradition will be referring to a specific case of pregnancy rather than the general norm thereof. Such a twelve-month pregnancy, al-Qarāfī argued, did occur and thus the purport of the prophetic tradition will be in conformity with reality and simultaneously with the medical views.[13]

. . .

The fourth section was dedicated to addressing a possible question that might tarnish the integrity of al-Qarāfī's way of reasoning, namely why do Muslim jurists need to base religious rulings in Islamic Law on views expressed by non-Muslims (in reference to the Greek and Jewish physicians)? In response, al-Qarāfī clarified that these views were expressed by specialists in human anatomical dissection (musharriḥūn) who dissected the pregnant

---

*Eds.: Ibn Mas'ūd was a companion of the Prophet Mohammed and eminent source of numerous hadith (traditions) about what the Prophet taught or did.

women that had been sentenced to death, and cut their bellies open. Medical views based on scientific experiments augmented by sensory perception and eye-observation, al-Qarāfī stressed, should be taken seriously by Muslim jurists even if these views came originally from non-Muslims.[14] Thus, al-Qarāfī held that these embryological views convey certainty because they are based on eye-observation and sensory perception. On the other hand, references in the Islamic scriptures are open to more than one possible interpretation. That is why the purport of the prophetic tradition should undergo metaphorical interpretation in order to accommodate the certainty conveyed by the medical views.

. . .

(B) Ibn al-Qayyim: The vulnerability of the empirical evidence

Ibn al-Qayyim's main ideas on embryological views and their relevance to Islamic Law can be consulted in two books by him, namely *Al-tibyān fī aqsām al-Qur'ān* (Clarifying the oaths of the Qur'ān) and *Tuḥfat al-Mawdūd bi aḥkām al-mawlūd* (The gift of the Loving [God] on the rulings pertaining to the newborn). Both books included chapters on the growth of the human being from the very beginning of his creation till death.[15] . . . He accepted the apparent meaning of this prophetic tradition; the unborn goes through three main stages inside the uterus, namely *nuṭfa* (sperm-drop) for forty days, *'alaqa* (a clot of congealed blood) for forty days and *muḍgha* (a little lump of flesh) also for forty days and after the completion of these three stages which take 120 days in total, the angel breaths the soul into the fetus.[16]

Like al-Qarāfī, Ibn al-Qayyim was aware of the possible conflict between the tradition of Ibn Mas'ūd and the medical views. Unlike al-Qarāfī, Ibn al-Qayyim stressed the primacy of the religious sources because their purport constitute divine revelation. Thus, he argued that information provided by the prophetic tradition on the growth of the unborn inside the uterus should be conceived as certain as if this information was gained through eye observation. Hence, Ibn al-Qayyim held that the contradicting medical views are 'definitely wrong'.[17] These medical views on embryology, he argued, were not based on eye-observation or any other conclusive evidence.

. . .

Ibn al-Qayyim concluded his critique of these medical views by arguing that the main source of information in this respect should be divine revelation rather than the medical works because the former is not susceptible to error whereas the latter is.[18]

It is also clear that Ibn al-Qayyim was aware of the possible conflicts inherent in the scriptural references to embryology and that not all these references are decisive in nature. This gave him space to make choices, which sometimes came close to the medical views. . . . If it ever happened that the unborn moves before 120 days of pregnancy, Ibn al-Qayyim hypothesized, this does not necessarily mean that the embryo was already ensouled at this early stage. He argued that one should distinguish between two types of movement that can be made by the unborn. The first type is a spontaneous and involuntary movement, which can happen before the ensoulement of the fetus. The second type is a voluntary and conscious movement which can be done by the fetus only after being ensouled. According to Ibn al-Qayyim, the Hippocratic medical views, if ever proven to be true, should be understood as referring to the first type of movement whereas the tradition of Ibn Masʿūd refers to the second type.[19]

. . .

Conclusion

On the basis of this micro-study on the religio-ethical discussions conducted by the two medieval Muslim jurists al-Qarāfī and Ibn al-Qayyim on embryology, one can construct some of the essential features of the premodern Islamic medical ethics and its relation to contemporary Islamic bioethics.

First of all, medical knowledge was an integral part of pre-modern Islamic medical ethics. Although the Islamic scriptures included information on the development of the unborn inside the uterus, these two jurists took note of Graeco-Islamic-Jewish medical views and none of them called for an outright rejection of these views just because they fell within the category of 'ancient sciences'. Their disagreement was rather on how to evaluate the empirical evidence at hand. Both jurists accepted the credibility of human anatomical dissection (*tashrīḥ*) as empirical evidence. Al-Qarāfī held that medical views on embryology are based on a systematic practice of *tashrīḥ* and that is why the contradicting references in the Islamic scriptures should be metaphorically interpreted. However, Ibn al-Qayyim insisted that the medical views are based on other evidences whose reliability remain doubtful and held that religious evidences should be the main source of information in this respect.

. . .

Secondly, pre-modern Islamic medical ethics is an integral part of contemporary Islamic bioethics. Contemporary discussions conducted by Muslim religious and biomedical scientists on the beginning of human life depended heavily on the views expressed by medieval Muslim jurists on embryology. As for the medical knowledge, the Graeco-Islamic-Jewish medical views were replaced by modern research on embryology conducted in American and European universities. However, the question of the (un) reliability of the empirical evidence, which already preoccupied the minds of the medieval jurists, also remained central to the contemporary discussions.

Notes

1. It is to be noted that the recent publications of Justin Stearns already forcefully demonstrated the significance of examining the contributions of Muslim jurists in general for the sake understanding the relation between Islam and science. See, for instance, Justin Stearns. 2011. *The Legal Status of Science in the Muslim World in the Early Modern Period: An Initial Consideration of Fatwas from Three Maghribi Sources*. In *The Islamic Scholarly Tradition Studies in History, Law, and Thought in Honor of Professor Michael Allan Cook*. Asad Q. Ahmed, Behnam Sadeghi and Michael Bonner, ed. Leiden: Brill: 265–290; Justin Stearns. 2011a. *Infectious Ideas: Contagion in Premodern Islamic and Christian Thought in the Western Mediterranean*. Baltimore: The Johns Hopkins University Press.
2. See Sherman Jackson. 1996. *Islamic Law and the State: The Constitutional Jurisprudence of Shihāb al-Dīn al-Qarāfī*. Leiden: Brill: 1–32; Sherman Jackson. Shihāb al-Dīn al- Ḳarāfī. *Encyclopaedia of Islam*. Second edn.
3. See H. Laoust. Ibn Ḳayyim al-Djawziyya. *Encyclopaedia of Islam*. Second edn.
4. A. Dietrich. Buḳrāṭ. *Encyclopaedia of Islam*. second ed.
5. It should be noted that academic research proved that not every work ascribed to Hippocrates was necessarily authored by him. It has already been realized in antiquity that works carrying the name of Hippocrates as author cannot be written by the same individual, much less by the

historical Hippocrates. See R. Hankinson. 2006. Hippocrates and the Hippocratic corpus. *Encyclopedia of Philosophy*. Second edn. Detroit: Thomson Gale; 4: 373–376; K. Kelly. 2009. The History of Medicine: The Middle Ages. New York: Facts on File Inc.: 107. For the authorship of *Nutriment* in specific, see W. Jones. 1957 [1923]. *Hippocrates*. London-Cambridge, Massachusetts: William Heinemann Ltd. Harvard University Press; 1: 337–341.

6. D. Dunlop. The translations of al-Biṭrīq and Yaḥyā (Yuḥannā) b. al-Biṭrīq, *Journal of the Royal Asiatic Society* 1959; 91: 141–142; J. Mattock. 1971. *Hippocrates: Humours, Hippocrates: On nutriment*. Cambridge: Heffer and Sons Ltd.: i–ii.

7. English translation is quoted from J. Mattock, op. cit. note 12, pp. 17–18.

8. Ibn Sīnā. 1970. *Al-shifāʾ, al-Ṭabīʾiyyāt, al-Ḥayawān*. Ed. ʿAbd al- alīm Muntaṣir, Saʿīd Zāyid and ʿAbd Allāh Ismāʾīl. Cairo: Al-Hayʾa al-Miṣriyya al-ʿĀmma li al-Taʾlīf wa al-Nashr: 173; Al-Baladī. 1980. *Kitāb tadbīr al-ḥabālā wa al-aṭ fāl wa al-ṣibyān wa ḥifẓ ṣiḥḥatihim wa mudāwāt al-amrāḍ al-ʿāriḍa lahum*. Baghdad: Dāral-Rashīd li al-Nashr: 115.

9. See H. Fähnrich. 1997. Ibn Jumayʾ. *Encyclopaedia of the History of Science, Technology, and Medicine in non-Western Culture*. Dordrecht-Boston-London: Kluwer Academic publishers: 421–422; Eliyahu Ashtor. 2007. Hibat Allah, Ibn Jumayʾ Ibn Zayn. *Encyclopaedia Judaica*. Second edn. Vol. 9. Detroit: Thomson Gale: 93.

10. See Bernard R. Goldstein. Maimonides. *Encyclopaedia Judaica*. Vol.13. Detroit: Thomson Gale: 381–397.

11. See Fred Rosner. Moses Maimonides the Physician. *Moses Maimonides*: 3–32; Lenn Goodman. 2009. Bahya and Maimonides on the Worth of Medicine. In *Maimonides and his Heritage*. Idit Dobbs-Weinstein, Lenn Goodman and James Grady, eds. New York: State University of New York Press: 62.

12. [Al-Qarāfī. No date. *Anwār al-burūq fī anwāʾ al-furūq*. Cairo: ʿĀlam al-Kutub], pp. 224–5.

13. Ibid., p. 224.

14. Ibid., p. 225.

15. Ibn al-Qayyim. No date. Al-tibyān fī aqsāmal-Qurʾān. Cairo: Maktabat al-Qāhira, pp. 237–305; Ibn al-Qayyim. 1999. *Tuḥ fat al-Mawdūd bi aḥkām al-mawlūd*. Manṣūra, Egypt: Dār Ibn Rajab: 301–69.

16. Ibn al-Qayyim, 1999, op. cit. note [15], p. 316.

17. Ibn al-Qayyim, No date, op. cit. note [15], p. 246; Ibn al-Qayyim. op. cit. note [15], p. 316.

18. Ibn al-Qayyim, op. cit. note [15], p. 317–318.

19. [Ibn al-Qayyim, No date, op. cit. note 15], p. 246; Ibn al-Qayyim. 1999, op. cit. note [15], p. 318.

Abortion and Law in the High Middle Ages

Ignacio Castuera

Ignacio Castuera, a Mexican American United Methodist minister, has his doctorate from Claremont School of Theology. He has been active in supporting reproductive rights, serving on the Clergy Advisory Board and as a chaplain for the Planned Parenthood Federation of America as well as a board member of the Religious Coalition for Reproductive Rights. In this excerpt Castuera summarizes a complex period of late medieval Western European history when abortion transitioned from the category of sin to that of a criminal act. We recommend to readers Castuera's complete essay, which surveys views of abortion from the early church to the present.

Historian Barbara Tuchman once described the Middle Ages as "a distant mirror," by which she meant a period that can help us understand the present, but not by drawing simplistic parallels. The modern West both has its roots in the earlier period, and yet it is quite different. We can see that tension reflected in our understanding of how European Christians regarded abortion, exposure, and infanticide in the High Middle Ages. We must use care in examining this question. Viewing legal developments in the Middle Ages through modern eyes is almost certain to yield anachronisms. Müller (2012: 4) explains why the effort to uncover the true meaning of abortion in medieval Europe poses enormous problems of interpretation:

Source: Ignacio Castuera, "A Social History of Christian Thought on Abortion: Ambiguity vs. Certainty in Moral Debate," *American Journal of Economics and Sociology* 76, no. 1 (2017): 121–227.

> Issues of juristic nomenclature and procedure . . . [in] the original source
> material render the retrieval of lived circumstances difficult, if not impossible,
> and a thick layer of formulaic language exposes readers to narratives shaped
> by normative requirements and at the expense of what actually happened on
> the ground, be it in the privacy of homes or during interrogations. *Abortion
> in medieval practice remains enigmatic and for the most part eludes our modern
> curiosity*. (emphasis added)

One aspect of ancient science on the subject of gestation that entered into
the legal system in the high Middle Ages was the Aristotelian view that the
animation or "ensoulment" of the fetus took place at 40 days for boys and
80 or 90 days for girls. In 1140, Johannes Gratian, an Italian monk, published
the first collection of canon law, after methodically compiling teachings and
pronouncements of church leaders over the previous millennium to create
a set of rules that held far greater internal consistency than any previous
work on church law. Gratian's *Decretum* became the basis for both canon law
and many features of secular law for many centuries. On the question of the
legality of abortion, the rule was clear. Citing Augustine and Jerome, Gratian
(*Decretum* C. 32, q. 2, c. 8) definitively states: "He is not a murderer who
brings about abortion before the soul is in the body."

Gratian's compilation and synthesis of papal pronouncements and other
decrees was highly influential on the scholars of his era. Müller (2012: 3)
summarizes the law in the 12th century more generally, as it pertained to
abortion:

> . . . The criterion of birth was of no significance to twelfth-century law
> teachers, who rather presented the moment of animation and formation,
> between forty and eighty days after conception, as the decisive prerequisite
> for charges of punishable manslaughter.

For most of the next eight centuries, the legal system of the Catholic Church
considered the six to twelve weeks after conception as a period before
ensoulment or animation took place. Before a fetus became animated, the
law and Catholic legal teaching did not regard it as a person. However, it
should be noted that this was a matter of Church legal discipline, which was
separate from its moral teaching.

Even in cases of late-term abortion or infanticide, the Middle Ages was a
time of lax enforcement by the standards of our own time. Although modern
legal systems in the West are descendants of medieval law, it is easy to get lost
and confused if one tries to follow the stream to its source. Law in the Middle
Ages was carried out differently from today and performed diverse social
functions, many of which were aimed at the cure of souls, not the protection

of bodies. The violation of social norms could result in both civil and ecclesiastical penalties. Criminal law was not clearly separated from civil law. No police force or prosecutor's office existed to investigate crimes. In the absence of an administrative state, most cases were brought before a judge by an aggrieved party. Physical evidence was rarely obtainable, so most cases were decided on the basis of confession or eyewitness accounts. However, as Müller (2012: 177) points out, contrary to a popular misconception in our time, physical ordeals and torture were rarely used in the High Middle Ages to extract confessions, except in "extraordinary" cases of heresy and witchcraft, which were deemed to threaten the social order—much like "terrorism" today.

. . .

Thus, in normal cases involving the death of a fetus or infant, the accused was normally protected, both then and now, by a presumption of innocence. That was true until the idea of abortion became mixed with fears of magic and witchcraft toward the end of the Middle Ages.

For hundreds of years following the decline of the Roman legal system, law became erratic and incoherent. Manor courts might apply rules inconsistently and arbitrarily that would deeply offend modern concepts of justice. The same offense might be tolerated in one instance and serve as the basis of execution in an equivalent case. Rules of evidence were based on local custom. As part of the 12th-century renaissance, legal scholars such as Gratian began to formulate new legal categories that were intended to apply similar rules and judgments in similar cases. Müller (2012: 22) explains the legal revolution that took place in this period:

> The twelfth century was decisive in distinguishing punishable acts from other forms of human misconduct. For the first time in Western history, scholastic teachers systematically explored the difference between crime and tort, between litigation in pursuit of material compensation and, alternatively, penal consequences for delinquents found to have disturbed the public peace and offended the common good. . . .

Despite this giant intellectual leap, it took several centuries for the new ideas about law and crime to be thoroughly integrated into the diverse courts.

It was during this fertile period of legal reform that abortion was first deemed a *crimen* in a juridical sense. That term understandably gives rise to an expectation that it means what we now think of as "crime." That is only partially true. Müller (2012: 4–5) explains that it had multiple meanings that are no longer considered part of the law:

> [D]epending on context, trained lawyers would have referred to *crimen* in not one, but up to four different senses. First, they would have spoken of it in

now familiar fashion in order to denote a punishable crime; second, as a variety of misconduct leading to *irregularitas*, or ineligibility to higher (sacramental) rank within the ecclesiastical hierarchy; third, as sin *(peccatum)* in the modern Catholic understanding of the term—that is, as a wrong redeemable through private confession and secretly imposed works of penance *(penitentia)*; and fourth, as another form of *peccatum* against God's justice, perpetrated publicly and worthy of atonement before everyone's eyes.

Therefore, the mere use of the term *crimen* does not necessarily tell us whether abortion was considered a crime in the modern sense. In fact, the determination of which meaning would be applied would be related to the type of court in which a case was heard.

. . . The closest approximation to a central authority at the time was the Vatican, but even the Vatican had only very loose control over the diverse ecclesiastical bodies that had the authority to make judgments about legal and spiritual matters, which were not always clearly differentiated. The secular courts included knights, nobility, and royalty, all vying for control over territory and people. Canon law began to be codified during this period, but secular law was more anarchic then systematic.

In ecclesiastical courts, a woman accused by neighbors of having killed a child or aborted a quickened fetus or a man accused of battering a pregnant woman and causing a miscarriage might be called to answer the charge. Failing to do so, the person's public reputation would be tarnished. In a highly communal society, reputation or honor had high value, and in any case, the court had the means of punishing recalcitrant defendants. If the issue was deemed a matter of *penitentia*, the accused was presumed guilty unless proven innocent, and the punishment consisted of acts of atonement, which included "prayer, fasting, . . . pilgrimage, . . . [or] flogging, commutation to monetary payment, and imprisonment of uncertain duration and duress" (Müller 2012: 6). No physical evidence of guilt was required in these cases, only the word of an anonymous accuser.

Throughout the Middle Ages, the secular courts *(ius commune)* also heard accusations against men or women reputed to have caused a miscarriage, a crime potentially punishable by death. Other cases were about women accused of causing their own miscarriage or of committing infanticide. In law, the death of a developed fetus was equivalent to the death of a child, which could carry a death sentence. However, in the absence of an admission of guilt or statements of two witnesses who actually observed the act in question, it was impossible to convict any party of this crime. . . . Müller (2012: 178) concludes:

With scenarios of birth normally unfolding in the privacy of homes and surrounded by an intimate circle of family and friends, it must have been easy for the respectable to conceal vestiges of pre- and postnatal infanticide forever from outside scrutiny.

For this reason, it was rare for anyone to be convicted in the Middle Ages in a secular court of abortion or infanticide. The protection of the rights of defendants was simply too high during this period for the legal system to infringe very much on individual behavior.

In conclusion, it seems that the high Middle Ages is a period of paradoxical change with respect to the Catholic Church's official view of abortion. On the one hand, the modern concept of law emerged from the rationalization of canon law, which gave a decisive boost to the legalistic way of thinking about the killing of an animated fetus. Indeed late-stage abortion was deemed murder and carried the penalty of death, in principle. This development would certainly seem to confirm to Christians in the 21st century that the Middle Ages was an era of harsh moral judgments on abortion that treated it unambiguously as a criminal act.

On the other hand, the actual behavior of courts in the Middle Ages, both ecclesiastical and secular, would lead one to the opposite conclusion that abortion was not regarded by authorities as a serious offense. First, the law did not apply at all to abortion in the early stages of a pregnancy. The idea that ensoulment took place long after conception became enshrined in canon law at this time. Furthermore, the relatively few cases regarding the death of a fetus that were brought before a magistrate were very difficult to prove, according to the evidentiary requirements, and were almost never punished severely, either in the form of penance or in the form of fines or other secular penalties. Despite the growing legalism of Church authorities during this period, the policy regarding abortion was very similar to the one-time policy of the U.S. military toward homosexuality: "don't ask, don't tell."

Reference

Müller, Wolfgang P. (2012). *The Criminalization of Abortion in the West: Its Origins in Medieval Law*. Ithaca, NY: Cornell University Press.

20

Contraception in Protestant Theology: A Brief and Incomplete History

Kathryn D. Blanchard

Kathryn Blanchard was the Charles A. Dana Professor of Religious Studies for many years at Alma College, Michigan. Her teaching and scholarship focus on gender, economic justice, and environmentalism. This original paper emerges in part from previous research on the history of contraception in the Reformed tradition and offers insight to some of the ways that Reformed theology of marriage and sexuality differed from Roman Catholic views. Her discussion of thinking about children as "gifts" offers a theological frame intended to challenge the hyper-consumerism and individualism of late capitalism.

When most Protestant couples marry they assume that they will use some form of birth control (if they are not doing so already) to put off having children until they feel personally and/or economically ready for parenthood. And a growing number of married couples are comfortable saying they do not feel called *ever* to become parents. The question for Protestants (as well as for Catholics who promote natural family planning) is not *whether* to control conception but *how*.[2]

It is, however, no longer safe to assume that all Protestants are pro-contraception. This came to light most notably in religious freedom cases against the Affordable Care Act (Obamacare); in 2014, the U.S. Supreme Court ruled in favor of the Protestant owners of Hobby Lobby, who objected to paying for some forms of their employees' birth control on religious grounds. According to the court, the owners had 'sincere Christian beliefs that life begins at conception and that it would violate their religion to facilitate access to contraceptive drugs or devices that operate after that point,' i.e., methods believed to be abortifacient, such as IUDs or pills.[3] Since when, many Americans responded in surprise, have Protestants been opposed to birth control?

16ᵗʰ Century: Marriage Is Only *Partly* for Procreation

John Calvin, a Catholic-scholar-turned-Protestant-pastor, provided theological roots for what has come to be known as the Reformed tradition. His early interest in marriage was mainly as a legal institution, useful for keeping order by contravening lust, and therefore properly governed by the earthly magistrates. But he later became convinced of the need to explain marriage more theologically, in order that Christians might approach it not merely as a civic duty but as a divine calling. Calvin thus turned to the biblical theme of *covenant*—between God and Israel, between Christ and the church—as a means of stressing that marriage was not just for keeping sex orderly but also for purposes of mutual love and support, as well as procreation and nurture of children.[4]

In his early discussions of sex, Calvin appeals to Paul (1 Cor. 7) for a no-nonsense approach: 'If they cannot exercise self-control, they should marry.'[5] The main backdrop was the medieval Catholicism in which both he and his parishioners had been trained, which (Calvin feared) caused them to see marriage as a lesser good than celibacy. While Calvin did not oppose celibacy in theory, he was deeply skeptical of it in practice, believing it to be an extremely difficult state to which few were called and fewer could attain perfectly. Calvin acknowledges that the human condition is to long for physical and emotional intimacy, and argues that God provided marriage to satisfy that longing.[6] 'Let no man [sic] rashly despise marriage as something unprofitable or superfluous to him . . . If his power to tame lust fails him, let him recognize that the Lord has now imposed the necessity of marriage upon him.'[7]

Calvin calls married couples (especially men) to enjoy sex 'soberly', modestly and moderately, not becoming 'adulterers' toward their spouses.[8]

Noteworthy is that nowhere in this passage does the topic of children enter the discussion, either as a deterrent or as that which makes marital sex permissible or beneficial. With regard to questions of sexual purity, the main thing that recommends marriage to Calvin is its usefulness in preventing the uncontrolled burning of fallen humanity. In many cases he might have brought up children as marriage's main purpose, or even a secondary purpose, but he does not.[9]

Rather, it is companionship that seems to take (a very close) second place on Calvin's list of purposes. In his commentary on Genesis, Calvin teaches that God gave Adam a companion of 'the same kind with himself' so he could have 'a suitable and proper help'.[10] Humans were made of the same stuff, specifically so as to create the mutual respect and understanding between them that comes from recognizing one's own likeness in another person. Adam 'obtained a faithful associate of life; for now he saw himself, who had before been imperfect, *rendered complete* in his wife'.[11] The human alone was apparently deficient; only in community were they made perfect.

Most important for Calvin is the notion that children are a gift rather than the product of human will. Take, for example, his commentary on the Jacob-Leah-Rachel story of Genesis 29; he thought Jacob was guilty of excessive lust for Rachel and an irresponsible lack of kindness and honor given to his first wife, Leah, so God saw fit to step in and 'vindicate' Leah, giving her many children as a means of getting Jacob to love her more. 'This passage teaches us, that offspring is a special gift of God . . . expressly ascribed to him'.[12] Children are *given* by God as a 'pledge' or 'seal' on a marriage, a means to enhancing companionship between spouses. The begetting of children for Calvin is a special act of providence, rather than a matter of biology or human design. The honor to be parents of creatures made in God's image is not something to be controlled, regretted, or gloated over, but to be humbly received.[13] He reemphasizes this idea later in his Genesis commentary, when Jacob 'acknowledges and confesses that children are not so produced by nature to subvert the truth of the declaration, that the fruit of the womb is a reward and gift of God. . . . Let parents then learn to consider, and to celebrate the singular kindness of God, in their offspring'.[14] This is the crux of Calvin's teaching on parenthood: because it is a gracious gift, it must be undertaken with both modesty and gratitude.

Given his condemnation of Rachel's attempt to control procreation, we might deduce Calvin's disapproval of birth control. What is implied becomes explicit in his comments on Onan and Tamar in Genesis 38, the only (and therefore oft-cited) biblical reference to a deliberate act of contraception.

Here Calvin seems to be focused on biology: 'since each man is born for the preservation of the whole race, if anyone dies without children, there seems to be here some defect of nature'.[15] But control and obedience are also parts of the equation: Onan was obligated to procreate for his brother, and Tamar was 'held under an obligation to the house of Judah, to procreate some seed'.[16] In this context, Calvin is concerned primarily with Onan's decision to 'pour out his seed' on the ground rather than raise up a child for his brother. 'For this means that one quenches the hope of his family, and kills the son, which could be expected, before he is born. . . . Moreover he thus has . . . tried to destroy a part of the human race'.[17] Scientific inaccuracies aside, Calvin follows the traditional (and traditionally sexist) interpretation of Onan's act as not only an offense against his late brother, but as a virtual homicide and a sin against humanity. He condemns it, addressing not only the injunction against a man who commits *coitus interruptus*, but also any woman who 'drives away the seed out of the womb, through aids'.[18]

So, although Calvin views fellowship and continence as two crucial purposes of marriage, there is no doubt in his mind that there is a third purpose—procreation—which should not be voluntarily hindered. The Reformed tradition is thus heir to the same disgust toward 'unnatural' forms of contraception as the Catholic tradition, for different reasons.[19] But Protestant theologies are multifaceted, carrying within themselves potential lines of critique of any case against contraception—inheritances such as the willingness to interpret Scripture appropriately to one's own time and culture, even to such an extent as to dismiss certain Old Testament prohibitions;[20] the beliefs in the priesthood of all believers and in Christian freedom in matters not explicitly laid out in scripture;[21] and especially the idea that marriage is significantly, if not primarily, a covenant that fosters companionship and continence in addition to procreation.

20th Century: *Sex* Is Only Partly for Procreation

The 1930 Lambeth Conference among the bishops of the Church of England marked a turning point in the Protestant world. Until then, virtually all Christian churches opposed all forms of artificial birth control. But at the conference, the Anglican bishops voted by a large majority to adopt the following landmark resolution:

Where there is a clearly felt moral obligation to limit or avoid parenthood the method must be decided on Christian principles. The primary and obvious method is complete abstinence from intercourse as far as may be necessary in a life of discipline and self-control lived in the power of the Holy Spirit. Nevertheless in those cases where there is such a clearly felt moral obligation to limit or avoid parenthood and where there is morally sound reason for avoiding complete abstinence, the conference agrees that other methods may be used, provided that this is done in the light of the same Christian principles. The conference records its strong condemnation of the use of any method of contraception control from motives of selfishness, luxury, or mere convenience.[22]

The bishops left open the possibility that faithful Christian marriage might include the limitation *or even avoidance* of parenthood through the use of artificial means, as long as it was for unselfish and Christian reasons. The Federal Council of Churches in the United States made a statement in 1931 that the use of contraceptives by married people was 'valid and moral', partly because sex between mates was 'right in itself'.[23] Lutheran churches were somewhat slower to join in, but in 1952 the Lutheran bishops of Sweden made a cautious move toward contraception: 'There is something wrong', they maintained, 'in any marriage where the couple are biologically normal but want no children. Yet children are not the sole purpose of marriage . . . Seriously considered this situation does lead us to concede that under certain circumstances contraceptives may be permitted'.[24]

Each of these churches expressed the conviction that parenthood is good, but marriage and sex are for more than just procreation; that 'certain circumstances' of particular couples may call for different yet equally responsible Christian choices regarding contraception. Protestants, whose polity tends to reflect an approach that allows for 'shared discernment'[25] of the word of God, thus made the move away from hierarchical church orders, generally trusting Christian couples to make their own decisions according to their consciences. It must be said, however, that each of these churches still deemed birth control a matter to be *carefully considered* rather than assumed, to be used only when necessary and not taken lightly.

It is remarkable that almost across the board, contraception itself (within the context of marriage) was viewed as morally neutral; the main warnings were against having ill *motives* for using contraceptives. By the late 1960s, Protestant discourse had largely moved past the question of contraception and was heavily into the debate concerning induced abortion—usually seen as a distinct question. (It would be a while longer before they seriously took up same-sex marriage.)

21st Century: From Birth Control to Reproductive Justice

Protestant women rarely write about contraception as such and have typically turned their attention to abortion, whether for or against. Some Protestant women have importantly turned to the framework of *reproductive justice* (RJ), originally introduced by Black feminists and now gaining wider traction.[26] This is the notion that "all people can exercise the rights and access the resources they need to thrive and to decide if, when, and how to create and sustain their families with dignity, free from discrimination, coercion, or violence."[27] Reproductive justice certainly includes issues of access to birth control, but it does not typically separate it from issues of abortion, women's health, and even broader topics like domestic violence, systemic misogyny and racism, and economic opportunity.[28]

By and large, today's Protestant writing about birth control comes from Evangelical men, who seem to have the most continuing anxiety about 'the sea change . . . that Protestantism underwent in the 20th century from staunch opposition to acceptance of contraception'.[29] Among those Protestants still talking specifically about contraception, many are at their root arguing about abortion. The Hobby Lobby decision wasn't about *all* birth control but only *abortive* birth control. Likewise, Focus on the Family, in a statement regarding (married) couples' use of contraceptives, writes, 'We don't believe that it's wrong to prevent fertilization, but we oppose any method of so-called birth control that functions as an abortifacient', which for them includes IUDs and the pill; 'contraception is an issue that should be approached with prayer and wise counsel from friends, parents, mentors, pastors, and trusted medical professionals'.[30]

But there are indeed a few Protestants today who still argue that contraception of *any* kind is an offense against 'the biblical understanding of sex and sexuality'. They argue that sex without 'the most serious consequence of sexual immorality' (i.e. unwanted pregnancy) has degraded moral standards and harmed 'the spiritual meaning' of marriage.[31] Furthermore, partners must keep pregnancy at the forefront of their minds or risk becoming sex objects for each other, otherwise men will cease to view women with proper 'reverence'. Without the necessary connection between sex, marriage, and children, Protestantism has tumbled down a slippery slope to unmarried cohabitation and same-sex marriage, and thus—perhaps worst of all—'Protestants find themselves following the larger culture in matters of marriage and family'.[32]

Other Protestants take a more nuanced view, Christian ethicist, Kenneth Magnuson takes pains to distinguish contraception and birth control ('"birth control" refers to any action that is taken to prevent the birth of a child', including abortion, while '"Contraception" refers to forms of birth control that prevent conception'), but nevertheless links them together in terms of their negative social consequences.[33] He concludes that contraception is a mixed blessing, the benefits of which 'come with a price', namely the tragic social consequences of 'a contraceptive mentality, in which children are simply seen as choices', and even risks, 'which, if not planned, may be an intrusion into our plans, hopes, and dreams'.[34] In a culture that treats sex, marriage, and children as little more than consumer options, he argues, Christians should seek to set themselves apart as people who see the workings of God in their lives and in the world.

Perhaps the most important contribution Christians can make in conversations about contraception is the deceptively simple description of children as *gifts*—gifts to the human community and not just to biological parents—rather than choices, risks, mistakes, burdens, or consumer goods. While this may seem obvious (at least to those who have not 'chosen' to be childless), the framing of children as gifts is a crucial corrective to the overwhelmingly economic, meritocratic, and utilitarian language that permeates discussions, even Christian discussions, of contraception and abortion. To speak solely in terms of cost-benefit analysis is to give in to the idea that children are either commodities for those who can afford them, or liabilities to be minimized. Terms like 'overpopulation', 'too many babies',[35] and 'excess children'[36] require that we ask: *which part* of the population, which babies, which children, represent the 'excess'? Which people are gifts, and who should never have been born? And who decides? Such rhetoric cannot help but lend support to hegemonic policies that discriminate on the basis of class, race, gender, or disability, and may defeat the very freedom of conscience they are trying to promote. Traci West puts her finger on this truth in her observation that fertility (often Black women's fertility) or 'the spreading of life', once seen as a good, can come to be seen as 'the spreading of pathology, of . . . a disease of catastrophic potential'.[37]

The relationship between grace and human will, between gift and decision, is not an either-or proposition.[38] With regard to parenting, the fact that Christians live their lives in response to the command of God means that they must inquire of God on (at least) whether or not they should try to have children, and if so, when and how many. The *methods by which they respond* to these commands are less important than their *free obedience* to their calling, which can take place only in a context of reproductive justice.[39]

Notes

1. An earlier version of this article appeared as 'The Gift of Contraception: Calvin, Barth, and a Lost Protestant Conversation,' *Journal of the Society of Christian Ethics* 27, no. 1 (2007): 225–49.
2. See Gloria H. Albrecht, 'Contraception and Abortion within Protestant Christianity', in *Sacred Rights: The Case for Contraception and Abortion in World Religions*, ed. Daniel C. Maguire (New York: Oxford University Press, 2003), 79-104; Gilbert Meilaender, 'Sweet Necessities: Food, Sex, and Saint Augustine', *Journal of Religious Ethics* 29, no. 1 (2001); 'Ru-486 Kills Again', *Christianity Today* (December 2003).
3. Supreme Court of the United States, *Burwell, Secretary of Health and Human Services, et al v. Hobby Lobby Stores Inc., et al* (June 30, 2014).
4. Calvin argues for three purposes of marriage: companionship (1.27, 2.18, 2.21); the blessing of procreation, in order to foster the creation of community among the human race (1.28); and the sober exercise of God-given sexuality (2.22). John Calvin, *Commentary on Genesis* (Albany, OR: AGES Software, 1998).
5. John Calvin, *Institutes of the Christian Religion*, ed. John T. McNeill, trans. Ford Lewis Battles (Philadelphia: Westminster, 1960), II.viii, 43. He cites 1 Cor. 7.9.
6. Ibid., 41.
7. Ibid., 43.
8. Ibid.
9. Barbara Pitkin, "'The Heritage of the Lord": Children in the Theology of John Calvin', in *The Child in Christian Thought*, ed. Marcia J. Bunge (Grand Rapids: Eerdmans, 2001), 189.
10. Calvin, *Genesis*, 72.
11. Ibid., 73. Emphasis added.
12. Calvin, *Genesis* (29.31), 521.
13. Ibid., (30.9-13), 528.
14. Ibid., 574 (Gen. 33.5).
15. Ibid., 627 (Gen. 38.8).
16. Ibid., 627.

17. Ibid., 627-8, (Gen. 38.10).
18. Ibid.
19. John Noonan, *Contraception* (Cambridge: Belknap Press of Harvard University Press, 1986), 353.
20. See Georgia Harkness, *John Calvin: The Man and His Ethics* (New York: Henry Holt, 1931), 206.
21. Calvin, *Institutes*, III.xix.2-8.
22. Alfred M. Rehwinkel, *Planned Parenthood and Birth Control in the Light of Christian Ethics* (St. Louis: Concordia, 1959), 39.
23. Ibid., 40.
24. Ibid., 41.
25. Albrecht, 83.
26. Rebecca Todd Peters, *Trust Women: A Progressive Christian Argument for Reproductive Justice* (Boston: Beacon, 2018).
27. If, When, How, 'What is Reproductive Justice?' (retrieved July 7, 2020): https://www.ifwhenhow.org/about/what-is-rj/.
28. E.g., Loretta Ross and Rickie Solinger, *Reproductive Justice: An Introduction* (Oakland: University of California Press, 2017).
29. W. Ross Blackburn, 'Sex and Fullness: A Rejoinder to Dennis Hollinger on Contraception', *Journal of the Evangelical Theological Society* (January 1, 2015), 117–130.
30. Focus on the Family, 'Use of Contraceptives in Marriage'.
31. Evan Lenow, 'Protestants and Contraception', *First Things* (January 2018), 16.
32. Ibid., 17.
33. Kenneth Magnuson, 'What Does Contraception Have to Do with Abortion? Evangelicals v. Augustine and *Roe v. Wade*', *The Southern Baptist Journal of Theology* 7, no. 2 (2003), 54.
34. Ibid., 64.
35. Daniel C. Maguire, *Sacred Choices: The Right to Contraception and Abortion in Ten World Religions* (Minneapolis: Fortress, 2001), 15.
36. Christine Gudorf, 'Contraception and Abortion in Roman Catholicism', in Maguire, *Sacred Rights*, 57.
37. Traci C. West, 'The Policing of Poor Black Women's Sexual Reproduction', in *God Forbid*, ed. Kathleen M. Sands (New York: Oxford, 2000).
38. Amy Laura Hall, 'Better Homes and Children', *Books & Culture* (2005): 20.
39. Loretta Ross and Rickie Solinger, *Reproductive Justice: An Introduction* (Oakland: University of California Press, 2017).

21

Reproduction in Bondage

Dorothy Roberts

Dorothy Roberts is a professor of law who has taught at Northwestern University and University of Pennsylvania. Her teaching and research focus on the intersections of criminal and family law, civil liberties, reproductive rights, gender, and critical race theory. The book from which this excerpt is taken is one of the most widely read accounts of the exploitation of Black women's bodies and offers an incisive analysis of how the reproductive realities of Black women today have deep and tangled roots in a system of chattel slavery.

The dual status of slave women as both producer and reproducer created tensions that perplexed their masters and injured their children. A slaveholder was caught in an impossible dilemma-how to maximize his immediate profits by extracting as much work as possible from his female slaves while at the same time protecting his long-term investment in the birth of a healthy child.[1] The two goals were simply incompatible. Pregnancy and infant care diminished time in the field or plantation house. Overwork hindered the chances of delivering a strong future workforce.

Bearing children who were their master's property only compounded the contradictions that scarred slave women's reproductive lives. It separated mothers from their children immediately upon conception. The division between mother and child did not exist for white women of that era. The notion that white mother and child were separable entities with contradictory interests was unthinkable, as was the idea of a white woman's work interfering

Dorothy E. Roberts, *Killing the Black Body: Race, Reproduction, and the Meaning of Liberty* (New York: Vintage, 1999).

with her maternal duties. Both violated the prevailing ideology of female domesticity that posited mothers as the natural caretakers for their children.

The First Maternal-Fetal Conflict

The conflict between mother and child was most dramatically expressed in the method of whipping pregnant slaves that was used throughout the South. Slaveholders forced women to lie face down in a depression in the ground while they were whipped. A former slave named Lizzie Williams recounted the beating of pregnant slave women on a Mississippi cotton plantation: ". . . Dey [the white folks] would dig a hole in de ground just big 'nuff fo' her stomach, make her lie face down an whip her on de back to keep from hurtin' de child."[2]

This description of the way in which pregnant slaves were beaten vividly illustrates the slaveowners' dual interest in Black women as both workers and childbearers. This was a procedure that enabled the master to protect the fetus while abusing the mother. It was the slave-holder's attempt to resolve the tough dilemma inherent in female bondage. As far as I can tell, the relationship between Black women and their unborn children created by slavery is the first example of maternal-fetal conflict in American history.

Feminists use the term "maternal-fetal conflict" to describe the way in which law, social policies, and medical practice sometimes treat a pregnant woman's interests in opposition to those of the fetus she is carrying. The miracles of modern medicine, for example, that empower doctors to treat the fetus apart from the pregnant woman make it possible to imagine a contradiction between the two. If the mother opposes the physician's suggestions for the care of the fetus, courts often treat the standoff as an adversarial relationship between the pregnant woman and her unborn child. Pitting the mother's interests against those of the fetus, in turn, gives the government a reason to restrict the autonomy of pregnant women.

Some feminist scholars have refuted the maternal-fetal conflict by pointing to its relatively recent origin. Ann Kaplan has explored, for example, how current representations of motherhood in popular materials, such as magazines, newspapers, television, and films, allow the public to imagine a separation between mother and fetus. She gives examples of the recent focus on the fetus as an independent subject- sensational pictures in *Life* magazine of fetal development during gestation or a *New York Times* enlarged image of the fetus floating in space, attached to an umbilical cord extending out of frame and disconnected from the mother's body, which is not seen.[3] . . .

But the beating of pregnant slaves reveals that slave masters created just such a conflict between Black women and their unborn children to support their own economic interests. The Black mother's act of bearing a child profited the system that subjugated her. Even without the benefit of perinatology and advanced medical technologies, slaveowners perceived the Black fetus as a separate entity that would produce future profits or that could be parceled out to another owner before its birth. The whipping of pregnant slaves is the most powerful image of maternal-fetal conflict I have ever come across in all my research on reproductive rights. It is the most striking metaphor I know for the evils of policies that seek to protect the fetus while disregarding the humanity of the mother. It is also a vivid symbol of the convergent oppressions inflicted on slave women: they were subjugated at once as Blacks and as females.

. . .

The Tigress Fights Back

Despite the absolute power the law granted them, whites failed to crush slave women's spirit. Black women struggled in numerous ways to resist slave masters' efforts to control their reproductive lives. They escaped from plantations, feigned illness, endured severe punishment, and fought back rather than submit to slave masters' sexual domination. Slave women's sexual resistance, note historians Darlene Hine and Kate Wittenstein, "attacked the very assumptions upon which the slave order was constructed and maintained."[4]

A common recollection of former slaves was the sight of a woman, often the reporter's mother, being beaten for defying her master's sexual advances. Clarinda received a terrible whipping when "she hit massa with de hoe 'cause he try to 'fere with her and she try stop him."[5] Minnie Folkes remembered watching her mother being flogged by her overseer when she refused "to be wife to dis man." Decades after her emancipation, Minnie repeated with pride her mother's teaching: "Don't let nobody bother yo principle; 'cause dat wuz all yo' had."[6]

A cook named Sukie Abbot was particularly successful at putting an end to her master's harassment. When Mr. Abbott accosted her in the kitchen while she was making soap, Sukie struck back by pushing him, rear end first, into a pot of boiling lye. "He got up holdin' his hindparts an' ran from de kitchen," another Abbott slave recounted, "nor darin' to yell, 'cause he didn't want Miss Sarah Ann [his wife] to know 'bout it.'"[7] Mr. Abbott sold Sukie at the slave market a few days later, but he reportedly "never did bother slave gals no mo." No doubt there were, as well, many cases of slave women poisoning their masters in retaliation for sexual molestation.

. . .

Refusing to Bear Children for the Slave Master

Even more controversial is slave women's rebellion against their role as reproducer. There is evidence that some female slaves refused to bear children by abstaining from sexual intercourse or by using contraceptives and abortives. It is impossible to tell how much of female infertility and miscarriage was self-induced and how much resulted from slaves' harsh living conditions. Healthy pregnancy was hardly possible with the strenuous labor, poor nutrition, and cruel punishment bonded women endured. Still, whites suspected that their slaves took deliberate steps to prevent or terminate pregnancy.

Southern medical journals occasionally documented the abortion practices that planters found so disturbing. Dr. E. M. Pendleton from Hancock County, Georgia, wrote in 1849 that his patients who were slaves had many more abortions and miscarriages than white women.[8] Although he attributed some prenatal deaths to the stress of hard work, he confirmed planters' frequent complaint that "the blacks are possessed of a secret by which they destroy the fetus at an early stage of gestation." John T. Morgan, a physician from Murfreesboro, Tennessee, reported similar findings in a paper read before the Rutherford County Medical Society in 1860. Morgan recorded a number of techniques slave women employed "to effect an abortion or to derange menstruation": they used "medicine," "violent exercise," and "external and internal manipulation"; one stuffed "a roll of rags about two or three inches long and as hard as a stick" into her vagina. But Morgan found that slave women preferred herbal remedies to these "mechanical" means of abortion, including "the infusion or decoction of tansy, rue, roots and seed, of the cotton plant, pennyroyal, cedar gum, and camphor, either in gum or spirits"—techniques slaves probably brought with them from Africa.[9] Midwives conspired with pregnant slaves to induce and cover up abortions.[10] Despite these birth control practices, slave women were less successful at avoiding pregnancy than white women, whose birth rate declined throughout the nineteenth century.[11]

Some male slaves also refused to father children destined to become their masters' property. J. W Loguen vowed he would never marry until he was free, for "slavery shall never own a wife or child of mine."[12] Henry Bibb similarly declared, "if there was any one act of my life while a slave that I have to lament over, it is that of being a father and a husband of slaves." Bibb tried to flee to freedom with his wife, Malinda, and young daughter, but the party was captured by a patrol. When Bibb later succeeded in escaping without his family, he determined that the daughter he left behind "was the first and shall be the last slave that ever I will father for chains and slavery on this earth."[13] Bibb relinquished his procreative role by eluding the bonds of slavery altogether, a solution far easier for men than women to accomplish.

Infanticide was the most extreme form of slave mothers' resistance. Some enslaved women killed their newborns to keep them from living as chattel. In 1831, a Missouri slave named Jane was convicted of murdering her infant child, Angeline.[14] Jane was charged with "knowingly, willfully, feloniously and of her malice aforethought" preparing a "certain deadly poison" and giving it to Angeline to drink on December 8 and 9. The indictment further alleged that on December 11, so "that she might more speedily kill and murder said Angeline," she wrapped the baby in bedclothes and then "choked, suffocated and smothered" her.

Historian and former federal judge A. Leon Higginbotham, Jr., asks two important questions about this case.[15] First, he questions Missouri's purpose in convicting Jane for murder:

> Did the state prosecute because it cared about the dignity and life of a child born into lifetime slavery with the concomitant disadvantages of Missouri's law? Or did the state prosecute because Jane's master was denied the profit that he would have someday earned from the sale or exploitation of Angeline?

Slavery's dehumanization of Black children leaves little doubt that the courts condemned slave mothers in order to protect whites' financial stake in the children, not out of respect for the children themselves.

Second, Judge Higginbotham questions Jane's purpose in killing her daughter: "Perhaps the mother felt that the taking of her daughter's life was an act of mercy compared to the cruelty she might confront in Missouri's jurisprudence." Jane's motivation may have been to protect her child from slavery's brutality—to spare, rather than harm, her child. Death may have appeared a more humane fate for her baby than the living hell of slavery.

Judge Higginbotham does not ask a more troubling question: What if Jane sacrificed her child as an act of defiance, one small step in bringing about slavery's demise? Although compelled to do so, slave mothers helped to sustain slavery by producing human chattel for their masters. By bearing children, female slaves perpetuated the very system that enslaved them and their offspring. Perhaps Jane killed Angeline because she refused to take any part in that horrible institution. This possibility raises a difficult moral question: When is taking a life justified by a noble social end? But before reaching that issue we are faced with factual questions we cannot answer without more information about slave women's reasoning.

The present state of research leaves too many uncertainties for us to discern a definitive picture of female slave resistance against reproduction.[16] We do not know, for example, whether slave mothers practiced abortion and infanticide selectively, terminating pregnancies or the lives of children that resulted from rape or forced mating. Moreover, while infanticide spared children from the horrors of slavery, it was not a desirable strategy for overthrowing the institution. Slave mothers must have realized that their sporadic practice of infanticide would have little effect and its widespread practice would annihilate the race. The low suicide rate of slaves-only one-third that of whites - suggests that they did not commonly view death as a good way to escape from slavery's horrors.[17] It seems more likely that some slave mothers acted in desperation to protect their children, not to sacrifice them in protest against slavery.

Notes

1. [Jacqueline Jones, *Labor of Love, Labor of Sorrow: Black Women, Work, and the Family from Slavery to the Present* (New York: Vintage, 1986)], p. 19.
2. Michael P. Johnson "Smothered Slave Infants: Were Slave Mothers at Fault?" *Journal of Southern History* 47 (1981), pp. 493, 513.
3. E. Ann Kaplan, "Sex, Work, and Motherhood: The Impossible Triangle," *Journal of Sex Research* 27 (1990), pp. 409, 417.

4. Darlene Hine and Kate Wittenstein, "Female Slave Resistance: The Economics of Sex," in Filomina C. Steady, ed., *The Black Woman Cross-Culturally* (Rochester, Vt.: Schenkman, 1981), pp. 289, 296. See also Stephanie Shaw, "Mothering Under Slavery in the Antebellum South," in Evelyn Nakano Glenn, Grace Chang, and Linda Rennie Forcey, eds., *Mothering: Ideology, Experience, and Agency* (New York: Routledge, 1993), p. 237.

5. [Herbert Gutman, *The Black Family in Slavery and Freedom, 1750-1925* (New York: Pantheon)], p. 80.

6. Brenda E. Stevenson, "Gender Convention, Ideals, and Identity Among Antebellum Virginia Slave Women," in [David Berry Gaspar and Darlene Clark Hine, eds., *More Than Chattel: Black Women and Slavery in the Americas* (Bloomington: Indiana University Press, 1996)], pp. 169, 171.

7. Charles L. Purdue, Thomas E. Barden, and Robert K. Phillips, eds. *Weevils in the Wheat: Interviews with Virginia Ex-Slaves* (Charlottesville: University Press of Virginia, 1976), pp. 48-49.

8. Gutman, *Black Family in Slavery and Freedom*, p. 80.

9. Ibid., p. 81.

10. [Deborah Gray White, *Ar'n't I a Woman? Female Slaves in the Plantation South* (New York: Norton, 1985),] pp. 125-26.

11. Ibid., p. 87.

12. Quoted in ibid., p. 147.

13. Henry Bibb, *Narrative of the Life and Adventures of Henry Bibb, an American Slave*, 3rd ed. (Miami: Mnemosyne, 1969 [1850]), p. 44.

14. *Jane (a slave) v. The State*, 3 Mo. 45 (1831).

15. A. Leon Higginbotham, Jr., "Race, Sex, Education, and Missouri Jurisprudence: *Shelley v. Kramer* in Historical Perspective," *Washington University Law Quarterly* 67 (1989), pp. 673, 694-95.

16. Elizabeth Fox-Genovese, "Strategies and Forms of Resistance: Focus on Slave Women in the United States," in Gary Y. Okihiro, ed., *In Resistance: Studies in African, Caribbean, and Afro-American History* (Amherst: University of Massachusetts Press, 1986), pp. 143, 158.

17. [Robert William Fogel and Stanley L. Engerman, *Time on the Cross: The Economics of American Negro Slavery* (Boston: Little, Brown, 1974)], pp. 124-25.

22

The AMA's Crusade against Abortion

Paul Saurette and Kelly Gordon

Paul Saurette and Kelly Gordon are both Canadian professors of political science. Their book analyzes over 200 years of North American history related to abortion debates, legislation, criminalization and decriminalization, and the activism on both sides of the issue. We chose their discussion of a very particular moment in nineteenth-century US history when the (white male) physicians of the nascent American Medical Association pursued the criminalization of abortion as a means to promote their medical authority and social status in the midst of changing social norms about medical care. Under the banner of Victorian morality, a small group of physicians led the charge that transformed a broad acceptance of abortion as a private means of birth control into a public rejection and criminalization of abortion.

By the mid-1800s, a number of elements were changing in American society that would have consequences for the practice of abortion. Abortion became one of the first medical specializations, with practitioners increasingly advertising their services publicly. The press was also beginning to demonstrate a new willingness to cover sensationalist trials involving allegedly botched abortions and professional abortion providers (Mohr 1978, 46). Combined, these two factors contributed to a growing social awareness of the reality of the widespread practice of abortion in the US, ultimately

Source: Paul Saurette and Kelly Gordon, *The Changing Voice of the Anti-abortion Movement: The Rise of "Pro-woman" Rhetoric in Canada and the United States* (Toronto: University of Toronto Press, 2016).

leading to the emergence of new critical questions about the legality and morality of abortion. By the mid-1800s, abortion was increasingly viewed by elites and the broader public as an issue worthy of their political and professional concern (ibid.).

Other social realities would also help transform the practice of abortion into a moralized and politicized issue during this period. The spread of much more rigid Victorian societal norms, including those relating to sexuality, meant that women who attempted to procure an abortion were increasingly portrayed as unmarried women of loose morals or victims of male lust (Reed 1978, 25). This portrait was far from accurate: aspiring upwardly mobile couples were some of the most frequent users of various forms of contraception and family planning. Regardless, this current of Victorian moralization fused with other ideological trends (particularly moral panics about the supposed falling birthrates of native-born white Americans and threats from "fast-reproducing" immigrants) and led to the emergence for the first time of an explicit debate around abortion. Increasingly, elites framed the issue of abortion in relationship to motherhood, asking what proper women should do to live up to their place as "true wives" and fulfil their maternal duties in the name of their gender, nation, and race (Reagan 1996, 12).

As is so often the case in politics, however, it was only once an influential and politically mobilized group began pushing for systematic change that abortion became a contested political and moral issue in the US. In what is an excellent historical lesson in the profound effects that a determined interest group with social and intellectual capital can have, the politicization and criminalization of abortion in the US is inextricably linked to the efforts of a small group of physicians and the self-interest and ambition of the newly formed American Medical Association (AMA) (Reed 1978, 27; Rose 2008).

Founded in 1847, the AMA sought to represent certain health care providers, consolidating them under its membership while excluding others (including midwives) (Haussman, 2005, 25). While the majority of physicians involved in the AMA did not oppose abortion, a small but very vocal group organized within the association to make the prohibition of this practice a key issue on the AMA's agenda (25). The primary mover behind this group was Dr. Horatio Storer, who was a recently graduated physician when he founded the Physicians' Crusade Against Abortion in 1857. Until this time, male physicians had had very little role in women's health. Until the mid-1800s, gynaecological practice was generally the providence of women, especially female midwives (as female physicians were rare) (Acevedo 1979, 162). By the mid-1800s, however, male physicians and the AMA were increasingly expanding into these areas. In this context, Storer was a pioneer and innovator in obstetrics and gynaecology in the formal field of medicine, teaching one of the first courses on women's diseases to be offered as distinct from midwifery in a university.

In 1857, Storer petitioned the AMA to create a Committee on Criminal Abortion. The AMA agreed, made him chairman, and gave the committee the mandate to prepare a report on the issue. Storer led this process, publishing no fewer than nine articles on abortion for physicians in 1859, and authoring the committee's *Report on Criminal Abortion*. Interestingly, Storer's texts did not use the religious and highly moralized language that would eventually come to characterize anti-abortion activism in the latter half of the twentieth century. Instead, he focused on redefining, on the basis of a scientific perspective, the pre-quickening period as fundamentally the same as post-quickening and post-birth. . . .

Storer's report to the AMA concluded that "while physicians have long been united in condemning the act of procuring an abortion, at every period of gestation, except as necessary for preserving the life of either the mother or child, it has become the duty of the association, in the view of the prevalence and increasing frequency of the crime, publicly to enter into an earnest and solemn protest against such unwarranted destruction of human life" (quoted in Rose 2008, 10). The report went much further, encouraging the AMA to formally petition governors and legislatures of states, as well as the president and Congress, to revise statutory and common law to ensure that they prohibited abortion, although usually with one exception: that physicians alone had the right to induce abortions when they deemed them necessary (Tatalovich 1997, 37; Reagan 1996, 13). In 1859, the AMA unanimously adopted the report, and this remained its official policy on abortion until 1967.

While this early history might appear to suggest that abortion was already a profoundly polarized moral and political issue in the US over 150 years ago, historians have instead suggested that the main reasons why this report gained wide support within the AMA were not particularly ideological, political, or even medical. Rather, they suggest that most doctors supported this move for reasons of professional self-interest. By using abortion as a wedge issue and publicly opposing it, the AMA was able to portray itself as morally and professionally superior to the practice of midwifery; this allowed the AMA to undercut the influence of midwives over the crucial realm of female reproductive health (Haussman 2005, 24; Rose 2008, 10). Physicians were sometimes quite explicit about their financial motives in this struggle

(Sanger 2004; Mohr 1978). In 1875, for example, the Southern Michigan Medical Society was reminded by one of its members that "regular physicians are still losing patients, even long-time patients, to competitors willing to 'prevent an increase in their families' by performing abortions" (quoted in Sanger 2004, 26). As historian Leslie Reagan has shown, the AMA's move against abortion also benefited its members in other important ways - for example, it increased their overall intellectual and social capital by elevating the scientific authority of doctors above the moral authority of religious leaders (Reagan 1996, 13). The push to criminalize birth control and abortion also was largely successful at eliminating midwives as legitimate medical practitioners. Over the latter half of the nineteenth century, physicians thus effectively took control of the domains of reproduction and women's health, including moving childbirth from midwife-supervised home births to (male) physician-supervised hospital births (Sanger 2004, 26).

Not surprisingly, the AMA's official discursive justifications for opposing abortion rarely made reference to the lucrative and self-interested underpinnings of its anti-abortion position. Instead, its public argumentation was grounded in scientific, medical, and (sometimes) moral rationales. In some ways, these early AMA arguments and efforts seem consistent with the "traditional image" of the anti-abortion movement. Storer and his colleagues were a group of white men who claimed to warrant control over women's bodies and reproductive lives on the basis of a variety of gendered and moralized norms. For example, using what would become a dominant anti-abortion strategy, Storer and the AMA's public discourse opposed abortion on the basis that it was analogous with murder. Physicians and religious leaders increasingly argued in tandem that there should be no difference in the treatment of a pre- or post-quickening fetus and that abortion should not be legally permissible except for therapeutic reasons (Sanger 2004, 26). With this shift, then, we can see the emergence of the early stages of the "fetal personhood" argument that would come to dominate the abortion debate in the 1970s and 1980s.

. . .

Criminalizing Abortion, 1840-1900

Although the AMA was not the only actor pushing for the criminalization of abortion, its discourse had a substantial effect on framing the debate over abortion in the US for the next sixty years. The group also played a very active role in inspiring, aiding, and intensifying legislative efforts to enact further anti-abortion laws. And as the century progressed, federal and state governments increasingly began to enact laws in line with the AMA's views on the illegality of abortion and the immorality of contraception.

In fact, in the mid- to late 1800s, the US witnessed an explosion of new and far more restrictive legislation that sought to fully outlaw abortion at the state level. According to historian James C. Mohr, the campaign against abortion reached its climax between 1860 and 1880, with a surge of at least forty anti-abortion statutes being enacted into law. In the period between 1866 and 1877 alone, over thirty anti-abortion pieces of legislation came into law, many completely outlawing the practice. A total of thirteen state jurisdictions entirely banned abortion for the first time, while twenty-one others revisited and further restricted their existing statutes regarding the permissibility of abortion (Mohr 1978, 200). These new and updated laws "regarded abortion in an entirely different light from common laws and statutes regulating abortifacients" that had existed in the first half of the century (Reagan 1996, 13). In particular, most of these new laws included two innovations: first, they eliminated the concept of quickening altogether, prohibiting abortion at any point of pregnancy; and second, many also introduced punishments for women who had abortions, something unheard of in the early part of the century (Reagan 1996, 10).

. . .

While the years between 1840 and 1880 "produced the most important burst of anti-abortion legislation in the nation's history," one exception continued to exist in many of the new anti-abortion laws (Mohr 1978, 200). Most of the legislation included a number of provisions that allowed for very restricted abortion access to protect the life and/or health of the woman, usually only in cases where it was authorized by more than one doctor. The inclusion of these life and health exceptions would prove to be notable for two reasons. First, the fact that physicians had both "won the criminalization of abortion and retained to themselves alone the right to induce abortion when they determined it necessary" underlines the degree to which control over women's reproductive decisions had been captured by the medical community (Reagan 1996, 13). Second, and even more importantly politically, although no one could have predicted it at the time, these exceptions created a legal context that would eventually allow doctors who were sympathetic to legalizing abortion to push for the reform and liberalization of abortion laws in the 1960s.

Although this time period was dominated by the creation of stringent anti-abortion legislation, many historians suggest that the practice and regulation of abortion remained far more complicated than it might appear. Leslie Reagan, for instance, contends that, even during this period, "the meaning of the law and the legality and illegality of abortion changed over time . . . Because laws governing abortion did not precisely define what was criminal and what was not, this had to be worked out in practice, in policing, and in the courts" (Reagan 1996, 4-5). Reagan also has shown that the role of physicians in the criminalization of abortion was also more complicated than it might appear, given the aggressive role of the AMA (3). On the one hand it would have been nearly impossible to enforce anti-abortion laws without the cooperation of physicians who, in many instances, acted as "an arm of the state" (3). On the other hand, many physicians displayed great sympathy for women who, for a wide variety of reasons, found themselves facing unplanned pregnancy. In this regard, "sympathy for their female patients drew physicians into the world of abortion in spite of legal and professional prohibitions" (3).

While there is no question that the AMA's influence and public discourse was a major factor in the growth of anti-abortion legislation, it is important to note that this surge was not simply the result of the medical profession's position against abortion. Nor was it the accomplishment of a unified, organized, and politically embedded anti-abortion movement. In reality, the campaign to ban abortion in the nineteenth century included many different groups, and anti-abortion discourse was itself quite diverse. Given the AMA's influence, its "scientific" perspectives on fetal life and arguments about women's health and well-being had an enormous impact on public opposition to abortion and defined the anti-abortion position in significant ways. However, historians insist that the move to ban "abortion was not solely based on a respect for unborn life at its earliest stages" but was rather part of a larger campaign that viewed women's reproductive freedom as "a threat to the power structure of nineteenth century America" on demographic, racial, and moral grounds (Sanger 2004, 25).

The AMAs' medicalized anti-abortion discourse was joined in the public sphere by a number of other discourses. There was, for example, highly nativist discourse that suggested that Protestant women's relatively easy access to birth control and abortion "threatened Anglo-Saxon Protestants who wanted to maintain control over American society" (Sanger 2004, 25). Fearing that, given the influx of Irish Catholic immigrants (largely between the years 1820 and 1880), native-born Protestants would soon be outnumbered—and outvoted—nativists grounded their opposition to abortion in the larger "goal to preserve the primacy of the Anglo-Saxon, Protestant religion, culture, and political power" in America (27). This argument was further buttressed by a distinctly racialized discourse, which represented an America under a larger threat from "non-white" immigrants. This heavily racialized discourse largely revolved around the falling birthrates of native-born white Americans and stoked racial and ethnic fears as an impetus to control women's reproduction. As one physician argued in 1874, "the annual destruction of fetuses has become so truly appalling among native[-born white] American women that the Puritanic blood of '76 will be but sparingly represented in the approaching centenary" (27).

References

Acevedo, Zoila. 1979. "Abortion in Early America." Women and Health 4 (2): 159–67.

Haussman, Melissa. 2005. *Abortion Politics in North America* Boulder, CO: Lynne Rienner Publishers.

Mohr, James C., 1978. *Abortion in America: The Origin and Evolution of National Policy, 1800–1900.* New York: Columbia University Press.

Reagan, Leslie, 1996. *When Abortion Was a Crime.* Berkeley: University of California Press.

Reed, James. 1978. *From Private Vice to Public Virtue: The Birth Control Movement and American Society Since 1830.* New York: Basic Books.

Rose, Melody. 2008. *Abortion: A Documentary and Reference Guide: A Documentary and Reference Guide.* Westport, CT: Greenwood.

Sanger, Alexander. 2004. *Beyond Choice: Reproductive Freedom in the 21st Century.* Cambridge: Perseus Books.

Tatalovich, Raymond. 1997. The Politics of Abortion in the United States and Canada. New York: M.W. Sharpe.

23

Reproductive Justice and Eugenics

Loretta J. Ross

One of the original twelve founders of the reproductive justice movement, Loretta Ross has been a leader in human rights and antiracism activism and research for decades. She co-founded the SisterSong Women of Color Reproductive Justice Collective in 1997 and is the author of numerous essays and a co-author and co-editor of several books on reproductive justice. We selected this excerpt for its attention to the ugly history of eugenics in the United States, which was a widespread and pervasive ideological movement in the early twentieth century that had a profound impact on the bodily autonomy and reproductive health of thousands of people. Ross highlights the resistance work of African American women and addresses the complexity of the work of Margaret Sanger in the Black community.

Reproductive justice is a critical theoretical framework promoted by activist women of color to more effectively describe how the intersections of gender, race, class, ability, nationality, and sexuality influence reproductive politics in the United States to produce a complex matrix of reproductive oppression. This theoretical framework is based on discussions among activist women of color about sex, reproduction, and sexuality, originating with African American women in 1994. Oppression is defined as an "unjust situation where, systemically and over a long period of time, one group denies another group access to the resources of society."[1] As an expression of collective social trauma,

Source: Loretta J. Ross, "Trust Black Women: Reproductive Justice and Eugenics," in *Radical Reproductive Justice: Foundations, Theory, Practice, Critique*, ed. Loretta J. Ross, Erika Derkas, Whitney Peoples, Lynn Roberts, and Pamela Bridgewater (New York: Feminist, 2017), 58–85.

reproductive oppression is experienced by women of color as the exploitation of our bodies, sexuality, labor, and fertility in order to achieve social and economic control of our communities and in violation of our human rights. A new theoretical framework for women of color was necessary because earlier analyses paid inadequate attention to our physical and emotional realities, and failed to analyze and criticize the immortalized eugenics ideologies and politics by which it is determined that some bodies matter and others do not.

In short, RJ has three core values: the right to have a child, to not have a child, and to parent the children we have in safe and healthy environments. As a departure from the privacy-based pro-choice framework, RJ activists recognize that in addition to supporting the pro-choice movement's goals of protecting abortion rights and securing safe and effective contraceptives, as people of color subjected to continuous population control strategies, we must fight equally as hard for the right to have children and to parent the children we have.

As people of color, we struggle for the recognition of our humanity against white prejudices not only through politics and economics but also through science, technology, and biomedicine. bell hooks posits that "the very concept of white supremacy relies on the perpetuation of a white race. It is in the interest of continued white racist domination of the planet for white patriarchy to maintain control over all women's bodies."[2] Racial and sociopolitical categories are "reproduced and reconstituted through techno-scientific practices that act on, with, and against human bodies."[3] These are additional sites of struggle around blood politics and the axes of domination that the predominantly white pro-choice movement either undervalues or understates. However, as women of color, our self-determination engages multiple dimensions of contention based on the intersections of race, gender, class, immigration, sexual orientation, gender identity, and religion. RJ asserts the human right to make personal decisions about one's life, and calls on the international legal regime and the norms and standards of the global human rights movement in our multi-issue, intersectionalized organizing strategy.

. . .

Eugenics and African American Women

The fight against white supremacy and patriarchal state violence never ends, as the ongoing struggle against eugenics demonstrates. Eugenics is also popularly known as population control, and includes any number of nonbiological measures. To understand the impact of eugenics and white supremacy in reproductive politics, it is necessary to understand the ubiquitous nature of internalized racism and its dependence on misogyny that is disturbingly normalized in US society. In the words of Ruha Benjamin:

> Racism is . . . not simply ignorance, or a *not* knowing. It is also (at the very least) a logic, a reason, a justification, and a way of knowing the world and other human beings that is always violent, routinely deadly, and brilliantly codified in the very thing we would turn to for justice. Until we come to grips with the *reasonableness* of racism, we will continue to look for it on the bloody floors of Charleston churches and the dashboard cameras of Texas highways, and overlook it in the smart sounding logics of textbooks, policy statements, court rulings, science journals, and cutting edge technologies.[4]

Eugenics as a philosophy and practice depends on the intersections of racism, sexism, and nativism. Eugenics had its origins in manipulating human reproduction, but its philosophical tentacles spread throughout a society that was already deeply stratified by race, gender, region, class, and religion. Proponents of eugenics sought to affect nearly every area of human endeavor by assigning values to different births, engineering society toward perfectability, and designating the benefits of society based on elite racial and class preferences.

Eugenics was a formal movement launched in the early part of the twentieth century by people who believed they could improve humanity through "scientifically" selective breeding. The term "eugenics" was coined by British scientist Francis Galton in 1883, to mean "nobility of birth;' at a time of British class upheaval due to industrialization. The middle and upper classes were determined to prevent revolutionary tendencies among the poor. Because elites benefited from the rapid industrialization, they did not perceive poverty and work dehumanization as an issue of social inequality, but rather one of heredity.

When elites migrated this ideology to the United States, they borrowed a "scientific" rationale for imposing limits on the births among populations they deemed undesirable, while they particularly encouraged white, middle- and upper-class Protestants to have more children. As part of a Victorian backlash against the growing sexual freedom of white women, religious and political leaders denounced birth control. The federal government had passed the Comstock Law in 1873 prohibiting the distribution of birth control information and devices, aiming to increase birth rates among white people. During this same period in the early twentieth century, thousands of African Americans fled the Jim Crow South and migrated to the North. These fast-paced demographic changes alarmed many nativist whites, who questioned birth control or sterilization for themselves but approved of it as a strategy of negative eugenics to contain people of color and immigrants. In contrast, northern European immigrants and their descendants were being encouraged to breed, as part of the positive eugenics ideology. Rapid population growth was one factor that helped overrun Native Americans, settle the West, and fulfill the mythical ideology of Manifest Destiny. The continuing sterilization of Indigenous women was a strategy of "reproductive disappearance."

It was in this context that Margaret Sanger began to campaign for women's birth control in the early 1900s. Sanger was a public health nurse who witnessed the tragic number of deaths in New York of women who sought to control their fertility using dangerous self-induced abortions or contraception techniques. She embarked on a personal and political crusade against maternal mortality to repeal the 1873 Comstock Law. To challenge the laws that unfairly punished sexually active women, she imported birth control information and devices from Europe and made it her personal mission to distribute them to poor white women. She opposed abortion, which at the time was unsafe due to prohibition and technological limitations, and believed contraception was the only practical way to decrease women's abortion mortality rates. She was arrested several times, but never desisted in her campaign to ensure that women could access birth control.

Sanger, eager to win the support of elites for her campaign, was endorsed by several leading eugenicists and permitted some of their articles to be printed in her magazine, *Birth Control Review*. The magazine contained a strange admixture of feminism, racism, and ableism. She has been accused by antiabortionists of promoting racialized genocide against African Americans, although she eventually repudiated the eugenics philosophy, largely because many eugenicists only supported birth control through a racist lens. Despite her distaste for eugenics, particularly after its association with Nazi philosophy, the damage to Sanger's reputation had already been done.

By also claiming genetic differences among races of people, eugenicists reinforced the justification for white supremacy as a politicized and publicly supported project. Indiana became the first state in 1907 to pass the first eugenically motivated sterilization law to promote the targeting of "confirmed criminals, idiots, imbeciles, and rapists." North Carolina was particularly aggressive in sterilizing African Americans: 65 percent of the procedures were performed on black women. By the 1970s, nearly one-quarter of Native American women in the United States had been sterilized.[5]

It was not ignorance about the humanity of poor people or nonwhite people that motivated these laws; it was indifference. Using the pseudoscience of eugenics, vulnerable people were targeted because of their race, mental and physical disabilities, economic status, ethnicity, immigration status, education level, religion, or age. It is important to point out that poor white women, particularly in Appalachia, were also targeted for forced sterilizations. Thus, eugenics was a race- and a class-based ideology of population control. Anyone whose freedom was impaired—those in prisons, jails, detention centers, and mental health institutions; Native American's undergoing forced assimilation at boarding schools were especially vulnerable to this selective, "reasonable" state sanctioned reproductive oppression.

People with disabilities were particularly singled out. Eugenics was as useful in defining disability as it was in defining race. People with disabilities were deemed inherently unfit to have and raise children, proving that parental capability was defined by social markers of disadvantage, not actual physical or biological characteristics. The definition of who should be sterilized expanded to include people who were homeless, alcoholics, or simply poor.

To promote the reproduction of self-defined "racially superior" people, eugenics proponents argued for both "positive methods," such as tax incentives and education for the desirable types, and "negative methods," such as sterilization, involuntary confinement, and immigration restrictions for the undesirables. The United States became the first nation in the world to permit mass sterilization as part of an effort to "purify the race." By the mid-1930s about twenty thousand Americans had been sterilized against their will, and most states had passed eugenics laws. Black people, Catholics, poor white women, and others such as the mentally or physically disabled were singled out for planned population reductions through both government and privately financed means.

The fiercest supporters of eugenics were not only the rabid haters in the Ku Klux Klan of the late nineteenth century, who practiced extra-legal executions like lynching but also mainstream white Americans troubled by the effects of urbanization, industrialization, and immigration-so that violent terrorism was enabled and shielded by public policies. After the Civil War, African Americans enjoyed a very brief period in which they could vote, participate in politics, acquire the land of former slave owners, start businesses, and use public accommodations. This aroused racist white panic throughout the country. Eugenics codified white American frenzy against African American progress during and after Reconstruction.

By the 1920s, more than five million white people openly belonged to the Ku Klux Klan, including several US Congressmen. President Theodore Roosevelt made dire predictions about "race suicide" in 1902 if the country continued to tolerate rising birth rates among black Americans and burgeoning "non-Yankee" immigration. Eugenics was endorsed by President Calvin Coolidge who said in 1924, "America must be kept American. Biological laws show . . . that Nordics deteriorate when mixed with other races."[6] Notably, state laws against miscegenation (or race mixing) increased after the Civil War until they were ruled unconstitutional by the Supreme Court in 1967.

In fact, the birth rate of African Americans was slower than that of whites after the Civil War and until World War II, but it suited the purposes of the white racial alarmists to distort the facts. At the height of the eugenics movement, thirty-two states enforced compulsory sterilizations through both legal and extralegal means. The United States was the first country in the world to undertake concerted compulsory sterilization programs, and inspired the Nazis during their genocidal reign of World War II.

. . .

African American Women Resist Eugenics

Despite the dominance of eugenics ideology and practices, black women of the early twentieth century wanted to determine the number and spacing of their children. At the same time, they resisted government and privately funded antinatalist (antibirth) population control campaigns. This dual value system seeded an expanded vision of reproductive justice that guides the work of women of color today.

Early African American activists understood the complex nature of black womanhood and believed that fertility control was an essential part of the movement to rise from the brutal legacy of slavery. Sanger, through her passion to establish birth control clinics, touched a responsive chord in African American women, many of whom were middle-class. In 1918 the Women's Political Association of Harlem announced a scheduled lecture on birth control, Alice Dunbar Nelson endorsed birth control in an article in 1927, and Adam Clayton Powell Jr. spoke at public meetings sponsored by women's groups in support of family planning. The NAACP openly supported family planning. The "racial uplift" view of the times was that African Americans needed to control family size to integrate into the American mainstream through education and jobs.

The National Urban League asked Sanger to open a family planning clinic in the Columbus Hill section of the Bronx. In 1930 Sanger opened a clinic in Harlem that sought to enlist support for contraceptive use and to bring the benefits of family planning to women who were denied access to their city's health and social services. Staffed by a black physician and black social worker, the clinic was endorsed by the *Amsterdam News* (a powerful local newspaper), the Abyssinian Baptist Church, the Urban League, and the black community's elder statesman, W E. B. DuBois.

Beginning in 1939, DuBois also served on the advisory council for Sanger's "Negro Project," which was a "unique experiment in race-building and humanitarian service to a race subjected to discrimination, hardship, and segregation"[7] designed to serve African Americans in the rural South. Sanger responded to requests by black women to offer services in the Deep South, which was most hostile to birth control, and where white people often discriminated against black women when they tried to obtain reproductive health services. Southern white men feared birth control access by white women, although they mostly masked their concerns in religious moralities rather than open racial animosity.

Other leaders of the African American community involved in the project included Mary McLeod Bethune, founder of the National Council of Negro Women, and Adam Clayton Powell Jr., pastor of the Abyssinian Baptist Church in Harlem. The Negro Project was also endorsed by prominent white Americans involved in social justice efforts at that time, including Eleanor Roosevelt, the most visible and compassionate supporter of racial equality in her era, and the medical philanthropists Albert and Mary Lasker, whose financial support made the pilot project possible. Funding for the project dried up in 1942 after Sanger clashed with the white men hired to run it. She had demanded African American doctors and nurses staff the project, but was denied.

Despite early missteps that resulted in her association with the eugenics movement, Sanger became a passionate opponent of racism. Sanger predicted in 1942 that the "Negro question" would be foremost on the country's domestic agenda after World War II. Her accomplishments on behalf of the African American community were unchallengeable during her lifetime and remain so today.

Charges of reproductive racism against Sanger are most often made by anti-choice activists unfamiliar with the history of black women's views on managing their fertility. They don't believe in the agency of black women and don't understand Sanger's collegial relationship with black leaders. Black women have never been dupes, but fierce defenders of our freedoms and our bodies, such as Fannie Lou Hamer calling sterilizations "Mississippi appendectomies" to protest sterilization abuse. The tangled fabric of lies and manipulation woven by anti-choice activists around the issues of class, race, and family planning continues to be embroidered today by the antiabortion movement using strategies like the antiabortion billboards, more than a century after the family planning movement began.

Notes

1. Patricia Hill Collins, *Black Feminist Thought: Knowledge, Consciousness, and the Politics of Empowerment* (New York: Routledge, 2000), 4.
2. bell hooks, *Feminist Theory: From Margin to Center* (Boston: South End Press, 1984), 52.
3. Ruha Benjamin, "Catching Our Breath: Critical Race STS and the Carceral Imagination," *Engaging Science, Technology, and Society* 2 (2016), 153.
4. Ibid., 148–9.
5. Kathryn Krase, "History of Forced Sterilization and Current US Abuses," Our Bodies Ourselves, October 1, 2014.
6. Alan L. Stoskopf, "Confronting the Forgotten History of the American Eugenics Movement," *Facing History and Ourselves News*, 1995, 7.
7. Ellen Chesler, *Woman of Valor: Margaret Sanger and the Birth Control Movement in America* (New York: Simon & Schuster), 1992, 388.

24

The Continuing Struggle against Genocide:

Indigenous Women's Reproductive Rights

D. Marie Ralstin-Lewis

D. Marie Ralstin-Lewis has an MS in sociology from the University of Oregon, where her research focused on race, ethnicity, disability, ethnic identity, social stratification, and reproductive technologies. She currently works as a special education teacher in Salem, Oregon, and is active in the district's Native education program. This essay examines historical, governmental, and legal documents that display the eugenicist tactics used against Native communities. "Genocide," Ralstin-Lewis argues, is an appropriate term to describe the results of this history, including sterilization campaigns; the imposition of Euro-American Christian views of gender, sexual mores, and family structures; and the seizing of Indian lands.

Women have always been the backbone and keepers of life of the indigenous nations of North America. Most precontact indigenous civilizations functioned as matriarchies, and women of those cultures did not espouse subordination to males, whether such males were Native or from the white/Euro-American culture. Considering their traditional significance in the continuation of Native cultures, it should not come as a surprise

Source: D. Marie Ralstin-Lewis, "The Continuing Struggle against Genocide: Indigenous Women's Reproductive Rights," *Wicazo Sa Review* 20, no. 1 (2005): 71–95.

that European colonizers often targeted Native[1] women. The assaults on Native women continue to be a goal of some descendants of these European colonizers.

. . .

Traditionally, Native women held positions of esteem in tribal societies and were thought to be born with certain dispositions toward spiritual guidance, and so could offer important knowledge in many matters. As Paula Gunn Allen states, they held a responsibility to maintain the life of the tribe:

> Women are . . . graced with certain inclinations that make them powerful and capable in certain ways . . . Their power includes bearing and rearing children . . . cooking and similar forms of "women's work"; decision making; dreaming and visioning; prophesying; divining, healing, locating people or things; harvesting, preserving, preparing, storing, or transporting food and healing stuffs; producing finished articles of clothing; making houses and laying them out in the proper village arrangement; making and using all sorts of technological equipment such as needles, scrapers, grinders, blenders, harvesters, diggers, fire makers, lathes, spindles, looms, knives, spoons, and ladles; locating and/or allocating virtually every resource used by the people.[2]

Within Native cultures, woman derived their influential and powerful status "by virtue of her femaleness, her natural and necessary fecundity, and her personal acquaintance with blood" (meaning menstruation). European settlers who came to North America embracing Christianity and a rigid system of patriarchy, however, had another view of women. In their quest for land and resources, they profoundly disrupted and dishonored the cooperation and balance between tribal men and women, as well as the agency of women.[3]

Native women did not fit into the classification systems of the Christian colonizers. Native communities often functioned harmoniously without the distinction of gendered social ranks that Christians expected. Patriarchy essentially left women dependent and vulnerable to male coercion. Many Native cultures, by contrast, recognized women as autonomous beings existing within a system of mutual responsibility. This equality of gender struck European settlers as odd, if not blasphemous.

At various times, the colonizers sought to transform Indians into mirror images of Europeans. As the nineteenth century progressed, federal policy demanded that Native women abandon their customary roles as familial anchors and accept a life in male-dominated households. These disruptions of Native cultures subsequently increased the power of Native men at the expense of the women, who not only lost influence in their own domestic sphere but formal voting authority in some tribes as well. Moreover, the influence of Christianity and its redefinition of gender hierarchies decreased women's autonomy by changing notions of sexual propriety.

. . .

Connecting Reproductive Abuses and Racism

In Europe during the late 1800s, Sir Francis Galton, cousin of Charles Darwin, coined the term "eugenics" (literally meaning "well-born"). Galton advocated the regulation of human breeding to ensure the propagation of the more "talented" (essentially members of the upper class and enterprising members of the middle class) of the species. Eugenics is defined as "the method of improving the intellectual, economic, and social level of humans by allowing differential reproduction of superior people to prevail over those designated as inferior." As the eugenics movement spread rapidly throughout Europe in the late nineteenth and early twentieth centuries, its followers established laboratories, international societies, and serial publications to promote their agenda.[4]

In the early 1900s, U.S. scientists focused their research on human heredity, encouraging the growth of the eugenics movement in the United States. Unfortunately, the predominant belief among geneticists was that a single gene controlled most human traits, but little consideration was given to how environment might influence behavioral traits. This nature-over-nurture theory led to the conclusion that those who [were] mentally ill, poor, criminal, retarded, or simply unsuccessful were not only socially but also biologically inferior. For eugenicists, then, improving society meant identifying and controlling inferior groups and their breeding practices. As eugenics grew in the United States, disagreement increased about whether the movement should focus solely on race or include other "inferiorities" such as insanity, criminality, and physical defects. Many eugenicists, feeling that whites were more advanced than other races in the evolutionary process, viewed higher birthrates among Native Americans and other people of color with alarm. Compounding matters, many whites saw declining birthrates of white women as the harbinger of "race suicide" for whites. Additionally, with the long history of racism in the United States even before the onset of the eugenics movement, eugenicists had little trouble influencing many whites that people of color were inferior.[5]

. . .

An astonishing number of doctors did not think that Native women were competent enough to effectively use birth control. A 1972 study found that six percent of doctors would recommend sterilization as a permanent form of birth control for their private white patients, while fourteen percent of doctors recommended sterilization for poor and minority patients on public assistance. In the case of welfare mothers with three or more children, ninety-seven percent of doctors either recommended or preferred sterilization. Numerous doctors favored punitive action toward women with several illegitimate children, such as withholding welfare benefits and compulsory sterilization. A study the following year revealed that many of these white doctors believed that they were helping society by limiting the births of low-income minority women, and alleviating their own tax burdens.[6]

. . .

Population Control or Generations of Genocide?

Deprived of their traditional ways of life through the twin effects of federal policy and U.S. expansion, Native peoples lost their self-sufficiency, experienced dramatic population losses, and were forced to depend on government subsidies and health care to survive. . . .

Facing poverty and having few options, many Native women remained almost entirely dependent on the federal government for health care through IHS. In fact, federal policies had left many Natives trapped in a cycle of poverty and landlessness. This dependence has placed them at greater risk than other minority groups for abuses by the medical profession. While other women also became victims of sterilization and reproductive rights abuses, Indian women constitute a unique class of victims. Different social and cultural realities set them apart from other women of color. Because of their dependence on IHS health care and various state medical programs, they were vulnerable to the health personnel practicing medicine in those public facilities. The federal government, through IHS physicians, increasingly targeted Indian women because of the women's high fertility rates. The 1970 census shows that, over a lifetime, Indian women had an average of 3.79 children. This rate was significantly higher than the median fertility rate of all other women in the United States, with only 1.79 children per mother. Apparently, because the government has a responsibility to provide services to those it recognizes as Native American, it would prefer to limit rather than increase that number. From 1970 to 1980 the birthrate for white women fell by .28 children while the birthrate for Native American women declined by 1.99 children.[7]

. . .

The Discovery of Sterilization Abuse in Indian Country

In 1974, Constance Redbird Pinkerton-Uri, a Choctaw/Cherokee physician, upon hearing complaints from women sterilized against their will, launched her own investigation into the forced and coerced sterilization of Native American women. After several years of examining IHS records and interviewing medical staff and victims, Dr. Uri convinced Senator James Abourezk (Democrat, South Dakota) of the Senate Interior Subcommittee on Indian Affairs to look into the matter. Senator Abourezk prompted a General Accounting Office (GAO) study of IHS records.

The GAO report (HRD-77-3) has been called "only the tip of the iceberg of United States government sponsored sterilizations conducted on American Indians,"[8] and it gave an idea of the severity of the problem, although it was plagued with limitations. Although the GAO report only investigated four of the twelve IHS hospitals, the number of sterilizations was still staggering. In just over three years (1973–1976) in these four hospitals, 3,406 women were sterilized. Senator Abourezk commented that, considering the small number of Native Americans in the population, sterilizing 3,406 Indian women would be comparable to sterilizing 452,000 white women. There is little doubt that the number would actually be larger if the investigation had covered all the IHS facilities (and private facilities with IHS contracts). Additionally, the GAO failed to interview women who had been sterilized, nor did it ask Indian communities for information regarding sterilizations. Its investigators only considered documents provided by IHS officials. The GAO conducted the investigation in an attempt to discredit Dr. Uri. However, the number of sterilized women was too significant to be coincidental.[9]

While the report never fully established that the IHS had actually coerced women into having sterilizations, it did stress that there were deficiencies in the informed consent process. The report revealed that IHS consent forms ignored problems of cultural and language differences. There is no indication that an appropriate explanation was given for sterilization, a word that does not exist in some tribal languages. The women often lacked an understanding of the finality of the procedure or even the nature of the procedure itself. Additionally, the report exposed that, while not forced, many women thought they *must agree* to the procedure. The report also found that the consent forms used by IHS *did not inform the women that they had the right to refuse to be sterilized*. Some of the sterilizations were performed on women under the age of twenty-one, some were done by way of an unnecessary complete hysterectomy rather than a simple tubal ligation, and many of the basic elements of voluntary, informed consent were missing from the consent forms the hospitals used.[10]

. . .

As news of the sterilizations spread, many Native American community leaders, including Cheyenne tribal judge Marie Sanchez, conducted their own inquiries. Sanchez and a Northern Cheyenne tribal member, Mary Ann Bear Comes Out, found that, over a three-year period, the IHS had sterilized 56 out of only 165 women of childbearing age on the Northern Cheyenne Reservation and Labre Mission grounds. They estimated that these sterilizations resulted in reducing births within this group by half or more over a five-year period. After spending much of his life investigating the sterilization campaign, Lehman Brightman (Lakota) estimated that forty percent of all Native women were sterilized.[11]

. . .

The reproductive capabilities and rights of women of color are at best overlooked by the government, and at worst blamed for everything from the rise in entitlement programs (such as welfare and Medicaid) to the national debt and the decline of the "native-born" population of the nation. In order to receive an equal access to the right of natality, women of color must be recognized for their innate humanity. Native women must be recognized for their traditional role as the keepers of life. By attacking the traditional status of women in indigenous nations, sterilization strikes at the very core of the value and uniqueness of women.

Notes

1. The terms "American Indian" and "Native American/Alaska Native" are glosses. They refer to the diverse aboriginal inhabitants of North America and are fraught with political and social quandaries. In this paper the terms "Native," "Native American," and "Indian" will be used for brevity's sake but are by no means meant to be all-inclusive or demeaning to the diversity within this admittedly broad grouping.
2. Paula Gunn Allen, *The Sacred Hoop: Recovering the Feminine in American Indian Traditions* (Boston, MA: Beacon Press Books, 1992), 254.
3. Ibid.
4. Michael Cummings, *Human Heredity: Principles and Issues* (New York: West Publishing, 1993), 9; Beverly Horsburg, "Schrödinger's Cat, Eugenics, and the Compulsory Sterilization of Welfare Mothers: Deconstructing an Old/New Rhetoric and Constructing the Reproductive Right to Natality for the Low-income Women of Color," *Cardozo Law Review* 17 (1996): 531–82.
5. Cummings, *Human Heredity*; Stefan Kuhl, *The Nazi Connection: Eugenics, American Racism, and German National Socialism* (New York: Oxford University Press, 1994); Nancy Ordover, *American Eugenics: Race, Queer Anatomy, and the Science of Nationalism* (Minneapolis: University of Minnesota Press, 2003).
6. Emily Diamond, "Coerced Sterilization under Federally Funded Family Planning Programs," *New England Law Review* 11 (1976): 589–614; [B. Dikens, "Forced Sterilization Is a Nice Name for Genocide," *Northwest Passage* 22, no. 9 (1982)]; [Jane Lawrence, "The Indian Health Service and the Sterilization of Native American Women," *American Indian Quarterly* 24, no. 3 (2000)].
7. The white birthrate was 2.42 children in 1970 and 2.14 children in 1980. See Anti-Genocide Committee of the Native American Solidarity Committee, "Genocide by Surgery," *Northwest Passage* (1978): 11; [Myla Carpio, "Lost Generation: The Involuntary Sterilization of American Indian Women," (Master's thesis, Arizona State University, Tempe, 1995)]; [M. Annette Jaimes and Theresa Halsey, "American Indian Women: At the Center of Indigenous Resistance in Contemporary North America," in

The State of Native America: Genocide, Colonization, and Resistance, ed. M. Annette Jaimes (Boston: South End Press, 1992)]; Lawrence, "The Indian Health Service"; [Sally Torpy, "Endangered Species: Native American Women's Struggle for Their Reproductive Rights and Racial Identity, 1970s to 1990s," (Master's thesis, University of Nebraska, Omaha, 1998)].

8. Brint Dillingham, "Sterilization Update," *American Indian Journal* 4, no. 9 (October 1977): 25.

9. Carpio, "Lost Generation"; Brint Dillingham, "Indian Women and IHS Sterilization Practices," American Indian Journal 3, no. 1(1977): 27–28; Brint Dillingham, "Sterilization of Native Americans," *American Indian Quarterly* 3, no. 7 (1977): 16–19; Torpy, "Endangered Species"; Western New York Educational Television Association, *Woman: Concerns of American Indian Women* (Washington, D.C.: Public Television Library, 1977).

10. Lawrence, "The Indian Health Service"; Torpy, "Endangered Species; [WARN, "The Theft of Life," Women of All Red Nations (WARN) Newsletter. We Will Remember Group, 1977].

11. Carpio, "Lost Generation"; [Bruce Johansen, "Reprise/Forced Sterilizations: Sterilization of Native American Women," 1998, http://www .ratical.org/ratville/sterilize.html]; Lawrence, "The Indian Health Service."

Part 4

Religious Arguments about Abortion

Introduction to Part 4

When most people think about the topic of religion and abortion, whether they self-identify as religious or not, their primary association is with dogmatic theological statements about the morality of abortion or normative positions that instruct believers about the permissibility or impermissibility of voluntarily ending a pregnancy. In short, many people reduce the topic of religion and abortion to a narrow consideration of what religious authorities say about whether abortion is right or wrong. This caricature of religious thinking about abortion, pregnancy, and reproduction is, in part, a reflection of media coverage that focuses on religious sound bites, often because the binary nature of "right or wrong" is easier to portray than the complex reality of reproductive management and the more nuanced positions that religions actually hold. In our efforts to show complexity and nuance, we have intentionally placed "Religious Arguments on Abortion" later in the volume because theological reflection is necessarily shaped by and responsive to, contextual realities, such as those discussed in the previous three parts. After examining women's experience (Part 1), social science evidence (Part 2), and historical context (Part 3), one is better prepared critically to read and analyze the normative positions associated with Judaism, Christianity, and Islam in this part. We believe you will find that these excerpts make evident the ways in which scholars and religious experts seek to weigh and balance a variety of factors in their consideration of the moral issues related to pregnancy, abortion, and childbearing.

Abortion is addressed in the historical documents, legal canons, theological texts, and ethical teachings of Islam, Christianity, and Judaism; however, considerable debate exists on how to interpret these references, who may interpret them, and what weight these interpretations should carry in each religion's authoritative moral teachings and legal rulings. Moreover, in addition to texts and traditions, additional factors considered in these normative arguments include: the moral standing and moral agency of the pregnant woman, questions of ensoulment and the moral status of the prenate, considerations about the life and health of the pregnant person, and the health status of the prenate, especially in cases of a diagnosis of severe disability or a condition incompatible with life.

In this section you will find Muslim, Jewish, and Christian views on abortion, ranging from conservative to progressive. We self-consciously have included a significant portion of progressive religious views in order to counterbalance the prevailing popular opinion that a religiously principled position on abortion will tend toward conservatism and that progressive or feminist positions are mostly secular.

Various branches or denominations within each religion are represented, since it would be erroneous to suggest that there is a singular Jewish, Christian, or Muslim position on abortion; indeed, these essays reveal some significant divergences within each religion. As readers will see, Islam's pronatalist orientation discourages abortion, particularly in situations of economic duress, but the legal considerations related to permissibility are predominately based on a determination of when a fetus receives its soul, which most schools of thought place at 120 days of gestation. While the Quran is fundamental for Shiites and Sunnis, the fact that adherents from these two branches rely on some different authoritative texts and have different juridical and institutional structures can result in divergences in moral and legal positions on abortion. Kiarash Aramesh discusses views of embryology and fetal ensoulment particular to Shiite scholarship and law (*sharia*). The essay by Abdulrahman Al-Matary and Jaffar Ali summarizes the position on pregnancy termination in the four Sunni schools of thought, with special attention to the role of an important *fiqh* (jurisprudence) council in Saudi Arabia. Judaism shares with Islam a traditionally strong pronatalist perspective, and this viewpoint is reflected in the essays of Conservative Jewish scholars David Feldman and David Kraemer. Judaism is unique among these three monotheisms in that it includes an explicit halakhic (legal) principle, as explained by Y. Michael Barilan, that specifies when the pregnant woman's life must be given precedence above that of her fetus.

The largest group of essays in this section addresses abortion and Christianity, which reflects two considerations. First, conservative Christian antiabortion rhetoric and activism plays a dominant role in conversations about abortion and religion in the public sphere in the United States; therefore, it is important to examine a broad range of arguments and positions within this particular tradition. Second, given the dominant role of Christianity in the public debate, there is a larger body of writings from Christian scholars and theologians, and notably this scholarship is dominanted by white male scholars. The essays by Norman Ford (focusing on papal documents) and Jason Eberl (focusing on Thomas Aquinas) present various ways fetal personhood has been debated in Roman Catholicism, which considers abortion an excommunicable sin. Abortion is not mentioned in the Bible, and Roy Bowen Ward's essay examines how key biblical texts have been misinterpreted to support a prolife position. Evangelical Protestant scholar C. Ben Mitchell makes the case that personhood at conception is a normative teaching rooted in early Christian texts. The statement from the Greek Orthodox Archdiocese of America affirms fetal personhood from conception but also allows abortion to save a woman's life.

In addition to these largely traditionalist perspectives, we have included feminist and womanist perspectives. These women scholars, in critical dialogue with their respective traditions, make the moral authority of pregnant persons a nonnegotiable factor for theological and ethical reflection on abortion. Dena Davis reflects on the subjective nature of halakhic casuistic reasoning, marked by the lack of female decisors (rabbinic authorities). Sa'diyya Shaikh makes a case for respecting the moral agency God gives humans and for gender justice regarding women's roles and reproductive burdens. Four progressive scholars engage aspects of the Christian tradition. Patricia Beattie Jung questions the morality of making bodily self-giving an obligation—especially in pregnancy. Toni Bond proposes a womanist theo-ethic based on the principles and values of reproductive justice. Rebecca Todd Peters takes a relational approach to understanding the pregnant person's moral obligations to the prenate. Sin, a concept often associated with abortion in Christian discourse, is analyzed by Margaret Kamitsuka, who gives reasons against seeing abortion as ipso facto sin.

As the essays in this section make clear, there is no univocal voice or position about the morality of abortion either within or across the traditions of Judaism, Islam, and Christianity. These texts are only representative of the range of arguments, positions, and perspectives available, but they offer a chance to engage with some of the key principles and values that are invoked in some important religious positions today.

As you read the essays in this section, we encourage you to consider the following:

1. In what ways does the knowledge you gained from the first three parts of the *Reader* related to experience, science, and tradition help inform how you read and understand these texts?

2. What similarities and differences can you identify between the arguments across traditions? What similarities and differences can you identify between the arguments within a tradition?

3. Identify and consider the form and method of each argument. How does each author engage with particular types of texts (e.g., halakhah, scripture, encyclicals, *fatwas*); authoritative interpreters (e.g., theologians of the early church, *fiqh* councils, eminent medieval rabbis); and philosophical or theological principles (e.g., ensoulment, the believer's God-given moral agency; human relationality; free will)? What elements hold authority and why? What counts as evidence or support for each position?

4. In what ways do these articles complicate the traditional prolife/prochoice binary? What do you see as more productive ways to frame the public discussion about abortion and what role might normative religious arguments play in the public sphere?

Judaism

25

Abortion:
The Jewish View

David M. Feldman

David Feldman (d. 2014) was the author of numerous books on Jewish thought and considered a respected expert on Jewish bioethics and medical halakhah. In addition to rabbinical duties in the congregations where he served, he was active in various medical and bioethics organizations, and taught at Jewish Theological Seminary of America, where he had received his PhD. This excerpt comes from a report he authored, which was adopted as a "majority opinion" by sixteen of the seventeen voting members at the August 23, 1983, meeting of the Rabbinical Assembly, which is the membership organization for Conservative rabbis.

The abortion question in talmudic law begins with an examination of the fetus' legal status. For this the Talmud has a phrase, *ubar yerekh imo*, a counterpart of the Latin *pars viscera matris*. The fetus is deemed a "part of its mother" rather than an independent entity. Of course, this designation says nothing about the right of abortion; this is found only in more theoretical contexts. In the case of an embryo found in a purchased animal, the embryo is intrinsic to its mother's body; its ownership is defined—it belongs to the buyer. Moreover, in the religious conversion of a pregnant woman, her unborn child is automatically included and requires no added ceremony. Nor does the fetus have power of acquisition. Gifts or transactions made on its behalf, except by its father, are not binding; it inherits from its father only, in a natural rather than transactional manner.

Source: David Feldman, "Abortion: The Jewish View," Rabbinical Assembly, 1983.

Germane as such information might seem to the question of abortion, it tells us little more than, in the words of a [modern] writer on Roman and Jewish law, that in both systems the fetus has no "juridical personality" of its own. The morality of abortion is a function, rather, of the legal attitude to feticide as distinguished from homicide or infanticide. The law of homicide in the Torah, in one of its several formulations, reads: *"Makkeh ish . . ."* (He who smites a man . . .) (Exodus 21:12). Does this include *any* "man," say, a day-old child? Yes, says the Talmud, citing another text: *"ki yakkeh kol nefesh adam"* (If one smite any *nefesh adam*) (Lev. 24:17), literally, any human person. The "any" is understood to *include* the day old child, but the *"nefesh adam"* is taken to *exclude* the fetus in the womb for the fetus in the womb is *lav nefesh hu* (not a person) until he is born. In the words of Rashi, only when the fetus "comes into the world" is it a "person."

The basis, then, for denying capital crime status to feticide in Jewish law, even for those rabbis who may have wanted to rule otherwise, is scriptural. Alongside the *nefesh adam* text is another basic one in Exodus 21:22, which provides:

> If men strive, and wound a pregnant woman so that her fruit be expelled, but no harm befell [her], then shall he be fined as her husband shall assess, and the matter placed before the judges. But if harm befell [her], then shall you give life for life.

The Talmud makes this verse's teaching explicit: only monetary compensation is exacted of him who causes a woman to miscarry. Though the abortion spoken of here is accidental, the verse is still a source for the teaching that feticide is not a capital crime (since even accidental homicide cannot be expiated by monetary fine).

. . .

In the rabbinic tradition, then, abortion remains a non-capital crime at worst. But a curious factor further complicates the question of the criminality of the act. This is the circumstance that one more biblical text (this one in Genesis and hence "before Sinai" and part of the Laws of the "Sons of Noah") served as the source for the teaching that feticide is indeed a capital crime— for non-Jews. Genesis 9:6 reads, "He who sheds the blood of man, through man (i.e., through the human court of law) shall *his* blood be shed." Since the Hebrew *(shofekh dam ha'adam ba'adam . . .)* allows for a translation of "man, in man," as well as "man, through man," the Talmud records the exposition of Rabbi Ishmael: "What is this 'man in man'? It refers to the fetus in its mother's womb." The locus of this text in Genesis, standing as it does without the qualifying balance of the Exodus (Sinaitic) passage, made feticide a capital crime for non-Jews (i.e., those not heir to the Sinaitic covenant) in Jewish law. Some modern scholars hold this exposition to be more sociological than textually inherent, representing a reaction against abuses among the heathen. In view of rampant abortion and infanticide, they claim, Rabbi Ishmael "forced" the above exegesis out of the Genesis text to render judgment against the Romans.

Regardless of its rationale, the doctrine remains part of theoretical Jewish law, as Maimonides systematically defines it:

> A "Son of Noah" who killed a person, even a fetus in its mother's womb, is capitally liable. . . . (The Jewish court is obliged to provide judges for the resident alien to adjudicate for them in accordance with these laws [of the Sons of Noah] so that society not corrupt itself. The judges may come either from their midst or from the Israelites.) (*Hilkhot Melakhim* 9:4; 10:11)

Therapeutic abortion is not, of course, included in this Noahide restriction. Nor is an abortion during the first forty days of pregnancy included, according to some. The implications of this anomaly of a different law for "Sons of Noah" were dealt with in a responsum of the eighteenth century:

> It is not to be supposed that the Torah would consider the embryo as a person (*nefesh*) for them (Sons of Noah) but not a person for us. The fetus is not a person for them either; the Torah merely was more severe in its practical ruling in their regard. Hence, therapeutic abortion would be permissible to them, too.[1]

In the rabbinic system, then, abortion is not murder. Nor is it more than murder, as would be the case if "ensoulment" were at issue. Talmudic discussions speak of the moment—conception, birth, post-birth, etc.—at which the soul joins the body. This is seen to be irrelevant to the abortion question, because the soul is immortal no matter when it enters or leaves the body. And, more important than being immortal, it is a pure soul, free of the taint of "original sin." In the sixth century, St. Fulgentius ruled that "original sin" is inherited by the soul of the fetus at conception, which made baptism in utero necessary in cases of miscarriage, and which made abortion worse than murder, in the sense that the fetus was being "killed in this world and the next." Judaism has no concept of "original sin" of this kind and, in the words of the Talmud and Daily Prayer Book, "My God, the soul with which Thou has endowed me is pure."

Murder (of the innocent) is forbidden even to save life. But with abortion removed from the category of murder, then therapeutic abortion becomes permissible and, in fact, mandated. The Mishnah sets forth the basic talmudic law in this regard:

> If a woman has [life-threatening] difficulty in childbirth, the embryo within her should be dismembered limb by limb, because her life takes precedence over its life. Once its head (or its greater part) has emerged, it may not be touched, for we do not set aside one life for another (*Ohalot* 7:6).

In analyzing such provisions, the Talmud suggested that the reason could well be that the fetus is in the category of an "aggressor"; its life is forfeit under the law which permits killing a "pursuer" in order to save the intended victim. The Talmud, however, dismisses this reasoning, since the fetus is an innocent being, and since one cannot know "who is pursuing whom"; the pursuit must therefore be deemed an "act of God," and this factor does not apply. In the Mishneh Torah, Maimonides also used the term "aggressor," but only figuratively; in truth he and his commentators concluded that the argument does not apply. It is either inapplicable or at best superfluous, because the fetus is not yet a person and murder is not involved. Maimonides formulates the talmudic law as follows:

> This, too, is a [negative] commandment: Not to take pity on the life of a pursuer. Therefore, the Sages ruled that when a woman has difficulty in giving birth, one may dismember the child in her womb, either with drugs or by surgery, *because it is like a pursuer seeking to kill her*. Once its head has emerged, it may not be touched, for we do not set aside one life for another; this is the natural course of the world (*Hilkhot Rotzeah U'Shemirat Nefesh* 1:9).

Some commentators of the Mishneh Torah suggest that although abortion is not technically murder, it is still so grave an offense that Maimonides resorted to the aggressor argument in order to buttress the permission for abortion; its justification is that the fetus is at least *like* an aggressor.

The subsequent rabbinic tradition seems to align itself either to the right, in the direction of Maimonides, or to the left, in the direction of Rashi. The first approach can be identified especially with the late Chief Rabbi of Israel, Issar Unterman, who sees any abortion as "akin to homicide" and therefore allowable only in cases of corresponding gravity, such as saving the life of the mother. This approach then builds down from that strict position to embrace a broader interpretation of life-saving situations, which include a threat to her health, for example, as well as a threat to her life. The second approach, associated with another former Chief Rabbi of Israel, Ben Zion Uziel, and others, assumes that no real prohibition against abortion exists and builds *up* from that lenient position to safeguard against indiscriminate abortion. This includes the example of Rabbi Yair Bachrach in the 17th century, whose classic responsum saw no legal bar to abortion, but would not permit it in the case before him. The case was one of a pregnancy conceived in adultery; the woman, in "deep remorse," wanted to destroy the fruit of her sin. The author concludes by refusing to sanction the abortion, not on legal grounds but on sociological ones, as a safeguard against further immorality. Other authorities disagreed on this point, affirming the legal sanction of abortion for the woman's welfare, whether life or health, or even avoidance of "great pain."

The criterion in both approaches becomes maternal rather than fetal. The principle in Jewish law is *tza'ar gufah kadim,* that her welfare is primary. Rabbinic rulings on abortion are thus amenable to the following generalization: If a possibility or probability exists that a child may be born defective, and the mother seeks abortion on the grounds of pity for a child whose life would be less than normal, the rabbi would decline permission. Since we do not know for sure that it will be born defective, and since we do not know how bad such a defective life will be for the child, and since no permission exists in Jewish law to kill born defectives, permission on those grounds would be denied. If, however, an abortion for the same potentially deformed child were sought on the grounds that the possibility is causing severe anguish to the mother, permission would be granted. The fetus is unknown, future, potential, part of the "secrets of God"; the mother is known, present, alive and asking for compassion.

. . .

In the current Tay-Sachs screening controversy, rabbinic authorities recommend screening before rather than during the pregnancy. This is because the alternative would be to resort to amniocentesis after the first trimester of pregnancy, with possible abortion on the basis of its results. This abortion for fetal rather than maternal indications would not ordinarily be sanctioned by Jewish law. True, rabbinic opinion permitting abortion for fetal reasons alone is not altogether lacking, but the normative rabbinic view is to permit it for maternal indications only. Yet, the one can blend into the other, as fetal risk can mean mental anguish on the part of the mother, so that the fetal indication becomes a maternal one. The woman's welfare is thus the key to warrant abortion.

Implicit in the Mishnah above is the teaching that the rights of the fetus are secondary to the rights of the mother all the way up until the moment of birth. This principle is obscured by the current phrase, "right to life." In the context of abortion questions, the issue is not the right to life, which is very clear in Jewish law, but the right to be born, which is not as clear. The right to be born is relative; the right to life for existing persons is absolute. "Life" may begin before birth, but it is not the life of a human person; animal life, plant life or even pre-human life are not the same as human life. Rabbinic law has determined that human life begins with birth. This is neither a medical nor a court judgment, but a metaphysical one. In the Jewish system, human life in this sense begins with birth. Of course, potential life already partakes of the potential sacredness of actual life, since the latter can have its inception only through the former.

Another slogan-like phrase is dealt with in the same Mishnah, wherein it is ruled that "once the fetus has emerged from the womb, it cannot be touched" even to save the life of the mother, "for we cannot set aside one life for another." The "quality of life" slogan or concept is thus inadmissible. The life of the mother has more "quality"; she is adult, has a husband, children, associations, while the newborn has none of these yet. Still, the sanctity of life principle means that life is sacred regardless of differences in quality; mother and newborn babe are equal from the moment of birth.

Talmudic statements do use the term "murder" in a figurative sense, of course, to describe even the neglect to conceive. Procreation is a positive mitzvah, and he who fails to fulfill this mitzvah is called "guilty of bloodshed." And much of the pro-natalist attitude of Judaism helps account for its abhorrence of casual abortion. There may be legal sanction for abortion where necessary, but the attitude remains one of hesitation before the sanctity of life and a pro-natalist respect for potential life.

Accordingly, abortion for "population control" is repugnant to the Jewish system. Abortion for economic reasons is also not admissible. Taking precaution by abortion or birth control against physical threat remains a mitzvah, but never to forestall financial difficulty. Material considerations are improper in this connection. In the Jewish community, today, with a conscious or unconscious drive to replenish ranks decimated by the Holocaust, contemporary rabbis invoke not the more lenient, but rather the more stringent responsa of the earlier authorities. The more permissive decisions, they point out, were in any case rendered against the background of far greater instinctive hesitation to resort to abortion. Against today's background of more casual abortion, rabbis are moving closer to the position associated with Maimonides and Unterman, allowing abortion only for the gravest of reasons.

Note

1. R. Isaac Schorr, *Responsa Koah Shor*, vol. I, no. 20; Kolomea 1888.

26

Jewish Ethics and Abortion

David Kraemer

David Kraemer is a longtime professor at the Jewish Theological Seminary in New York, the flagship school of Conservative Judaism in the United States, where he also received his PhD. Kraemer has published biblical commentaries and has written extensively on the Talmud and on topics ranging from suffering to a history of Jewish eating. Kraemer discusses the difference between a traditional halakhic and a modern (though still conservative) ethical approach to abortion and Judaism.

Contemporary Jewish commentators have written repeatedly on the question of Jewish law/values/ethics and abortion, some supporting it and others voicing condemnation. But virtually without exception, even when they have claimed to be speaking of values or ethics, their discourse shows that they have really meant Jewish law (Halacha). For those who are primarily concerned with ethics as such (henceforth: "ethicists"), there is no reason to grant that the two are the same—and considerable reason to argue they are not.

The crucial differences between Halacha and ethics are fourfold. Halacha defines a narrow canon, ethics should not. Halachists believe "Torah" (broadly defined) is eternal, contemporary; ethicists will understand the tradition contextually. Halachists submit to the final authority of their sources, ethicists exercise their judgment. Perhaps most crucially, halachists prefer clear, definitive conclusions, whereas ethicists will understand that complex ethical questions often do not yield univocal, overarching answers. It is obvious that the two are radically different enterprises, and the standards and assumptions of Halacha are obviously not appropriate for the ethicist.

Source: David Kraemer, "Jewish Ethics and Abortion," *Tikkun* 8, no. 1 (1993): 55–8.

At the same time, rejection of halachic discourse does not require the abandonment of traditional Jewish sources; it is possible to do ethics with traditional sources without accepting the ways of Halacha. In what follows, I hope to show how this can be done, first by reviewing and critiquing the common halachic approach to abortion and then illustrating the alternative.

The biblical text most often cited in connection with the abortion question is Exodus 21:22-3. The verses describe a case of two men who, in the course of a scuffle, unintentionally strike a pregnant woman, who then miscarries. The text continues: "If there be no catastrophe, he shall be punished according to what the woman's husband shall exact from him, it shall be determined through adjudication. But if there be catastrophe, then you shall give life for life. . . ."

Rabbinic tradition understood "catastrophe" to mean harm to the mother. Thus, if the mother's life was lost, so too should the life of the perpetrator be taken. But if the fetus was lost, no such "life for life" penalty was demanded. On this basis, halachists have argued that the fetus was not valued as a life; feticide is not a capital crime.

Citations of rabbinic literature relevant to this question begin with Mishna Ohalot 7.6:

> If a woman has difficulty in childbirth, we cut up the offspring in her womb and remove it limb by limb, because her life comes before its life. If most of it [the child; the Talmud's version is "most of the head"] has come out, we do not touch it, because we do not push aside one life for another.

This Mishna clearly teaches that, at least at certain times, the fetus's life must be taken in order to save the endangered life of the mother. Based upon the Mishna's stated reason ("her life comes before its life"), it may even be argued that this applies to any point in the pregnancy. The direction of the law as delineated here is permissive at least in cases of therapeutic abortion.

The Talmud suggests a new and possibly crucial justification for the mishnaic law quoted above. At Sanhedrin 72b, the text proposes that, even if most of the baby (or the baby's head) has already emerged, it should still be proper to save the mother's life by taking the baby's life because the child would be in the category of "pursuer"—according to rabbinic law, if one pursues another with intent to murder, a Jew is required to save the pursued even by taking the life of the pursuer. (The Talmud rejects the proposed reasoning, claiming that in this case it is actually "Heaven" that is doing the pursuing.) Maimonides and others understand this to suggest that, in the earlier mishnaic case, where the child is still mostly in the womb, the child is indeed categorized as a "pursuer" and for that reason its life may be taken. Following this reasoning, the conclusion regarding therapeutic abortion suggested above would appear unimpeachable and, indeed, most halachic authorities have ruled that such abortion is legitimate.

. . .

The problem with this whole discussion, from the perspective of modern ethics, is that none of these sources has been subjected to the necessary critique. For example, there are several problems with the verse from Exodus. First, its reference is ambiguous. While it is possible that the "catastrophe" it speaks of is the mother's death, it might also be the death of the child; if this were so, of course, radically different conclusions would be required. Second, even assuming that the ambiguous term refers to the mother, it is not clear that this text is relevant to the abortion debate. It speaks, after all, of the unintentional taking of fetal life, not of direct intervention to terminate such life. At best, the text implies that the killing of a fetus is not considered murder and even this is not clear since murder is intentional, and the killing described in the passage is unintentional.

The relevance of Mishna Ohalot is also questionable. In fact, the Mishna speaks not about danger to a mother's life early in pregnancy, but rather about danger to her life during childbirth. If by "abortion" we mean taking the life of a fetus mostly during the early months of a pregnancy, then this text has no direct bearing on the abortion question.

It is not surprising that classic rabbinic sources contain scant reference to abortion and focus instead on the dilemmas of childbirth. Danger to a mother's life in childbirth was extremely common in premodern society. For a variety of reasons (children were a financial asset; infant- and child-mortality rates were extremely high; medical procedures were dangerous or unreliable), abortion must have been uncommon. For related reasons (children as a financial liability; low infant mortality; safe and effective medical procedures), abortion is a common and reasonable option for us. What this all means, of course, is that the halachic authorities of old were not asking our questions about abortion. Can we justify deriving instruction when the analogies are so inexact and the circumstances so different?

For these same reasons, the talmudic discussion of Mishna Ohalot is also not substantively relevant. Nor, however, is its theoretical extension of much use. To begin with, it is not clear that Maimonides is correct in applying the principle of "pursuer" to the fetus before birth. But even if Maimonides is correct, we learn nothing about abortion in general. As stated, according to rabbinic law, even an adult "pursuer" may legitimately be stopped through the taking of his life. Thus, it is possible that the fetus could be judged a legally protected life and still be subject to the law outlined in the Mishna. In fact, there are multiple reasonable interpretations, and while these sources speak clearly about a common problem (danger in childbirth), they convey nothing unambiguous about abortion as such.

. . .

Considered from the perspective of modern ethics, the conventional, halachic approach to abortion leads to a dead end. But what is the alternative? If the task is not primarily deciding what is permissible and what prohibited, but discovering fundamental values embedded in the tradition that pertain to a given question, then our approach must change in several essential respects.

First, we must frame new questions—questions that relate not only to the former concern, Halacha, but also to the latter, ethics. Naturally, different questions will sometimes lead us to different texts—to precedents whose relevance is not simply in the analogues they offer but in the values and attitudes they assume. Second, we must look beyond the canon as defined by Halacha. Third, we must feel free to critique and question the teachings that the tradition records. And, finally, we must insist that general conclusions are not always possible; we must be open to ambivalence where the complexity of an issue so warrants.

In the case of abortion, our questions must include, but not be limited to, how Jewish traditions view the life or potential life of a fetus, the relationship of the fetus to the mother (and father), and the prerogatives of a mother (and father) with respect to the fetus. These questions will lead us back to some of the texts reviewed above, but other texts will also suggest themselves. More important, we will find that the nature of discourse and analysis changes. What follows is intended to illustrate the alternative for which I am arguing.

We begin with two traditions commonly cited in connection with the question of abortion, the first because of the light it sheds on the status of the fetus. The Talmud, at Yebamot 69b, declares that "until the fortieth day, the fetus is mere water." The attitude of the author is clear: During the earliest stage of fetal development the fetus is not yet considered human life in any genuine sense.

For the halachist, the consequence of this statement may be obvious; "mere water," after all, should not be protected by the law. Nevertheless, we recognize that this "mere water" will soon be far more; how do we factor in our concern for the ultimate potential of this primitive substance? Is such potential irrelevant (to my mind, an unreasonable position), or does it call upon us to respect this water more than other "mere water?" And, if we judge that potential is an important consideration, how does this balance against the mother's wishes and needs? Thus, this talmudic precept enables us to begin formulating essential questions. Despite its relative clarity, it does not direct us to a singular answer.

The second much-cited tradition, scattered through a related cluster of texts, relates to the question of the relationship between a fetus and its mother. The tradition records a dispute concerning whether a fetus is considered "its mother's thigh limb" or not. Certain texts seem to prefer the view that a fetus is indeed considered a limb of its mother, but this position is not clearly supported by the Talmud as a whole. On the contrary, what distinguishes these discussions—and what has gone unnoticed (or, at least, unnoted) by halachists—is that both opinions persist and that neither is deemed obviously superior to the other. The talmudic deliberations tend to explore the consequences of each without privileging one over the other.

From the ethicist's perspective, the Talmud's inconclusiveness in this matter is its most notable feature. The inability of the sages to support one position firmly shows their dilemma in assessing the status of the fetus vis-a-vis the mother. If the fetus were "its mother's limb" it would be judged to have no independent existence and therefore no independent rights. But the talmudic sages are not willing to grant the necessary correctness of that opinion. Nor, however, are they confident of the opposite opinion.

This indecision is evidence of ambivalence—an ambivalence with which we readily identify. The fetus is not quite a person; it is (for most of a pregnancy) unable to survive independent of the mother's body. Thus, it is reasonable to conclude that its life is in no significant way separate from that of the mother. On the other hand, there is no doubting the fetus's essential personhood, at least in potentia. The fetus, for a large part of its development, looks like a person and, one day soon, it will be a person. (Remember, each of us began as a fetus.) Thus, we also feel strongly that at some stage—a stage earlier than birth itself—the fetus has attained at least existential personhood. The positions recorded by the rabbis mark the two poles of our own confused reflections on this matter. If I understand them correctly, the rabbis support such confusion, confirming that there are no simple answers to these questions.

A text that has, to the best of my knowledge, never been cited in this connection is the Talmudic deliberation (Bava Batra 141b-142b) that considers whether one may give a gift to a fetus. The issue is the degree to which a fetus may be considered a legal entity: If it is such an entity, then it should be possible to give it a gift; the more distant it is thought to be from real personhood, the more difficult it should be to support the validity of such a gift. The discussion begins with the opinion that a fetus may not acquire property, but the Mishna which this deliberation accompanies suggests the opposite. In fact, although the first stated law is supported to the end, the deliberation goes out of its way to review the many parties who support the contrary opinion, believing that a fetus may acquire property.

Most interestingly, for our purposes, is the last minute modification of the first tradition by R. Yohanan: Yes, he agrees, a fetus may not acquire a gift, but there is an exception for one's own fetus (in the womb of one's wife), for "a person's feelings are especially close to his own child." In other words, while it might generally be true that a fetus is not "person" enough for another to have full and proper intent to give it a gift, one's own baby, even before birth, is certainly person enough. There are differences in our feelings for our own fetus and that of another—differences which have real consequences.

This Talmudic text is important to our deliberation for several reasons. First, it again records and gives credence to two contradictory views, suggesting that the question of a fetus's personhood does not yield unambiguous answers. Perhaps more important, it recommends that the personhood of a fetus may change as a function of our emotional connections to it; our own child, in utero, is indeed a person as far as we are concerned. It has a reality—a presence—that creates a genuinely human relationship even before birth. The relationship just described is not, in the estimation of the Talmud, limited to the mother. The deliberation speaks from the perspective of the father, showing that, in the opinion of its authors, the father as well as the mother may relate in significant ways to the fetus before birth.

. . .

It is difficult to build a case for actually outlawing abortion based upon these traditions. In certain cases, they clearly support both the legality and the morality of such an option. Yet we are also meant to recognize and regard at least the fetus's potential personhood, and this requires our personal renunciation of abortion as a ready option. To borrow Bill Clinton's formulation in the 1992 presidential campaign, we should be prochoice, not pro-abortion. Undoubtedly, there will be limited circumstances in which we will support abortion without hesitation. But hesitation should otherwise be the hallmark of our approach to this difficult issue.

27

Her Pain Prevails and Her Judgment Respected— Abortion in Judaism

Y. Michael Barilan

Y. Michael Barilan is a practicing physician and professor of medical law and ethics at the Sackler Faculty of Medicine, Tel Aviv University. He publishes widely on the intersections among bioethics, law and religion, especially Jewish religious law (halakhah). Barilan's much longer complete essay discusses an in-depth range of historical, ethical, and legal issues regarding the status of the fetus and the reproductive autonomy of Jewish women. In this excerpt, Barilan considers how the dictum of "her pain prevails" arises as a moral and legal principle based on rabbinic writings about pregnancy and birthing, which adds weight to the notion that a pregnant woman's life takes precedence of that of her fetus—even in light of the Jewish reverence for developing life in the womb.

[T]he Torah cherishes fetal life and places respect for developing life of any kind at the heart of its virtue ethics; indeed, *Halakhah* rescinds almost all purely religious taboos for the sake of saving human fetal life. On the other hand, . . . fetuses have no *legal* claim for life and that as long as they depend on the mother and threaten her well-being, they cannot be considered moral persons. Rather, maternal-fetal conflicts are typically settled following the dictum "her pain prevails," without weighing the proportionality of the fetal interest against her own.[1] Maimonides coined this dictum,

---

Source: Y. Michael Barilan, "Her Pain Prevails and Her Judgment Respected—Abortion in Judaism," *Journal of Law and Religion* 25, no. 1 (2009): 97–186.

> [If] they determined the foods that are proper for her, and she craves to eat
> more, or to eat other foods, due to the disease of craving that she has in her
> belly, she [should] eat as she will, whatever she wants, and the husband cannot
> deter her by saying that, if she eats too much or if she eats bad food, the child
> will die, because the pain of her body prevails.[2]

(In Hebrew, *tza'ar* means "pain," sorrow; *guffa* means "her body" as well as
"her own self").

. . .

Maimonides's bold assertion of the right of a pregnant woman who craves
food to eat excessively has raised much consternation among later rabbis,
though the rabbinic code of law, Shulhan Arukh, incorporates it along with
a dissenting opinion.[3]

Others have followed Maimonides in arguing that women are not
obligated to undergo suffering to save their fetuses. Rabbi Avraham, citing
Rabbi Auerbach, explains why an Israeli woman in the 1970s has no
obligation to undergo the travails of surgery in order to save the life of her
sick fetus,

> The woman is under no obligation to subject herself to the danger of a
> Cesarean section, when she is afraid of the operation, in order to save her
> fetus. What she is obligated to do, by virtue of her marital commitment to her
> husband, is to subject herself to the danger of pregnancy and an ordinary
> delivery, because she took that upon herself, and accordingly married.[4]

. . . Once more in his ruling, we can see that the nature and interests of the
fetus play no role whatsoever in the equation; the only parties who count are
the woman and her husband.[5]

. . .

Obstructed Labor and the Incorporation of Self-Defense

We have seen that the high value accorded human life in *Halakhah* is
derived from the paradigmatic case[6] of a pregnant woman who is seized
by irrational food cravings, highlighting the interdependence of fetal and
maternal life and the special sensitivity of *Halakhah* to even "irrational"
maternal suffering and any threat, even if small, to human life. If we explore
later rulings, however, we will see that the case of a woman seized with food

cravings sets the basis for the high legal standing of human life when purely religious laws (e.g., the laws of Shabbat and kosher food) must be violated to save it. However, the paradigmatic case of obstructed labor (discussed in this section) as a case of self-defense sets the basis for the legal standing of human life in situations of interpersonal conflicts. Some modem rabbis extrapolate the law on self-defense toward a stricter stance toward abortion.

The Mishnah states:

> If a woman has difficulty in childbirth, one dismembers the embryo within her, limb by limb, because her life takes precedence over its life. Once its greater part has emerged, it may not be touched, for we do not set aside one life for another.[7]

Rashi, in his commentary on this passage, writes: "As long as it has not come out into the light of day, it is not a soul, and it is permissible to kill it in order to save its mother."[8] His words are well in line with the principles laid out in Arakhin[9] regarding the execution of a pregnant woman, which makes the only relevant milestone in the pregnancy the moment on the birthstool, when the fetus has "moved from its place [in the womb]" *(akkar mimkomo)* and thus becomes "another body" *(guffa aharina).*[10] Whereas Rashi understands the Talmud to hold that even after the fetus has moved from its place, it is not a legal person until it is born, Maimonides writes:

> This is a negative precept, not to have compassion for the soul of the persecutor (rodef). Accordingly, the sages instructed that, if a pregnant woman has difficulty in childbirth, it is permissible to cut up the fetus in her vitals, whether by use of a medicine or by hand, because it is like a persecutor which runs after her in order to kill her. But after its head has emerged, it may not be touched, for we do not set aside one life for another, and this is the way of the world.[11]

Maimonides explains that the duty to kill persecutors when necessary to save the victims also applies to an innocent persecutor who has legal standing equal to other humans, such as an infant.[12]

It would appear that for the pre-moderns, the persecutor principle applies only at the moment when a fetus "is another body" on the birthstool and not to any abortion at a previous time; and indeed, none of the pre-modern *posqim** used it in this way.[13] However, a responsum given by eighteenth-century Austrian, Rabbi Shor, appears to be the line of demarcation between pre-modern and modern rulings, which are much more restrictive of

---

*Eds.: *Posek*, pl. *poskim*, is the Hebrew term for a "decisor" or legal scholar.

abortions, though his summary does appear to be in line with Rabbi Joseph of Trani.[14] Shor ignores the birth-moment as decisive in conferring the legal status of a person,[15] and instead discusses the relevance of the "persecutor" principle to abortions for medical reasons.[16]

I believe these rulings can be reconciled to some extent: the very fact that the Mishnah chooses the moment of birth as paradigmatic on the conflict between the mother and the fetus is meant to underscore that, up to that stage, there can be no doubt that the mother's life takes precedence over the fetus's life, even when the mother's interests are only to fend off suffering. By contrast, when the fetus is in the liminal stage—it "has moved from its place" but "the greater part has [not yet] emerged,"—it has a special status and must not be killed other than to save the mother's life (as Rabbi Zweig[17] specifies in his commentary on Rashi). Indeed, it is hard to think of any other reasonable justification for killing it at that stage.

Cutting the Fetus (embryotomy) or Cutting the Mother (cesarean surgery)

In order to understand the abortion debate historically, particularly when it comes to the discussions of the fetus as a pursuer, which we will next engage, we must suspend our mental imagery of modern pregnancy, which involves gynecological ultrasounds, safe obstetric clinics and other privileges of those in affluent parts of the world, and reconnect mentally to the realities of pregnancy and childbirth as our foremothers lived them in the past. Approximately seven percent of women died as a result of pregnancy and childbirth, and approximately one-fourth of mortality among women between the ages of fifteen and fifty resulted from obstetrical causes.[18] This grim situation is the daily reality of millions of women from sub-Saharan Africa to Nepal.[19]

In the previous section, we have seen that the two most prominent medieval authorities, Rashi and Maimonides, offered somewhat different wording to explain the law on difficult birth. Many commentators study this issue as a dispute between Rashi and Maimonides. According to Rashi, the fetus "is not a soul";[20] if the mother is a "soul," and the fetus is not, her life easily takes precedence over its life, even if it is not a "persecutor." According to Maimonides, the fetus "is a soul"—otherwise, there would be no need to invoke the law permitting the elimination of a persecutor.[21]

If we follow this line of thinking historically, we inevitably find the source of the contemporary debate on the moral standing of the fetus, and whether it is a person, in the heart of Jewish medieval scholasticism. Followers of Maimonides would assume that the fetus is a person and consequently would permit abortion *only* for the sake of saving the life of the mother from a direct threat originating from the fetus, whereas Rashi' s followers would not consider the fetus a person and consequently would be receptive to abortion for other reasons, including the maternal sense of suffering and shame described in the case of a woman sentenced to death.[22]

In my view, a close reading of both texts yields clues indicating that both rabbis are working within the paradigm of self-defense. Once the woman has sat down on the birthstool and the fetus has moved from its place, "it is another body." At that point, the image of the fetus as persecutor becomes much more concrete—we can conceptualize one entity moving against the life of another. Indeed, a literal translation of Rashi's work would be: "it has uprooted from its place and is moving forward."[23] Such conceptualization of the process of labor is in line with the contemporary philosophical literature on self-defense. Those authors who endorse killing the innocent in self-defense do so only if the so-called "aggressor" constitutes an *active threat* (e.g., moving toward the victim) and not merely a passive bystander.[24]

Even though Rashi's words fit smoothly into a self-defense paradigm, we must ask why, unlike Maimonides, he does not simply resort to that argument, but rather sees the need to focus on the non-personhood status of the fetus. Some commentators seem to think that Rashi's addition is necessary, pointing out that the analogy between childbirth and other situations of self-defense is not compelling.[25] But it is evident that Maimonides regards the fetus as a typical aggressor.

I would argue that the law of the *Mishna* on the dismemberment of fetuses during "difficult labor" necessitates *both* paradigms—the one on self-defense and the one on the non-person status of the fetus—because, ultimately, Jewish law not only permits but mandates the death of the "persecuting" fetus. The legal paradigm of self-defense typically creates only *permission* or an *excuse* to kill. In Common Law, a similar defense is known as the "defense of necessity."[26] But the *Mishna* does not describe this situation as calling for an excuse for a doctor or mother who elects to kill the fetus; rather, it prescribes a positive duty to kill the aggressor. A duty to kill more properly applies in Jewish law to *non-human* "aggressors"; for example, the Talmud clearly mandates the destruction of property that threatens human life.[27] Even though the fetus is not "property," Rashi reminds us that it is also not a person.

Notes

1. This is possibly due to the influence of the laws on self-defense, which, until today, take one of either two formats—the "proportionality principle" (weighing the interest at risk against the harm done during the act of defense or diversion of harm) and the "discrete" (holding that any unjust infringement of a basic right merits repulsion by the mildest means necessary, regardless of the consequences to the aggressor). G. P. Fletcher, *Proportionality and the Psychotic Aggressor: A Vignette in Comparative Criminal Theory,* 8 ISRAEL L. REV. 367 (1973).
2. Maimonides, Mishneh Torah, Hilkhoth Ishut 21, 11 (Hebrew).
3. For a discussion, *see* AVRAHAM SOFER AVRAHAM, NISHMATHH AVRAHAM, YOREH D'EA vol. B, 66 (Falk-Schlesinger Inst. 1985) (Hebrew).
4. AVRAHAM SOFER AVRAHAM, 5 NISHMATH AVRAHAM, ORAH HAIM § 330 (Falk Schlesinger Inst. 1997) (Hebrew). The woman is anyhow entitled to no-fault divorce, but this idea bears educational value (the construction of the role of a pious wife) and pecuniary consequences (divorce without a good reason, may cost her money).
5. In the case of "the pregnant woman who smelled [food and was seized by cravings] on Yom Kippur." Talmud, Yoma 82a, . . . the Shulhan Arukh stipulates: "[If] a pregnant woman smelled [food], they whisper in her ear that it is Yom Kippur. If she calms down when she remembers that, this is best; and if she does not, they feed her." Shulhan Arukh, Orah Haim 617:2. According to Rashi on *Yoma,* it is the fetus which craves and the fetus which becomes persuaded (not to eat), and it may even persecute her with its cravings.
6. *See* Talmud, Yoma 82a.
7. Mishnah, Oholoth 7:6.
8. Rashi on Talmud, Sanhedrin 72b.
9. [Talmud, Arakhin, 7a. According to the physiology of the time, labor begins when the fetus becomes detached from its "place" in the womb and embarks on its journey as "another body." From this stage on, it must not be allowed to perish along with its mother.]
10. Rashi on Talmud, Arakhin, 7a.
11. Maimonides, Mishneh Torah, Hilchoth Rotzei'ah 1:9.

12. *Id.* at l :6. A few rabbis try to argue that it is forbidden to kill an innocent persecutor person (as opposed to a fetus whose birth has not been completed) *unless* the persecution is direct such as in the case of a rapist jumping on a victim. U. Jungreis, *Organ Donations for the Sake of Saving Life,* 3 Atereth Shlomo 214-24 (1998) (Hebrew). Similar interpretations are given in the names of Rabbi Auerbach and Rabbi Haim of Brisk. I have found only one rabbinic source who objects to the killing of an innocent persecutor. I. Schepansky, *Studies in the Laws of Persecutor,* 20 (69(1)) OR HA-MIZRAH 15 (1971) (Hebrew). SAUL NATHANSON, RESPONSA SHO'EL U'MESHIV, Pt. 2, Mark 50 (4th ed. Lemberg 1877) (Hebrew). This responsum, however, restricts the permission to kill the persecutor only to the persecuted person.

13. One possible exception is Lamproneti (Italy, eighteenth cent.). Elsewhere I have argued that his discussion is not relevant to abortion. Y. Michael Barilan, *The Sorrows of her Body takes Precedence: Induced Abortions in Halakhah and in Israeli Law, in* THE RIGHT TO LIFE WITH NO MALFORMATIONS 81 (J. Davis & A. Sahar eds., Dionon 2007) (Hebrew).

14. [Joseph Trani, Responsa Maharit, Pt. A, Mark 97. While the condemned mother is alive, Rabbi Joseph of Trani is even more lenient in permitting abortion "because of its mother's need." He notes, "And there is no vacillation whatsoever on the grounds of loss of souls." *Id.* at Mark 99.]

15. I. Shor, *Responsa "Koah Shor,"* Pt. l, Mark 20 (Cracow 1903) (Hebrew).

16. *Id.*

17. See M. L. Zweig, *On Abortion,* 1 NOAM 37, 45, 56 (1964) (Hebrew).

18. Robert Schofield, *Did the Mothers Really Die? Three Centuries of Maternal Mortality in "The World We Have Lost," in* THE WORLD WE HAVE GAINED: HISTORIES OF POPULATION AND SOCIAL STRUCTURE 231 (Lloyd Bonfield et. al, eds., Basil Blackwell Ltd. 1986); Vincent De Brouwere, *The Comparative Study of Maternal Mortality Over Time: The Role of the Professionalisation of Childbirth,* 20 SOC. HIST. MED. 541 (2007); EDWARD SHORTER, A HISTORY OF WOMEN'S BODIES ch. 7, 160–64 (Basic Books 1982).

19. Kenneth Hill et al., *Estimates of Maternal Mortality Worldwide Between 1990 and 2005: An Assessment of Available Data,* 370 LANCET 1311 (2007).

20. Rashi, *supra* note [10].

21. Maimonides, *supra* note [11].

22. In another place, Rashi takes a more lenient ruling in a debate on bastard fetuses supporting his position by the assumption that they are not persons ("souls"). Rashi & Tosafoth, *"Me'ube'ret atzmo"* on Talmud, Sotta 26a (Hebrew).

23. Rashi on Talmud, Arakhin 7a. This is also the reading of H. O. Grodzinsky, *Responsa " Ahi'ezer,"* Pt. 3, Mark 72 (early twentieth cent., Vilnius) (Hebrew).

24. Larry Alexander, *Self-defense, Justification and Excuse,* 22 PHIL. PUB. AFFAIRS 53–66 (1993).

25. Rabbi Jacob Shor (in the anthology of nineteenth-century *Responsa Teshuvot Ge'onim Batrai,* Mark 45) points out that Maimonides' exact words were "like a persecutor" and not "a persecutor." On the other hand, it should be recalled that Maimonides cites "the woman having difficulty in childbirth" as a paradigmatic case of the law permitting the execution of a persecutor, which is part of the law of murderers. The *halakhic* ruling given by Maimonides starts with the word "Accordingly."

26. A. W. Brian Simpson, *Cannibalism and the Common Law* (Univ. Chi. Press 1984).

27. Talmud, Baba Kamma 117b.

28

Abortion in Jewish Thought:
A Study in Casuistry

Dena S. Davis

Holding a JD and a PhD in religion, Dena Davis teaches bioethics with
an interest in religion and law at Lehigh University. She has published
widely on reproductive and other biomedical ethics, legal issues related
to medical decisions, and Jewish bioethics. This essay on abortion,
written by Davis in 1992, still stands as a clear explication of the casuistry
in traditional Jewish halakhah (legal writings). Casuistry is a type of
ethical reasoning that appeals to cases (rather than moral principles) and
then argues analogically to apply past precedents to a new ethical
dilemma. Davis analyzes the interpretative and subjective nature of this
casuistry approach in Jewish rulings on miscarriage and abortion.

Casuistry—the mode of ethical reasoning that focuses on paradigm cases
rather than principles—has been lately rehabilitated. In 1982, Toulmin
pointed to a shift in medical ethics away from relating cases to general
ethical theories, and toward "direct analysis of the practical cases themselves,
using methods more like that of traditional 'case morality'" (749). More
recently, Jonsen and Toulmin have produced a monumental work on the
uses of casuistry. Their basic claim is that "the primary locus of moral
understanding [lies] in the recognition of *paradigmatic examples* of good
and evil, right and wrong." In other words, *"moral knowledge is essentially
particular*, so that sound resolutions of moral problems must always be
rooted in a concrete understanding of specific cases and circumstances" (330,
emphasis in original). They distinguish this claim from the weaker assertion

Source: Dena S. Davis, "Abortion in Jewish Thought: A Study in Casuistry," *Journal of the American
Academy of Religion* 60, no. 2 (1992): 313–24.

that casuistry is unavoidable because general principles must eventually be applied to actual cases.

My position is that cases are more than clever teaching tools or devices to spice up an otherwise dry discussion. While moral knowledge is particular, in that we must act in particular instances, I still want to argue that ethics is grounded in universal principles. I take an intermediate tack: Cases are powerful influences on our ethical thinking, which shape our understanding of principles at the same time that those principles inform our understanding of cases.

. . .

One tradition in which casuistry has always been central is the *halakha* that provides the structure of ethical and legal thinking in the Orthodox and Conservative Jewish communities (and at least the "background music" for the Reform movement as well). This essay examines the role played by casuistry in the discussion of abortion within the halakhic tradition.

. . .

The passage in Exodus is the most authoritative because it is biblical rather than rabbinic. It reads:

> If men strive, and wound a pregnant woman so that her fruit be expelled, but no harm befall [her], then shall he be fined. But if harm befall [her], then shalt thou give life for life. (Feldman 1974:254)

In this case, accidentally causing a woman to miscarry is a civil injury, and the perpetrator must pay a fine. But accidentally killing the woman is a criminal case, and the wrongdoer is subject to death. The fetus is not considered a *nefesh adam* (human person) in Jewish law at any stage in pregnancy (Green 1985a:260; Feldman 1974:253-4). Unlike the woman, the fetus has neither the moral nor juridical status of a person. Consequently, when the woman's life is endangered by pregnancy or childbirth, she has the right to protect herself by destroying the fetus. In halakha this is not only her right but her obligation because the duty to protect one's life and health outweighs all others (the principle of *pikuach nefesh*) (Feldman 1986:26-7).

The Exodus passage does not imply that fetal life is held lightly as if it were simply property. David Bleich speaks for the tradition when he says (35), "Judaism regards all forms of human life as sacred . . . Fetal life is regarded as precious and may not be destroyed wantonly." Judaism holds that human life is intrinsically sacred because humans are created in God's image. Sherwin (175) identifies three claims of Jewish theology regarding human life: that each person is unique, that each human life is therefore irreplaceable, and that because of that unique and irreplaceable character, each human life "embodies intrinsic sanctity." Furthermore, when a fetus is destroyed, *its* possible offspring are destroyed as well (Feldman 1974:285).

Thus, the Exodus passage on the one hand, and the intense concern for the preservation of human life on the other, set the ontological boundaries within which halakhists can make decisions. Within these boundaries cases exert their gravitational pull, governing the ebb and flow of argument, as halakhists make their points by orienting specific questions to paradigmatic cases. The passage in *Mishnah Oholot* reads as follows:

> If a woman is having difficulty giving birth, one cuts up the fetus within her and takes it out limb by limb because her life takes precedence over its life. Once its greater part has emerged, you do not touch it, because you may not set aside one life for another. (Biale 1984: 221)

This passage presents the paradigm case to which the principles inferred from the Exodus narrative are applied. The mother's life is threatened (however innocently) by the fetus. Since we know from Exodus that the fetus is not a *nefesh* and can never be preferred over the mother, it follows that the fetus must be destroyed to protect her. The second half of the passage is puzzling, because it is impossible to imagine a situation to which it would apply. If the head has emerged (or its larger part, in the case of a breech presentation) the mother's life may still be in danger, but not in any way that would be diminished by destroying the fetus. The second half of the passage describes a null set, even in ancient times. The practical result is, "An abortion must be performed any time it is necessary, and may not be performed in those instances in which it would be pointless in any case." So the thrust of this passage, as it relates to abortion, is to remind us of the absolute precedence of the woman's life.

There are certain principles for which this case stands. It would be impossible to tug the case in a radically different direction, for example to argue that fetal life has a claim equal to the mother's. But within its directional thrust, there are many interpretive moves to be made. What is meant by "difficulty in childbirth," i.e. what kinds of threats are serious enough to come under the rubric of this case? A wide range of interpretation is possible. Even Immanuel Jakobovits, one of the most conservative commentators, states that the threat to the mother need not be either immediate or absolutely certain (130). Further, a grave psychological threat is considered by many decisors to be as weighty as a physical hazard (Jakobovits:124; Feldman 1974:287).

. . .

Rabbi Uziel, a twentieth-century halakhist, uses this precedent to argue for a very lenient view (Feldman 1974: 291):

> It is clear that abortion is not permitted without reason. That would be destructive and frustrative of the possibility of life. But for a *reason*, even if it is a *slim reason*, such as to prevent her *nivvul* [disgrace], then we have precedent and authority to permit it.

. . .

These cases all point to the centrality of the subjective experience of the individual sufferer. This is a felicitous point at which to end this part of my essay, for I wish to move now to a discussion of the role of subjectivity in halakhic reasoning.

As we shall see, the roles of subjectivity and of analogy are well recognized by some modern scholars of halakha. The issue that has been ignored, however, is the interaction between subjectivity, analogy, and the identity of the interpreters themselves. If one part of the community has been left out of the interpretive process, there is a good reason to question the credibility of the results.

To argue casuistically is to argue analogically. We take the case before us, sort out its component parts, and attempt to find its geographical place in the "moral taxomony." Is this case more "like" this precedent-narrative, or more "like" that one? In issues of bioethics, we are dealing with emotions and with uncertainty. Thus, analogic argument is necessarily subjective.

. . .

Louis E. Newman, in an extremely perceptive essay, argues that most contemporary halakhists make the error of assuming that the texts virtually interpret themselves, with the decisors acting almost like passive conduits, and the "right" answers a foregone conclusion. In fact, as he shows, the role of interpretation cannot be ignored.

> All contemporary Jewish authorities look to the same body of literature as a source of precedents, that is, they are committed to the same canon. All would acknowledge that the history of previous interpretation of these sources must be given some weight and that the principles embodied in these sources (and not merely the words of the texts themselves) must be interpreted. It is within these parameters that each interpreter works, rendering a personal, but constrained and therefore objective, judgment as to the meaning of these texts when applied to a contemporary moral problem. (Newman:32)

. . .

If one accepts Newman's approach, it follows that different people, with radically different experiences and status in a society, may very well have different "interpretive assumptions" that will be reflected in the "conclusions we draw." Newman focuses on the difficulty of applying ancient texts to the modem dilemmas posed by medical technology. But there is a deeper, prior problem: *who* is allowed into the interpretive process and whose subjective experience is to count? Newman, Green and other liberal critics fail to notice that women have been excluded almost completely from the halakhic process (Davis). Just as, in American law, feminist jurisprudence and critical race theory present the view that excluding women and people of color from casuistic scholarship has resulted in an ideological interpretation of law that reflects the bias of white males who flourish under the *status quo,* so I argue that in a culture as powerfully gender-oriented as Judaism, it is reasonable to assume that the body of law would be different had women been part of the interpretive process.

One example will serve to highlight the problem. In Jewish law, the Biblical commandment "Be fruitful and multiply" is understood to apply to men but not to women. This talmudic ruling allows women greater latitude in birth control devices and family planning than is allowed to men. Rachel Biale comments:

> Although the exact rational for this exemption is only alluded to, it is clear that the Rabbis felt it necessary not to require women to do something that "puts their lives on the line." The Rabbis were concerned primarily with the physical dangers of childbirth, but they were also aware of the emotional and social dimensions: the way in which women's lives were devoted to and determined by childbearing. (1988:28)

Biale's comment raises a number of questions. If the Rabbis' "awareness" of the emotional and social dimensions of childbearing played a part in their decisions, one can only wonder if that awareness might have been even more sensitive, more accurate, if some of the Rabbis had been women. Perhaps women view the burdens of childrearing very differently than do men; perhaps they would take different emotional and social factors into account or weigh them differently. (Perhaps they might want to limit their number of progeny so as to give women the time and energy to become talmudic scholars!) Our contemporary awareness of the exclusion of female scholars at the time of talmudic rulings on contraception causes us to question whether the rulings might not be the products of a flawed process. Thus, we wonder if a contemporary reevaluation of the various rulings on contraception might not be in order. The halakhic debate, we suspect, would result in a more sensitive set of decisions today, if women and their interpretations were part of the discussion. But then we confront the reality that few women have been trained to be Talmudic scholars and that there is still intense male resistance to sharing with women this most powerful role in Jewish culture.

In other words, halakhic reasoning is analogical, interpretive and ineluctably subjective, but only half the people expected to adhere to it are allowed into the process. This presents problems for its credibility both within and without its own community. True, decisors are enjoined to take women's suffering into account, even to put it first, but it is male "understanding" of female experiences, percolated through the male experience of Jewish culture in which they occupy a very different position. To say that all interpretation is ideological is not to say that women's is any less so, but only to make the point that a casuistic enterprise which invited all its constituents into the process has a better chance of arriving at fair and sensitive conclusions.

Within the community, as women begin to challenge their exclusion from the study and interpretation of halakhah, they inevitably question the credibility of rulings handed down by a male rabbinate which speaks *to* them rather than *with* them. Blu Greenberg (1976:204) describes even her very orthodox community as one in which few Jews look to rabbinic leadership on matters of contraception, family size, and abortion. Greenberg (1981:9-10) asserts that halakhic education is the single most important area for the equalization of women in Judaism.

. . .

Greenberg (1976:204-206), who struggles with the question of whether it is possible to be a traditional Jew and a feminist, imagines a halakha that would broaden the interpretation of therapeutic abortion, "to extend the principle of precedence of the mother's actual life and health to include serious regard for the quality of life as well." Factors she would consider include the need to support herself or her husband through school, overwhelming responsibilities to existing children, and so on. From the Jewish emphasis on love and sexuality as positive values, Greenberg draws the conclusion that abortion might be acceptable for the wife who becomes pregnant before the couple has a chance to develop a good relationship. Greenberg's suggestions are so "liberal" that it is difficult to imagine that they could persuade commentators like Bleich or Jakobowits. But that is not the point. If women were trained in the halakhah and invited to be full participants in the interpretive process, their voices would be part of the discussion. If women's experiences of childbearing and childraising were part of the halakhic data, taken on their own terms and not mediated through male sensibilities, then the results would be more credible to the women (and men) who are expected to live by them.

References

Biale, Rachel 1984 *Women and Jewish Law*. New York: Shocken Books.

Biale, Rachel 1988 "Abortion in Jewish Law." *Tikkun* 4:26–28.

Bleich, J. David 1979 "Abortion in Halakhic literature." In *Jewish Bioethics*, 134–177. Ed. by Fred Rosner and J. David Bleich. New York: Hebrew Publishing Company.

Feldman, David 1974 *Marital Relations, Abortion and Birth Control in Jewish Law*. New York: New York University Press.

Feldman, David 1986 *Health and Medicine in the Jewish Tradition*. New York: The Crossroad Publishing Company.

Green, Ronald M. 1985a "Contemporary Jewish bioethics: a critical assessment." In *Theory and Bioethics*, 245–266. Ed. by E. E. Shelp. Amsterdam: D. Reidel Publishing Company, 1985.

Greenberg, Blu 1981 *On Women and Judaism: A View from Tradition*. Philadelphia: The Jewish Publication Society of America.

Greenberg, Blu 1976 "Abortion: a challenge to halakhah." *Judaism* 201–208.

Jakobovits, Immanuel 1979 "Jewish views on abortion." In Jewish Bioethics, 118–133. Ed. by Fred Rosner and J. David Bleich. New York: Hebrew Publishing Company.

Jonsen, Albert and Toulmin, Stephen 1988 *The Abuse of Casuistry: A History of Moral Reasoning*. Berkeley: University of California Press.

Newman, Louis E. 1990 "Woodchoppers and respirators: the problem of interpretation in contemporary Jewish ethics." *Modern Judaism* 10 (1990): 17–42.

Sherwin, Byron 1990 *In Partnership with God: Contemporary Jewish Law and Ethics*. Syracuse, NY: Syracuse University Press.

Toulmin, Stephen 1982 "How medicine saved the life of ethics." *Perspectives in Biology and Medicine* 25 (Summer): 746–750.

Christianity

29

The Human Embryo as Person in Catholic Teaching

Norman Ford, S.D.B.

Australian emeritus professor of Catholic moral theology and Catholic priest Norman Ford (d. 2022) taught and wrote widely on healthcare ethics. In this essay, Ford delves into the various meanings of prenatal life in Catholic moral teachings, showing that the Vatican's strong claims about protection of new human life from the moment of fertilization stand alongside its cautious reticence about pronouncing definitively when an ensouled person begins. Take note of how the Vatican documents Ford discusses weave together the language of morality and science in order to mount arguments in support of protecting life from conception.

At least from the Middle Ages until 1869 it was commonly accepted in the West that the human person did not begin until several weeks after conception. This is admitted by the Church:

> It is true that in the Middle Ages, when the opinion was generally held that the spiritual soul was not present until after the first few weeks, a distinction was made in the evaluation of the sin and the gravity of the penal sanctions . . . But it was never denied at that time that procured abortion, even during the first few days, was objectively a grave sin. This condemnation was in fact unanimous.[1]

In 1869 Pius IX, in the light of the growing consensus among scientists and philosophers, dropped these distinctions and extended the excommunication for abortion to all stages of pregnancy.[2] The view that a human individual and person begins at conception grew steadily over the next century.

Source: Norman Ford, S.D.B., "The Human Embryo as Person in Catholic Teaching," *The National Catholic Bioethics Quarterly* 1, no. 2 (2001): 155–60.

Second Vatican Council

By the time of the Second Vatican Council the original works of scholars like Karl Rahner, Peter Schoonenberg, and in English, Joseph Donceel, had begun to question whether a human individual and person begins at fertilization.[3] In its major Pastoral Constitution, *Gaudium et Spes,* the Council made the following significant statement: "Life once conceived must be protected with the utmost care; abortion and infanticide are abominable crimes."[4] It is interesting to note the previous draft of this text: "Life already conceived in the womb must be protected with the utmost care; abortion and infanticide are abominable crimes."[5] Some nineteen speakers requested that the phrase "in the womb" be deleted since the fertilized egg, even if not yet in the womb, is something sacred.[6] The document's drafting commission agreed that the fertilized egg in the fallopian tube ought to be respected and proposed the definitive text quoted above, stating that there was no intention of elaborating on when ensoulment occurs.[7]

It is obvious that the Vatican Council unequivocally declared there is a moral obligation to protect human life from conception even though it was not prepared to commit itself to any statement on precisely when the spiritual soul is creatively infused to constitute a person. The Council did not attempt to specify the meaning of conception beyond the common assumption that human life begins at fertilization. In other words, the Council taught that human life once conceived ought to be respected and protected, regardless of when the individual human person begins.

Declaration on Procured Abortion

The Church has continued to take for granted that human life and the human individual begin at fertilization. However, in the 1974 *Declaration on Procured Abortion,* footnote 19 says that it does not formally address when ensoulment occurs nor when the fruit of conception is constituted into a person. The Church was primarily interested in offering sound moral advice on the absolute due respect for human life from conception:

> This declaration expressly leaves aside the question of the moment when the spiritual soul is infused. There is not a unanimous tradition on this point and authors are as yet in disagreement. For some it dates from the first instant, for others it could not at least precede nidation. It is not within the competence

of science to decide between these two views, because the existence of an immortal soul is not a question in its field. It is a philosophical problem from which our moral affirmation remains independent. . . .[8]

It is to be noted that the question of when ensoulment occurs, and consequently of when a human person begins, pertains to the competence of philosophy and not of the biological sciences.

Donum Vitae

After the birth of Louise Brown, the first baby born through *in vitro* fertilization techniques (IVF), on 25 July 1978, IVF embryos were soon being manipulated and discarded around the world. The Church was concerned about this gross lack of respect for human embryos, and gave its first official response to new reproductive technologies in the 1987 document *Donum Vitae*.[9] Questions naturally arose about the moral status of human life in the fertilised egg or the zygote: is this human life a human individual and a person?

The Congregation for the Doctrine of the Faith openly admitted it was

. . . aware of the current debates concerning the beginning of human life, concerning the individuality of the human being and concerning the identity of the human person.[10]

The Congregation, however, found no convincing arguments in support of claims that a human person begins at any time other than conception, understood as fertilization. A line of prudent caution was adopted by the Congregation in acting on the moral principle that any reasonable doubts about the personal status of human life from conception should be resolved in practice in favor of the zygote. . . .

. . . recent findings of human biological science . . . recognize that in the zygote (the zygote is the cell resulting from the fusion of two gametes) resulting from fertilization the biological identity of a new human individual is already constituted.

Certainly no experimental datum can be in itself sufficient to bring us to the recognition of a spiritual soul; nevertheless, the conclusions of science regarding the human embryo provide a valuable indication for discerning by the use of reason a personal presence from this first appearance of a human life: how could a living human creature not be a human person? The Magisterium has not expressly committed its authority to this affirmation of a philosophical nature, but it constantly reaffirms the moral condemnation of any kind of procured abortion. . . .[11]

For practical and moral purposes, the Church teaches that the fruit of human generation, from fertilization onwards, should be treated as a personal being, but at the same time stopped short of making an express philosophical commitment to the personal status of the zygote.

Evangelium Vitae

In *Evangelium Vitae*, his 1995 encyclical letter on ethical issues concerning human life, Pope John Paul II addressed the status of early human embryo and quoted liberally from the 1974 *Declaration* and *Donum Vitae,* thereby personally endorsing the passages cited:

> . . . Even if the presence of a spiritual soul cannot be ascertained by empirical data, the results themselves of scientific research on the human embryo provide "a valuable indication for discerning by the use of reason, a personal presence at the moment of the first appearance of a human life: how could a living human creature [*vivens creatura humana*] not also [*etiam*] be a human person?"[12]
>
> Furthermore, what is at stake is so important that, from the standpoint of moral obligation, the mere probability that a person is involved would suffice to justify an absolutely clear prohibition of any intervention aimed at killing a human embryo . . . "*The human creature [creatura humana] is to be respected and treated as a person from conception;* and therefore from that same moment his rights as a person must be recognized, among which in the first place is the inviolable right of every innocent human creature [*creatura*] to life."[13]

John Paul II makes it clear that the Magisterium made no decision for or against the common opinion held for centuries that ensoulment and the beginning of the person did not occur for several weeks after conception. In *Evangelium Vitae* he teaches that scientific studies on the human embryo provide grounds to discern rationally a personal presence once human life is present in an embryo [*creatura humana*]. The Magisterium holds there are sufficient reasons to support this position and to warrant presuming its truth and to treat human embryos as persons, that is, with absolute moral respect in private life and in public policy. Hence the Magisterium speaks and writes about human embryos as though they were persons.

The use of the Latin term for *man or human being* in Church documents is *homo*. The theory of "delayed hominization" refers to the human person being formed when the spiritual soul is created within the embryo at some time after conception. In the 1974 *Declaration* the term *homo*, however, is used to refer to the fruit of human generation both before and after animation by a spiritual soul. It says that it suffices that

> this presence of the soul be probable (and one can never prove the contrary) in order that the taking of life involve accepting the risk of killing a man [*homo*], not only waiting for, but already in possession of his soul.[14]

A biological human organism is a human entity, but cannot be a person if a spiritual soul has not yet been created within to constitute a personal being. The Pope did not use the term *homo* in this context and instead spoke of a personal presence in a "human creature."

. . .

While there are good reasons to believe the early human embryo is an individual and person from conception, it is difficult to establish this with the certitude required for the Church to formally teach this. The Church has a duty to protect human embryos, but not to the detriment of the truth. The Church cannot teach something to be true unless the Magisterium is convinced this is so beyond reasonable doubt. Hence the Church acted wisely, neither overstating nor understating the truth based on the evidence available.

The Arguments on the Status of the Early Embryo

The Church accepts the commonly held view that a human being and person begins at fertilization when the fusion of sperm and egg gives rise to a zygote, a single-cell human embryo whose genetic individuality and uniqueness remain unchanged during normal development. Cell divisions and differentiation are programmed for the organization and growth of the same developing human individual already present in the zygote. From conception, the ongoing unity of the embryo is demonstrated by its unidirectional development and growth as one and the same living human being. According to this account the zygote is an actual human person and not simply a potential human person in much the same way as an infant is an actual human person with potential to develop to maturity. This view is simple, easy to grasp, and is supported by eminent scientists and philosophers.

This position may be coherent but not necessarily true. A fetus, with its millions of cells, is definitely an organized human individual with potential for further development as the same living individual. But is the fetus the same organized living individual as the zygote? Put another way, when the zygote divides during normal development to form two cells, do we have a *two-cell individual* or simply two individual cells? Each of the first two cells has its own organization, nutrients, and life cycle. It seems more likely that there are just two distinct cells even though their membranes touch each other. If this is so, it is hard to claim that the first two or four cells already constitute one organized human individual and person.

It can be replied, however, that the genetic code of the zygote, which is purposefully programmed to produce a human individual, is found in each of the first two cells and then four cells, and so on. This would mean that the genetic code of these early cells work in tandem from the first division onwards to continue to form a human individual.

To this it can be replied that the genetic code is first programmed to produce the external membranes and only then does it form a definitive, organized human individual (or two in the case of identical twins). In short, it can be argued, the presence of the genetic code itself does not suffice to constitute a human individual, but that only its activation does, whereby specialized cells and membranes are produced to form and enclose an organized human individual about fourteen days after fertilization. If this argument is accepted, fertilization is not the beginning of the development *of* the human individual but the beginning of the formative process and development *into* one (or more human individuals). Ultimately this issue cannot be resolved in the first instance by appealing to the teaching of the Church, but only by reflection and critical analysis on all the relevant scientific information interpreted in the light of sound philosophical principles.

Respect Due to Human Embryos

In the meantime, the Church rightly stands firm on the principle that the fruit of human generation, the *creatura humana* of Pope John Paul II, is morally inviolable from conception and human embryos should be treated as persons. The obligation to show moral respect for human embryos is a profoundly human insight and reflects the respect due to our *shared humanity*. It arises in the heart and mind—not only from religious sources.

We have a moral duty to protect human embryos, but no dominion over embryonic human life. We should not settle for the reductionism that sees embryonic human life as no more than mere genetic material, devoid of significance and value. Ethical respect for human embryos should take precedence over pragmatic and utilitarian considerations.

Notes

1. S. Congregation for the Doctrine of the Faith, *Declaration on Procured Abortion, Acta Apostolicae Sedis* 66 (1974), n. 7; for more historical details see Norman Ford, *When Did I Begin? Conception of the Human Individual in History, Philosophy and Science* (Cambridge: University Press, 1991) 28–59.
2. Ford, ibid., 58.
3. Ibid., 51–52 for references: Karl Rahner, *Theological Investigations*, Vol. 9 (London: Darton, Longman & Todd, 1972) 226, 236; Peter Schoonenberg, *God's World in the Making* (Dublin: Gill and Son, 1965), 49–50; Joseph Donceel, "Immediate Animation and Delayed Hominization," *Theological Studies* 31 (1970) 76–105.
4. Pastoral Constitution, *Gaudium et Spes*, 51.
5. *Acta Synodalia Sacrosanti Concillii Oecumenici Vaticani II*, Vol. IV, Pars VI, (Rome: Vatican Polyglot Press, 1978) 478 (my translation).
6. *Acta Synodalia Sacrosanti Concilii Oecumenici Vaticani II*, Vol. IV, Pars VII, (Rome:Vatican Polyglot Press, 1978) 501.
7. *Ibid., 501.*
8. *Declaration on Procured Abortion*, footnote 19.
9. *L'Osservatore Romano*, 11 March 1987, Supplement. The Latin text was published in *Acta Apostolicae Sedis* 80 (12 Jan. 1988) 70–102.
10. *Donum Vitae*, I,1.
11. Instruction *Donum Vitae*, I,1.
12. *Donum Vitae* I,1.
13. Pope John Paul II, *Encyclical Letter, Evangelium Vitae*, (Vatican City: Libreria Editrice Vaticana, 1995) n. 60. See also Ford, *When Did I Begin?* 68–84.
14. *Declaration* n. 19: for the Latin text see *Acta Apostolicae Sedis* (1974) 738. n. 19.

30

Aquinas's Account of Human Embryogenesis and Recent Interpretations

Jason T. Eberl

Jason Eberl is a professor of healthcare ethics. In this essay, he displays the ongoing significance of the thought of medieval theologian Thomas Aquinas in Catholic debates about personhood and the ethics of abortion. This excerpt gives a summary of Aquinas' view of embryogenesis, followed by Eberl's critique of the position of another Thomist scholar (Robert Pasnau), who reads Aquinas as favoring delayed hominization. Eberl claims that current embryological science supports the idea of ensoulment at conception.

In addressing bioethical issues at the beginning of human life, such as abortion, *in vitro* fertilization, and embryonic stem cell research, one primary concern is to establish when a developing human embryo or fetus can be considered a *person*; for it is generally held that only persons are the subjects of rights, such as a "right to life." An important metaphysical viewpoint to consider in this regard is that of the 13ᵗʰ century philosopher and theologian, Thomas Aquinas.

. . .

Aquinas argues that all human beings are persons (*Summa theologiae* [ST] IIIa 16.12.*ad* 1), but that an embryo or fetus is not a human being until

Source: Jason T. Eberl, "Aquinas's Account of Human Embryogenesis and Recent Interpretations," *Journal of Medicine and Philosophy* 30, no. 4 (2005): 379–94.

its body is informed by a *rational soul*.[1] Aquinas's explicit account of human embryogenesis has been generally rejected by contemporary scholars due to its dependence upon medieval biological data, which has been far surpassed by current scientific research. Aquinas, following Aristotle, understands conception to involve male semen acting upon female menstrual blood to form an embryo; semen is the *agent* of conception and the female contribution is simply the matter that *passively* receives semen's activity to be formed into an embryo (ST Ia 118.1.*ad* 4; Aristotle, *De generatione animalium* [DGA] II 3, 736a24-737b6). The contemporary understanding of conception characterizes *both* the male and female gametes—sperm and ovum instead of semen and menstrual blood—as active components insofar as each contribute half the genetic code that serves as the formal and efficient cause of an embryo's formation.

A number of scholars, however, have attempted to combine Aquinas's basic metaphysical account of human nature with current embryological data to develop a contemporary Thomistic account of a human being's beginning.[2] The issue at hand in developing such an account is the distinction between "immediate"—when fertilization of an ovum by a sperm cell is complete— and "delayed"—sometime after fertilization—*hominization*. The term "hominization" refers to when a developing embryo first has a specifically "human" rational soul as its substantial form, that is, organizing principle.[3] The debate among scholars who argue for either immediate or delayed hominization centers on the application of Aquinas's metaphysical principle that only an *appropriate* body may be informed by a rational soul to constitute a human being. Those who favor immediate hominization, such as Benedict Ashley (1976), claim that there is nothing about the biological nature of a human embryo from the moment the process of fertilization is complete that disallows its being informed by a rational soul. This account purports to satisfy the above Thomistic principle while denying Aquinas's own conclusion, based on the embryological data at his disposal, that an early embryo's body is not appropriate for being informed by a rational soul; I will elaborate on Aquinas's principle and conclusion in the following section.

Scholars who favor delayed hominization, such as Joseph Donceel (1970), Robert Pasnau (2002), and Norman Ford (1988), argue that there are certain intrinsic qualities of an early embryo which indicate that it is not an "individual substance of a rational nature"[4] until it reaches a certain point in its biological development.

. . .

Aquinas's account of human embryogenesis begins with his understanding of a human being as constituted by a rational soul informing a material body (Eberl, 2004). In defining the necessary and sufficient conditions for something to be informed by a soul—which may be either vegetative, sensitive, or rational[5]—Aquinas first notes Aristotle's definition of "soul" as "the actuality of a physical organic body having life potentially" (ST Ia 76.4. *ad* 1; cf. Aristotle, *De anima* [DA] II 1, 412a20-2). Aquinas then asserts that "such potentiality does not reject the soul" (ST Ia 76.4.*ad* 1). Aquinas explains this definition and assertion as follows:

> It is said that the soul is the actuality of a body, etc., because through the soul it is a body, is organic, and has life potentially. But the first actuality is said to be in potentiality with respect to the second actuality, which is the operation. For such a potentiality does not reject, that is, does not exclude the soul (ST Ia 76.4.*ad* 1; cf. *In Aristotelis librum De anima commentarium* [In DA] II 2).

Aquinas holds that a soul's potentiality to perform its definitive operations—whether life, sensation, or rational thought—is necessary for it to exist (*Quaestio disputata de anima* [QDA] XII.*ad* 7). The actualization of such potentiality, however, is *accidental* to the soul's existence: "To be actually thinking or sensing is not substantial being, but accidental" (QDA XII).

Of course, a developing human embryo or fetus, and even a newborn infant, does not actually exercise all the operations proper to a human being, including rational activity. Nonetheless, Aquinas denies that this lack implies that a rational soul does not inform the matter of a developing human embryo, fetus, or newborn infant. All that is required for the presence of a rational soul, and thus the existence of a human being, is a human body that has the potentiality for the operations proper to a rational soul:

> If a human being derives his species by being rational and having an intellect, whoever is within the human species is rational and has an intellect. But a child, even before leaving the womb, is within the human species; although there are yet no phantasms in it that are actually intelligible (*Summa contra Gentiles* [SCG] II 59).

Concerning the question of when the potentiality for the operations proper to a rational soul is first present in a developing human body, Aquinas asserts that a body must have the proper *organic structure* if it is to have a rational soul as its substantial form: "Since the soul is the act of an organic body, before the body has organs in any way whatever, it cannot be receptive of the soul" (*Quaestiones disputatae de potentia dei* [QDP] III 12). The appropriate organs for a rational soul are those associated with sensation, because it is through sensation of particular things that the mind comes to possess intelligible forms, which are the natures of things understood as abstracted from any particular material conditions (ST Ia 84.6; Eberl, 2004; Stump, 2003, pp. 244-76; Pasnau, 2002, pp. 278-95, 310-29; Kretzmann, 1999, pp. 350-64). The abstraction of intelligible forms from the products of sensation—the "phantasms" referred to in the above passage from SCG—is the essence of rational thought as Aquinas defines it: "Therefore, the rational soul ought to be united to a body which may be a suitable organ of sensation" (ST Ia 76.5; cf. ST Ia 55.2). This understanding leads Aquinas to develop an account of *successive ensoulment* in a human embryo's formation. After conception—the action of semen upon menstrual blood—occurs, a material body exists that has a vegetative soul as its substantial form, i.e., an entity that has life at its most basic level. As the early embryo develops and its organic structure increases in complexity to the point where it can support sensitive operations, the embryo's vegetative soul is annihilated and its matter is informed by a sensitive soul. Since, according to Aquinas, a thing's identity is determined by its having the same substantial form (Eberl, 2004), the early vegetative embryo has ceased to exist and a new embryo has come into existence that is an animal life form, due to its having the capacity for sensation.

The final stage of embryonic development occurs when the embryo has developed to a point where it has a sufficiently complex organic structure to allow for rational operations.[6] At this point, the sensitive soul is annihilated and the animal embryo goes out of existence as its matter becomes informed by a rational soul.

. . .

Pasnau (2002, p. 115) argues that a zygote or early embryo does not have an active potentiality for rational thought by asserting that Aquinas defines an active potentiality as having a capacity in hand to perform some action, and thereby denies that a natural potentiality, as defined above by Kretzmann, is a type of active potentiality. Pasnau utilizes a distinction between an assembled hammer, which has a capacity in hand to drive nails, versus unassembled pieces of metal and wood, which lack a capacity in hand to drive nails. In the first case, no further change is required to the hammer's constitution in order for it actually to drive nails; whereas, in the second case, an external agent must assemble the metal and wood pieces for them to have a capacity in hand to drive nails. Pasnau concludes that a zygote or early embryo is akin to the unassembled parts of a hammer. It has only a passive potentiality to develop into an organism with a capacity in hand for rational thought.

Pasnau is correct in holding that, for Aquinas, if the development of a zygote or early embryo depends upon the assembling powers of some external agent, then it does not have an active internal principle for developing into a being that actually thinks rationally. It thus would have merely a passive potentiality for rational thought and could not be considered as informed by a rational soul. Contemporary genetic understanding, however, indicates that a zygote or early embryo has an active internal principle guiding its development into a being that actually thinks rationally; it has an active potentiality for rational thought in the sense of a natural potentiality. A zygote or early embryo is not akin to the unassembled pieces of a hammer; while such pieces depend upon an external agent to assemble them in the proper fashion, a zygote or early embryo has no such need. Given a supportive environment—one that provides simply nutrition, oxygen, and protection from harmful external influences—a zygote or early embryo will develop into a being that has a capacity in hand for rational thought and that actually thinks rationally. That the actualization of this natural potentiality requires time and internal development does not count against its being an active potentiality.

. . .

I conclude that the interpretations offered by . . . Pasnau, while they closely follow what Aquinas explicitly says concerning embryogenesis, do not correctly take account of the role Aquinas's nuanced concept of "active potentiality" plays in defining the nature of a zygote or early embryo in the light of contemporary genetic understanding. Evidence that a zygote or early embryo has an active internal principle guiding its ordered natural development into a being that actually thinks rationally is sufficient, I contend, to conclude that it is already a rational being. It has an active potentiality for rational thought and is thus informed by a rational soul.

Notes

1. All translations of Aquinas's works are my own and, for the most part, are taken from the Leonine critical edition published by the Vatican (Commissio Leonina, 1882–). The following are editions of Aquinas's works cited in this article that have not yet appeared in the Leonine critical edition: Cathala & Spiazzi (1950), Mandonnet & Moos (1929–1947), and Spiazzi (1949a,b).

2. Since Aquinas holds that all human beings are persons, I will utilize the terms "human being" and "person" interchangeably.
3. As a substantial form, a human rational soul is responsible for (1) the existence of a human being, (2) the actualization of the matter composing a human being, and (3) the unity of existence and activity in a human being (SCG II 68; In DA II 2).
4. This is Aquinas's definition of "person," which applies to, among others types of beings, a body informed by a rational soul (ST Ia 29.1). This definition of "person" was originally formulated by Boethius (*Contra Eutychen et Nestorium* III).
5. Following Aristotle (DA II 3, 414a29-415a13), Aquinas defines a "rational" soul as having the relevant capacities for life, sensation, and rational thought and being the type of soul proper to the human species. A "sensitive" soul, on the other hand, has the relevant capacities for only life and sensation, and is the type of soul proper to all non-human species of the animal genus. A "vegetative" soul has the relevant capacities for only life and is proper to all non-animal living organisms.
6. Since, according to Aquinas, rational operations do not require the use of a bodily organ (QDA II), the requisite organic complexity here is that which allows for the operations of sensation and imagination such that the mind can abstract intelligible forms from phantasms.

References

Aristotle (1984). *De anima and De generatione animalium*. In J. Barnes (ed.), *The complete works of Aristotle* 2 vols Princeton, NJ: Princeton University Press.

Ashley, B. (1976). A critique of the theory of delayed hominization. In D. McCarthy & A. Moraczewski (eds.), *An ethical evaluation of fetal experimentation: An interdisciplinary study* (pp. 115–129). St. Louismo: Pope John XXIII Center.

Boethius (1918). Contra Eutychen et Nestorium. In H.F. Stewart, E.K. Rand, and S.J.Tester (trans.), *Tractates and the consolation of philosophy*. Cambridge, MA: Harvard University Press.

Cathala, R. & Spiazzi, R. (eds.) (1950). *In duodecim libros metaphysicorum Aristotelis expositio*. Turin: Marietti.

Commissio Leonina (ed.) (1882–). *S. Thomae Aquinatis Doctoris Angelici Opera Omnia*. Rome: Vatican Polyglot Press.

Donceel, J. (1970). Immediate animation and delayed hominization. *Theological Studies*, 31(1), 76–105.

Eberl, J.T. (2004). Aquinas on the nature of human beings. *Review of Metaphysics*, 58(2), 333–365.

Ford, N. (1988). *When did I begin? Conception of the human individual in history, philosophy and science*. New York: Cambridge University Press.

Kretzmann, N. (1999). *The metaphysics of creation: Aquinas's natural theology in* Summa contra Gentiles II. Oxford: Clarendon Press.

Mandonnet, P. & Moos, M. (eds.) (1929–1947). *Scriptum super sententiis magistri Petri Lombardi*. 4 vols. Paris: Lethielleux

Pasnau, R. (2002). *Thomas Aquinas on human nature*. New York: Cambridge University Press.

Spiazzi, R. (ed.) (1949a). *De spiritualibus creaturis*. In *Quaestiones disputatae*, vol. 2. Turin: Marietti.

Spiazzi, R. (ed.) (1949b). *Quaestiones disputatae de potentia dei*. In *Quaestiones disputatae*, vol. 2. Turin: Marietti.

Stump, E. (2003). *Aquinas*. New York: Routledge.

31

The Use of the Bible in the Abortion Debate

Roy Bowen Ward

Roy Bowen Ward (d. 2012) was a longtime professor of comparative religion and biblical studies at Miami University, Ohio, where he also helped found a women's studies program and LGBTQ organizations. This essay was circulated for many years by the Religious Coalition for Reproductive Choice and still stands as one of the few scholarly pieces comprehensively treating the abortion issue in the Bible from a prochoice perspective.

The most obvious answer to the question of what the Bible says about abortion is "nothing." There is no commandment, "Thou shall not abort." There is no passage that describes anyone having an abortion. John T. Noonan, an antiabortion Roman Catholic scholar writing in 1970, simply admits, "The Old Testament has nothing to say on abortion."[1] Writing soon after *Roe v. Wade,* the Jesuit scholar John Connery, in his history of the abortion issue, writes: "If anyone expects to find an explicit condemnation of abortion in the New Testament, he will be disappointed. The silence of the New Testament regarding abortion surpasses even that of the Old Testament."[2]

. . .

There were several methods used for abortion in the ancient world: surgical procedures, manipulative procedures, abortifacients applied as suppositories, and oral abortifacients. The Ebers Medical Papyrus from Egypt, dated between 1550 and 1500 B.C.E., reads, "The Beginning of Recipes that are made for women to cause a woman to stop pregnancy in the

Source: Roy Bowen Ward, "The Use of the Bible in the Abortion Debate," *St. Louis University Public Law Review* 13 (1993): 391–408.

first, second or third period."[3] There follows a list of herbal recipes to be applied as suppositories; most of the herbs listed are known and attested abortifacient.[4] John M. Riddle, in his extensive study on contraception and abortion, concludes that drug abortifacient administered orally or as suppositories became the normal means of abortion from early Greek medicine down to the 19th century.[5] Certainly when Christianity began, plant and herb abortifacient were known, and such information was published in *De materia medica* by Dioscorides who lived under the emperors Claudius and Nero in the first century C.E.[6] But Riddle argues that such information was the result of centuries of folk experimentation, primarily by women. "People observed the effect that plants had on animals and on themselves and learned what to take to prevent or end pregnancy at the same time that they learned how to avoid unwanted terminations."[7] The silence of the Bible on abortion was not because abortion wasn't practiced. Effective (and safe) abortifacient were available and used.

. . .

Even when admitting that there are no explicit references to abortion in the Bible, those who oppose abortion will often cite the commandment "Thou shall not kill."[8] No direct object is supplied for the verb "to kill." Does the prohibition also cover feticide?

It is important to look at the commandment in context. Certainly the commandment does not indiscriminately refer to killing anything alive - the Israelites were expected to kill animals, both to eat and to sacrifice.[9] They were also expected to kill Philistines and other enemies in war.[10] And they were even expected to kill their children under certain situations: whoever cursed his father or mother was to be killed.[11] The command not to kill was certainly not "pro-life" in an unqualified way.[12]

. . .

Old Testament

Long before the abortion debate, scholars of the Old Testament agreed that the most important Hebrew word describing a human being was *nephesh,* a word that occurs 755 times in the Hebrew Bible. As E. Jacob puts it, *nephesh* is "the usual term for a man's total nature."[13] As Hans Walter Wolff puts it, *nephesh* is "a living being, a living person, a living individual."[14] The defining characteristic of a *nephesh* is breath. In fact, Jacob argues that the etymology of *nephesh* goes back to a root that means "to breathe."[15]

The classic text is *Genesis* 2:7: "The Yahweh God formed the earthling ['*adam*] of dust from the earth ['*adamah*], and breathed into its nostrils the breath [*ruach*] of life; and the earthling ['*adam*] became a living *nephesh*."[16]

. . .

If *nephesh* is the fundamental term for the living being, the "person," in Hebrew thought, and if *nephesh* is basically understood as a creature that breathes, then a fetus is not a *nephesh*, not a living person until birth.

This conclusion is consistent with the one law in the Bible that refers to miscarriage. When men were fighting and they caused a pregnant woman to miscarry, the penalty was a fine; if the mother was harmed, it was "life for life" *(nephesh* for *nephesh)*.[17] It is generally accepted that this passage shows that the fetus did not have the same status as the mother in ancient Hebrew law.[18]

Since *Roe v. Wade*, some conservative Protestant scholars, attempting to support an antiabortion position, have called into question the long-standing interpretation that *Exodus* 21:22-25 refers to miscarriage.[19] They argue it refers instead to premature birth.[20] According to this line of interpretation, if both the premature child and the mother are unharmed, a fine is levied, but if either the premature child or the mother is harmed, the penalty is life for life, eye for eye, and so forth.[21]

But this new interpretation is not plausible. The law in *Exodus* 21 is worded quite similarly to that in the 19th or 18th century B.C.E. Code of Hammurabi, 209 and 210: "If a seignior struck a(nother) seignior's daughter and has caused her to have a miscarriage [literally, caused her to drop that of her womb], he shall pay ten shekels of silver for her fetus. If that woman had died, they shall put his daughter to death."[22] A similar parallel is found in the Hittite Laws, 1:17: "If anyone causes a free woman to miscarry [literally, drives out the embryo]—if (it is) the 10th month, he shall give 10 shekels of silver, if (it is) the 5th month, he shall give 5 shekels of silver and pledge his estate as security."[23]

. . .

Some writers, in their attempt to find passages in the Bible with which to argue that the fetus is a person, turn to several texts that refer to the womb, passages such as the 139th Psalm; *Isaiah*, chapter 49; and *Jeremiah*, chapter 1.[24] However, these writers fail to take into account the details and context of these passages.

The psalmist of *Psalm* 139 has been accused by his enemies,[25] and he closes with a plea to God to search him to see whether there is any wickedness in him.[26] But before making that plea, the psalmist proclaims that God already knows him and his innocence,[27] and his words even before he speaks them.[28] God will always be with him, even in the grave.[29] Then the psalmist says in *Psalm* 139:13-16, "It is you who did form my kidneys, who did weave me together in my mother's womb. . . . My bones were not hidden from you when I was being made in secret, colorfully wrought in the depths of the earth. Your eyes have seen my embryo. In your books were written, every one of them, the days that were formed form me, when as yet there were none of them."[30]

The emphasis in this passage is "that the Creator of mankind is also the Creator of every individual person"[31] and therefore knows all things about the person *before* they exist. The Creator knows a man's word before it is on his lips,[32] his days before they take place[33] and this man when he is but an embryo (Hebrew *golem,* that which is formless)[34] that the Creator is weaving together. This in no way suggests that he was a *nephesh* before he was born, but that the Creator knows things and people before they exist.

The same notion of God's foreknowledge is found in the calling of Israel as his servant in *Isaiah* 49:1-6. In verse 1 it states that God "has called me from birth; from the womb of my mother he pronounced my name."[35] And in verse 5 it refers to God "who formed me from the womb to be his servant."[36] The accent is on the foreknowledge and planning of the calling of his servant.

. . .

None of the womb passages mentioned above provide a basis for arguing that the fetus is a person *(nephesh);* they provide a basis only for the faith that God is creator of all and that in his sovereignty he knows people before they exist, even as he knows words before they are uttered or days before they occur.

New Testament

. . .

Some who want to argue that the fetus is a "person" point to the birth stories of John the Baptist and Jesus in the *Gospel according to Luke,* chapter 1.[37] An angel appears to Zechariah to announce the future birth of John,[38] and says, *inter alia,* "and he will be filled with the Holy Spirit, even from his mother's womb."[39] This translation from the Revised Standard Version is ambiguous, but the Jesuit scholar, Joseph A. Fitzmyer, translates the verse, "but even from his birth he will be filled with a holy Spirit."[40] The expression *ek koilias,* "from the womb," ordinarily refers to birth,[41] and this fits the context better. The angel says that many will rejoice at his birth[42] and then speaks of what he will be and do after his birth—and that he will be filled with the Holy Spirit.[43]

It is also worth noting that the angel says that Elizabeth will bear Zechariah a son, and *then* Zechariah will give the child a name.[44] There is a parallel in the angelic announcement to Mary: "You will conceive in your womb and bear a son and you shall call his name Jesus."[45] There is also a parallel in the angelic announcement to Joseph in the *Gospel according to Matthew* 1:21: "[S]he shall bear a son, and you shall call his name Jesus."[46] At the end of the Matthaean story it says: "[H]e knew her not until she had borne a son; and he called his name Jesus."[47] The giving of the name after the birth suggests an implicit distinction between the fetus and the person after birth. In the Matthaean story the naming is especially important because it grafts Jesus by adoption into the Davidic genealogy, an important theological point for this gospel.[48]

Later in the first chapter of the *Gospel According to Luke,* Elizabeth is five months' pregnant[49] when the newly pregnant Mary went to visit Elizabeth.[50] When Mary greeted Elizabeth, the fetus[51] in Elizabeth's womb moved.[52] Elizabeth is filled with the Holy Spirit and acknowledges Mary as "the mother of my Lord."[53] As Fitzmyer says, "Elizabeth is filled with Spirit and inspired to interpret the sign thus given to her."[54] In this text the key actors are Elizabeth and Mary. It would be over-interpretation to read into this verse (and verse 44) the basis for regarding the as yet unnamed fetus who moved as a "person."

. . .

The silence of the New Testament on abortion makes it impossible to prove whether, in the time that the New Testament writings were written, Christian women did or did not terminate their pregnancies. However, in that time there was encouragement not to marry and not to procreate. Because of the imminent end of the world and coming of the Kingdom and the return of Christ, heirs were not needed, and thus procreation was not needed. Such teachings might have led married, Christian women to use drug abortifacient as soon as they became aware that they were pregnant, especially since, as I have argued, there was nothing in the Bible that would suggest that using such abortifacient was morally wrong.

The argument against abortion arose from Platonic dualism, which was opposed to the body and especially bodily pleasure, including sex. Reducing the purpose of sex to procreation only, all unprocreative sex was condemned. Contraception came to be condemned. Abortion and infanticide were condemned because these actions showed that the intercourse was not intended for procreation. This basic argument is seen in the writings of the first century C.E. Alexandrian Jew, Philo, and it appears in Christian writings outside of the New Testament. But in the New Testament no such argument is articulated.[55]

Notes

1. John T. Noonan, Jr., *An Almost Absolute Value in History, in* THE MORALITY OF ABORTION 1, 6 (John T. Noonan, Jr. ed., 1970).
2. JOHN CONNERY, SJ., ABORTION: THE DEVELOPMENT OF THE ROMAN CATHOLIC PERSPECTIVE 34 (1977).
3. JOHN M. RIDDLE, CONTRACEPTION AND ABORTION FROM THE ANCIENT WORLD TO THE RENAISSANCE 69 (1992).
4. *Id.* at 69-72.
5. *Id.* at 64.
6. *Id.* at 31-45. See [MICHAEL J. GORMAN, ABORTION & THE EARLY CHURCH 48 (1982)] at 15, where he states, "Chemical or medicinal abortifacient of various compositions were common."
7. RIDDLE, *supra* note [3], at 164.
8. *Exodus* 20:13; *Matthew* 5:21.
9. *Leviticus* 1:1-27:34.
10. *Joshua* 1:1-24:33, *Judges* 1:1-21:25, and 1 *Samuel* 1:1-31:13.
11. *Exodus* 21:17; *Leviticus* 20:9.
12. See Raymond F. Collins, *Ten Commandments*, [THE ANCHOR BIBLE DICTIONARY (David Noel Freedman ed., 1992)] at 386: "The commandment is addressed to free, landholding Israelites and affords protection for the life of the Israelite."
13. Edmond Jacob, *Psuche, KTL, in* IX THEOLOGICAL DICTIONARY OF THE NEW TESTAMENT 620 (Gerhard Friederich ed., 1970).
14. HANS WALTER WOLFF, ANTHROPOLOGY OF THE OLD TESTAMENT 22 (1974).
15. Jacob, *supra* note [13], at 620.

16. *Genesis* 2:7; *see also* PHYLLIS TRIBLE, GOD AND THE RHETORIC OF SEXUALITY 75 (1978), and CAROL MEYERS, DISCOVERING EVE: ANCIENT ISRAELITE WOMEN IN CONTEXT 81-82 (1988).

17. *Exodus* 21:22, 23.

18. *See* CONNERY, *supra* note [2] at 11.

19. *Id.*

20. Jack W. Cottrell, *Abortion and the Mosaic Law,* 17 CHRISTIANITY TODAY 602 (1973).

21. *Id.*

22. *Code of Hammurabi* (T.J. Meek trans.), *in* THE ANCIENT NEAR EASTERN TEXTS 175 (J.B. Pritchard ed., 1955) [hereinafter *ANET*].

23. *Hittite Law,* (A. Goetze trans.) in ANET, *supra* note [22], at 190.

24. [GLEASON L. ARCHER, ENCYCLOPEDIA OF BIBLE DIFFICULTIES 246 (1982)], at 246, 247. Michael J. Gorman, *Why Is the New Testament Silent about Abortion?* J. AM. FAM. ASSOC., July 1993, at 16, 17 [hereinafter Gorman, *New Testament*]. Although Gorman's article makes no mention of the womb-passages, a drawing accompanies the article with quotations of *Psalms* 139:13, *Isaiah* 49:1, and *Jeremiah* 1:5.

25. *Psalm* 139:19.

26. *Id.* at vv. 23, 24.

27. *Id.* at vv. 1ff.

28. *Id.* at v. 4.

29. *Id.* at vv. 7f.

30. *See* WOLFF, *supra* note [14], at 96, 97; HANS-JOACHIM KRAUS, PSALMS 60-150, 509, 516, 517 (H.C. Oswald trans., 1989).

31. WOLFF, *supra* note [14], at 96.

32. *Psalm* 139:4.

33. *Id.* at v. 16.

34. KRAUS, *supra* note [30], at 511; WOLFF, *supra* note [14], at 240, n.17.

35. *Second Isaiah,* 20 THE ANCHOR BIBLE, 103 (John L. McKenzie, SJ., trans., 1968). The Hebrew *mibeten,* literally "from the womb," usually refers to birth, e.g., in Job 1:21; hence McKenzie translates it "from birth."

36. *Id.*

37. ARCHER, *supra* note [24], at 247.

38. Luke 1:11-13.

39. *Id.* at v. 15.

40. Joseph A. Fitzmyer, S.J., *The Gospel According to Luke* I-IX, 28 THE ANCHOR BIBLE, 304 (1981).

41. *See* THE SEPTUAGINT at *Judges* 16:17; 2 *Samuel* 7:12; *Job* 1:21, 10:18; *Psalms* 21(22):10, 70(71):6, 131(132):11, *Isaiah* 46:3, 48:8. *Contra* Fitzmyer, *supra* note [40], at 326.

42. *Luke* 1:14.
43. *Id.* at v. 15.
44. *Id.* at v. 13.
45. *Id.* at v. 31.
46. *Matthew* 1:21.
47. *Id.* at v. 24.
48. See KRISTER STENDAHL, MEANINGS: THE BIBLE AS DOCUMENT AND AS GUIDE 75-78 (1984).
49. *Luke* 1:24. 86. *Id.* at 1:39.
50. Id. at 1:39.
51. The common meaning of *brephos* is "fetus," although according to context it can mean a "new-born babe." The verb *brephoo* means to "form into a fetus."
52. *Luke* l :41.
53. *Id.* at vv. 41-43.
54. Fitzmyer, *supra* note [40], at 363.
55. Gorman makes a curious argument by arguing that three Christian writings—the Didache, Barnabas, and the Apocalypse of Peter—have prohibitions of abortion and that these three were sometimes included in canonical lists. This is beside the point, with respect to the use of the New Testament today, a New Testament that does not include these works. Gorman argues, "These three texts bear witness to the general Jewish and Jewish-Christian attitude of the first and second centuries, thus confirming that the earliest Christians shared the antiabortion position of their Jewish forebears." Rather, these writings show a connection with the kind of Judaism reflected by Philo, and when they were considered by some to be canonical in the third and fourth centuries, many Christians had accepted a platonic stance and were opposing abortion on sexual grounds. Gorman, *New Testament, supra* note [24], at 17-18.

32

The Value of Every Human Life

C. Ben Mitchell

C. Ben Mitchell is a recently retired professor of moral theology. He is ordained and has many years of active involvement in the Southern Baptist Convention and in organizations promoting Christian bioethical values. Mitchell's essay provides an evangelical perspective on how the Bible speaks to the value of unborn life and what various early Christian thinkers said about abortion. He concludes that there is a biblical and theological consensus in the early church that is echoed in the prolife commitments of evangelicals today.

Contemporary debates about abortion invoke terms such as "the right to life" and "the sanctity of human life." Admittedly, neither of these expressions is found per se in the Bible. Rather, the biblical witness testifies to the uniqueness of human life among other living things. Specifically, the Bible maintains that only human beings are made in the image of God (the *imago Dei*). Carl F. H. Henry, one of the leading theologians of the evangelical movement in the twentieth century, believed that "the importance of a proper understanding of the *imago Dei* can hardly be overstated. The answer given to the *imago-inquiry* soon becomes determinative for the entire gamut of doctrinal affirmation. The ramifications are not only theological, but [for] every phase of the . . . cultural enterprise as a whole."[1] Thus the image of God is a good place to begin this discussion.

C. Ben Mitchell, "The Vulnerable—Abortion and Disability," in *The Oxford Handbook of Evangelical Theology*, ed. Gerald R. McDermott (New York: Oxford University Press, 2010), 481–96.

The *imago Dei*

Genesis 1 declares that at the zenith of God's creative activity he made Adam a "living soul" (Genesis 1:24) in God's own "image" and "likeness" (Genesis 1:27). While other animals have souls as well, only humankind is made in God's image. The image of God, then, is the source of human exceptionalism, the notion that human beings occupy a unique place in the created order.

Furthermore, the creation covenant between God and his human handiwork included the mandate, "Be fruitful and multiply, and fill the earth and subdue it; and have dominion over the fish of the sea and over the birds of the air and over every living thing that moves upon the earth" (Genesis 1:28). One could hardly imagine the other animals needing an imperative to reproduce. Fecundity comes naturally, as it were. Humans, on the other hand, can choose sexual abstinence and potentially forego populating the earth. The divine imperative to multiply establishes a presumption in favor of procreation. Subsequently, the Bible makes it very clear that offspring are a reward from God. Children are seen as a spiritual and economic blessing (e.g., Psalm 127:3-5), pregnancies are welcomed with great joy and singing (e.g., Genesis 21:6-7; 1 Samuel 1-2; Luke 1), and infertility is seen as a terrible plight (e.g., Genesis 25:21; 30:1). So from the opening of the biblical narrative, human beings are singled out as sui generis and instructed to procreate.

The locus classicus for human exceptionalism is the prohibition against murdering humans (i.e., homicide) found in Genesis 9:1-6. After the devastating flood, God renewed the creation covenant with Noah and his children:

> God blessed Noah and his sons, and said to them, "Be fruitful and multiply, and fill the earth. . . . Every moving thing that lives shall be food for you; and just as I gave you the green plants, I give you everything. Only, you shall not eat flesh with its life, that is, its blood. For your own lifeblood I will surely require a reckoning: from every animal I will require it and from human beings, each one for the blood of another, I will require a reckoning for human life. Whoever sheds the blood of a human, by a human shall that person's blood be shed; for in his own image God made humankind. And you, be fruitful and multiply, abound on the earth and multiply in it." (NRSV)

Several features of the covenant renewal are notable. First, the covenant is identical to the creation covenant with respect to the positive commands to be fruitful, reproduce, and be good stewards over the earth and its resources.

Second, permission to kill animals for sustenance is added to the Noahic covenant. Third, animal life is thereby tacitly distinguished from human life by the prohibition of homicide. Finally, the rationale given for this prohibition is that humankind is made in God's own image. The conclusion seems to follow that since only members of the species *Homo sapiens* are imagers of God, human life deserves greater, or a different kind of, respect than animal life.[2]

Interpreters have varied widely in their opinions about what exactly constitutes the *imago Dei*. Numerous options have been offered: (1) humankind's erect bodily form, (2) human dominion over nature, (3) human reason. . . .[3] Nevertheless, one thing seems clear even from the history of interpretation; namely, that the *imago Dei* is attributed solely to human beings, notably including Jesus Christ—fully divine and fully human—who is "the image of the invisible God" (Colossians 1:15), the prototypical image of what it means to be one of us.[4] Thus, what it means to be human is to image God, and what it means to image God is to be human, as Jesus Christ is human.

Early Jewish and Christian Witnesses on Abortion

From the vantage point of biblical anthropology informed by the doctrine of the image of God, the rationale for the early Jewish community's views on abortion becomes clearer. As Michael J. Gorman has shown, despite the lack of a specific prohibition against abortion in the Hebrew Bible, the Jewish witness against the practice is fairly consistent. "Though rare cases of abortion may have occurred in Judaism," observes Gorman, "the witness of antiquity is that Jews, unlike pagans, did not practice deliberate abortion."[5] Philo of Alexandria (25 B.C.E.–41C.E.), for example, included a brief discussion of abortion under the heading of the commandment "Thou shalt not kill." He concluded that if a man should strike a pregnant woman causing her to miscarry, and the offspring was unshaped or undeveloped, a fine should accrue, but if the offspring was already shaped—with identifiable limbs—the man should be put to death.[6]

Similarly, the *Sentences of Pseudo-Phocylides* (c. 50 B.C.E.–50 C.E.), an early Jewish text based on the Septuagint, says that "a woman should not destroy the unborn in her belly, nor after its birth throw it before the dogs and vultures as a prey."[7] The Jewish apocalyptic *Sibylline Oracle* (c. second century C.E.) included among the "wicked" women who "produce abortions and unlawfully cast their offspring away" and sorcerers who dispense abortion-causing drugs.[8] Likewise, the apocryphal book *1 Enoch* (first or second century B.C.E.) declared that an evil angel taught humans how to "smash the embryo in the womb." Finally, the first-century historian and apologist for Judaism Josephus wrote in *Against Apion* that "The law orders all the offspring to be brought up, and forbids women either to cause abortion or to make away with the foetus; a woman convicted of this is regarded as an infanticide, because she destroys a soul and diminishes the race."[9] Contrast these injunctions with the barbarism of Roman culture. Cicero (106-43 B.C.E.) indicated that according to the Twelve Tables of Roman Law, "deformed infants shall be killed."[10] Plutarch (c. 46-120 C.E.) spoke of those whom he said "offered up their own children [for sacrifice], and those who had no children would buy little ones from poor people and cut their throats as if they were so many lambs or young birds; meanwhile the mother stood by without a tear or moan."[11] According to an inscription at Delphi, because of the infanticide of female newborns only 1 percent of six hundred families had raised two daughters. European historian W.E.H. Lecky called infanticide "one of the deepest stains of the ancient civilizations."[12]

Against this bleak backdrop, the Hebrew tradition provided a robust moral framework for early Christian condemnation of both abortion and infanticide. For instance, the *Didache* (c. 85-110) commanded, "Thou shalt not murder a child by abortion nor kill them when born." The *Epistle of Barnabas* (c. 130 C.E.), commanded, "You shall not abort a child nor, again, commit infanticide." Additional examples of Christian condemnation of both infanticide and abortion can be cited. In fact, some biblical scholars have argued that the New Testament's silence on abortion per se is due to the fact that it was simply beyond the pale of early Christian practice.

The Christian Apologists

The Christian apologists of the second and third centuries also spoke on the subject of abortion. Among them, Athenagoras and Tertullian stand out. Formerly a Greek philosopher who converted to Christianity, Athenagoras addressed his *Plea for Christians* (c. 177) to Roman Emperor Marcus Aurelius to defend followers of Christ against the charge that they were atheists (because they would not worship Caesar), incestuous (because they called one another "brother" and "sister" and then married one another), and cannibals (because they ate the body and drank the blood of Christ in the Eucharist). As evidence that Christians were not cannibals, Athenagoras maintained that Christians could not bear to watch the death of another human being, even at the gladiatorial games. His illustration of Christian respect for human life was telling: "What reason would we have to commit murder when we say that women who induce abortions are murderers, and will have to give account of it to God?"[13]

Raised in Carthage and trained as a lawyer, Tertullian offered a similar defense against the charge that Christians sacrificed their children in his *Apology* to Emperor Septimus Severus (197 C.E.): "In our case, murder being once for all forbidden, we may not destroy even the fetus in the womb, while as yet the human being derives blood from other parts of the body for its sustenance. To hinder a birth is merely a speedier man-killing."[14] The disapproval of abortion was clearly used as a sign of the virtue of the Christian community.

The Fathers and Augustine

Among the Church Fathers, Basil, Jerome, Ambrose, Augustine, and Chrysostom commented on abortion. Although there were clearly nuanced distinctions among them, they were univocal in their condemnation of the practice. Basil of Caesarea (c. 330-379) called abortion "murder," but just as clearly pointed out that it was not an unforgiveable sin and prescribed penance for the sin.[15] The rhetorician and Bishop of Milan, Ambrose (c. 339-397), repudiated the use of "parricidal mixtures" because they "snuff out the fruit" of the womb.[16] Jerome (c. 342-420) lamented that "some, when they learn they are with child through sin, practice abortion by the use of drugs. Frequently they die themselves and are brought before the rulers of the lower world guilty of three crimes: suicide, adultery against Christ, and murder of an unborn child."[17]

More than merely proscribing abortion and infanticide, however, early Christian communities provided alternatives, adopting children who were destined to be abandoned. For instance, Callistus (d. c. 223) provided refuge to abandoned children by placing them in Christian homes; Benignus of Dijon (third century) offered nourishment and protection to abandoned children, including some with disabilities caused by failed abortions.

Like his predecessors, Augustine of Hippo (354-430) was an ardent opponent of deliberate abortion. Gorman points out that no Church Father gave more attention to the subject than Augustine, not least because much of his own theologizing was about the origin and transmission of the soul, the doctrine of original sin, and the role of sex within marriage. For instance, in his discussion of the resurrection, Augustine asked whether an unborn fetus would be raised from the dead. He reasoned that in order for a person to be raised from the dead, he or she must first have lived. Can a fetus be reckoned to have lived? While his answer was somewhat modest about the nature of unborn human life, he preferred erring on the side of life. "On this score a corollary question may be most carefully discussed by the learned men, and still I do not know that any man can answer it, namely: When does a human being begin to live in the womb? Is there some form of hidden life, not yet apparent in the motions of a living thing? To deny, for example, that those fetuses ever lived at all which are cut away limb by limb and cast out of the wombs of pregnant women, lest the mothers die also if the fetuses were left there dead, would seem much too rash."[18]

In sum, the witness of Scripture and the consensus of the early church is that every human being, from conception through natural death is to be respected as an imager of God whose life has special dignity in virtue of his or her relationship to the Creator. The community of faithful Christians was marked by its rejection of abortion because it was seen as a violation of the command not to murder.

The Reformers

Although the topic of abortion did not result in a significant body of writing among the Reformers, Luther and Calvin had some pointed things to say about it. Luther, for instance, saw a correlation between contraception and abortion: "How great, therefore, the wickedness of [fallen] human nature is! How many girls there are who prevent conception and kill and expel tender fetuses, although procreation is the work of God! Indeed, some spouses who marry and live together . . . have various ends in mind, but rarely children."[19] Calvin decried abortion as a "monstrous crime to rob [the preborn child] of the life which it has not yet begun to enjoy. If it seems more horrible to kill a man in his own house than in a field, because a man's house is his place of most secure refuge, it ought surely to be deemed more atrocious to destroy a fetus in the womb before it has come to light."[20]

. . .

Conclusion

Although it is certainly true that evangelicalism is not monolithic and that there is diversity among those who claim the label, evangelicals are legatees of a great tradition, so that today "evangelical" and "prolife" have become nearly synonymous. For at the heart of the evangelical ethos is dependence on the revelation of God in the scriptures of the Old and New Testaments and in the person of Jesus the Christ. Because of their biblicism, anthropology, and Christology, evangelicals seek to preserve the lives of all of those who are made in God's image.

Notes

1. Carl F. H. Henry, "Man," in Everett F. Harrison, Geoffrey W. Bromiley, and Carl F. H. Henry, eds., *Baker's Dictionary of Theology* (Grand Rapids: Baker, 1973), 339.
2. This does not mean, however, that animals may be abused. Stewardship of the animals entails that they not be treated cruelly nor destroyed willy-nilly. . . .
3. James Leo Garrett, *Systematic Theology: Biblical, Historical, and Evangelical,* vol 1 (Grand Rapids: Eerdmans, 1990), 394-403. A benchmark essay on the image of God is D.J.A. Clines, "The Image of God in Man," *Tyndale Bulletin* 19 (1968), 53-103.
4. Or who, in the language of the Nicene Creed (325 C.E.), "came down and was incarnate and was made man."
5. Michael J. Gorman, *Abortion and the Early Church: Christian, Jewish and Pagan Attitudes in the Greco-Roman World* (Downers Grove, Ill.: InterVarsity Press, 1982), 34.
6. This is probably a reference to Exodus 21:22-25. For excellent treatments of this text vis-à-vis abortion, see Jack W. Cottrell, "Abortion and the Mosaic Law," *Christianity Today* 17 (March 16, 1973), 6-9, and James K. Hoffmeir, "Abortion and the Old Testament Law," James K. Hoffmeir, ed., *Abortion: A Christian Understanding and Response* (Grand Rapids: Baker, 1987), 49- 63.

7. *Sentences* 184-185.
8. *The Sibylline Oracles,* Book II.345.
9. Flavius Josephus, *Against Apion* 2.202.
10. Cicero, *De Legibus* 3.8.
11. Plutarch, *Moralia* 2.171D.
12. W.E.H. Lecky, *History of European Morals: From Augustus to Charlemagne,* vol. 2 (New York: D. Appleton, 1897), 24.
13. Athengoras, *Legatio* 35; cited in Gorman, *Abortion and the Early Church,* 54.
14. Tertullian, *Apology* 9.6, cited ibid., 55.
15. Basil, *Letter* 188, to Ampilochius, cited ibid., 67.
16. Ambrose, *Hexameron* 5.18.58 (the eighth homily, on day five); cited ibid., 68.
17. *Letter* 22.13 (to Eustochium), in T. C. Lawler, ed., *The Letters of St. Jerome,* trans. C. C. Mierow, (Westminster, Md.: Newman Press, 1963); cited ibid., 68.
18. St. Augustine, *Augustine: Confessions and Enchiridion*, trans. Albert C. Outler (Louisville, Ky.: Westminster/John Knox, 2006), 23.85.
19. Martin Luther, *Lectures on Genesis* 4.304-305.
20. John Calvin, *Commentaries on the Four Last Books of Moses,* vol. 3 (Grand Rapids: Eerdmans, 1950), 41-42.

33

For the Life of the World:

Toward a Social Ethos of the Orthodox Church

Greek Orthodox Archdiocese of America

This document was commissioned by Bartholomew I, who holds the title of Ecumenical Patriarch and Archbishop of Constantinople and is the spiritual leader of all Orthodox Christians. It is promoted by the Greek Orthodox Church in America, where it is published on their website. Orthodox churches in America are officially autocephalous (independent), but this document carries significant weight for Orthodox Christians globally. The statement is not a legal document or a dogmatic decree. This excerpt focuses on issues having to do with marriage, contraception, and abortion, and is considered as taking a less conservative position than prior teachings from Orthodox church leaders.

The Course of Human Life

§15 The course of a human life on earth—if it reaches its natural conclusion—begins in the moment of conception in the womb, extends from childhood to adulthood, and culminates at last in the sleep of bodily death. But the

Source: Greek Orthodox Archdiocese of America, "For the Life of the World: Toward a Social Ethos of the Orthodox Church," 2020. https://www.goarch.org/social-ethos.

stages of human life differ for each soul, and every path that any given person might take, whether chosen or unchosen, leads to possibilities either of sanctity or of spiritual slavery. . . . The Church seeks to accompany the Christian soul all along its way in this world, providing not only counsel but also the means of achieving holiness. And, at every stage, the Church proposes diverse models of life in Christ, diverse vocations for Christian living embraced within the one supreme vocation to seek the Kingdom of God and its justice.

. . .

§24 It is not the case that a man and a woman united in sacramental marriage become "one flesh" only in the bearing of children, even if (historically speaking) that may have been the chief connotation of the term as it was employed in the book of Genesis. From a very early period, Orthodox tradition has affirmed the sacramental completeness of every marriage that the Church blesses, even those that do not produce offspring. As St. John Chrysostom observed, "But suppose there is no child; do they remain two and not one? No; their intercourse effects the joining of their bodies, and they are made one, just as when perfume is mixed with ointment."[1] The Church anticipates, of course, that most marriages will be open to conception; but it also understands that there are situations in which spiritual, physical, psychological, or financial impediments arise that make it wise—at least, for a time—to delay or forego the bearing of children. The Orthodox Church has no dogmatic objection to the use of safe and non-abortifacient contraceptives within the context of married life, not as an ideal or as a permanent arrangement, but as a provisional concession to necessity. The sexual union of a couple is an intrinsic good that serves to deepen the love of each for the other and their devotion to a shared life. By the same token, the Church has no objection to the use of certain modern and still-evolving reproductive technologies for couples who earnestly desire children, but who are unable to conceive without aid. But the Church cannot approve of methods that result in the destruction of "supernumerary" fertilized ova. The necessary touchstone for assessing whether any given reproductive technology is licit must be the inalienable dignity and incomparable value of every human life. As medical science in this area continues to advance, Orthodox Christians—lay believers and clergy alike—must consult this touchstone in every instance in which a new method appears for helping couples to conceive and bear children, and must also consider whether that method honors the sacred relationship between the two spouses.

§25 Orthodox tradition, on the Feast of the Annunciation, celebrates the conception of Christ in his mother's womb, and on the Feast of the Visitation recalls John the Baptist leaping with joy in his mother's womb at the sound of the voice of the pregnant Mother of God. Already in the womb each of us is a spiritual creature, a person formed in God's image and created to rejoice in God's presence. From the first generations of Christians, therefore, the Church has abhorred the practice of elective abortion as infanticide. As early as the *Didache*, the first-century record of Church practices and ordinances, rejection of abortion was an express principle of the new faith,[2] one that— alongside the rejection of infant-exposure and capital punishment— demonstrated that Christian confession was opposed to the taking of human life, even in those cases in which pagan culture had regarded it as licit or even necessary. A human being is more than the gradually emergent result of a physical process; life begins at the moment of conception. A child's claim upon our moral regard then is absolute from that first moment, and Christians are forbidden from shedding innocent blood at every stage of human development. The Church recognizes, of course, that pregnancies are often terminated as a result of poverty, despair, coercion, or abuse, and it seeks to provide a way of reconciliation for those who have succumbed to these terrible pressures. Inasmuch, however, as the act of abortion is always objectively a tragedy, one that takes an innocent human life, reconciliation must involve the acknowledgment of this truth before complete repentance, reconciliation, and healing are possible. Moreover, the Church must be ready at all times—inasmuch as it truly wishes to affirm the goodness of every life—to come to the aid of women in situations of unintended pregnancy, whether as the result of rape or of consensual sexual union, and to come also to the aid of expectant mothers suffering from penury, abuse, or other adverse conditions, by providing them material and emotional support, spiritual succor, and every assurance of God's love, both during and after pregnancy.

§26 In the Orthodox marriage rite, the Church prays that the newly married couple might "be made glad with the sight of sons and daughters." The joy thus anticipated is unqualified; it is elicited not only by infants or children who meet a specific standard of fitness or health. All children are known and loved by God, all are bearers of his image and likeness, and all are due the same respect, reverence, and care. In the eyes of the Church, each of us is born as we are, "so that the works of God might be made manifest in [us]" (John 9:3). Therefore, the Orthodox Church recognizes no legitimate resort to the eugenic termination of new human life; and it welcomes every new medical advance that can preserve and improve the lives of children afflicted by disease and disability. The Church does recognize, however, that in the course of some pregnancies there arise tragic and insoluble medical situations in which the life of the unborn child cannot be preserved or prolonged without grave danger to the life of the mother, and that the only medical remedy may result in or hasten the death of the unborn child, contrary to all that the parents had desired. In such situations, the Church cannot pretend to be competent to know the best way of proceeding in every instance, and must commend the matter to the prayerful deliberations of parents and their physicians. It can, however, offer counsel, as well as prayers for the healing and salvation of all the lives involved. Furthermore, the Church laments the ubiquity of the loss of life *in utero* through miscarriage and stillbirth, understanding these experiences as particularly powerful forms of bereavement for the family, and it must revise those of its prayers that suggest otherwise, and rise to the sensitive and loving pastoral care that loss of pregnancy requires.

Notes

1. John Chrysostom, *Homily 12 on Colossians* 4:18. PG 62.388C. See *On Marriage and Family Life*, Crestwood, NY: St. Vladimir's Seminary Press, 2003, 76.
2. *Didache* 2. See *Early Christian Writings: The Apostolic Fathers*, London: Penguin Classics, 1987.

34

Abortion and Organ Donation:

Christian Reflections on Bodily Life Support

Patricia Beattie Jung

Patricia Beattie Jung is one of the foremost feminist Catholic ethicists in the United States, having written or co-edited eight volumes on issues of gender, sexuality, and bioethics, and having co-edited one book specifically on abortion and the Catholic tradition. This essay, originally published in 1988, is a classic argument for considering the ethics of pregnancy as analogous to the bodily self-gifting of live organ donation. From this perspective, the necessity of consent and agency in both circumstances becomes starkly apparent. Jung affirms the centrality of self-giving for the Christian faith but calls into question the notion that completing a pregnancy is always the pregnant person's moral duty.

All human beings have an obligation or duty to give some minimal degree of assistance to others in life threatening situations. Conversely, by virtue of a person's humanity, he or she may lay claim to or have a moral right to minimal assistance from others in perpetuating his or her own life. This thesis is put forward in order to distinguish my position from others. It is at least intelligible (though I believe erroneous) to delimit the responsibility

Source: Patricia Beattie Jung, "Abortion and Organ Donation: Christian Reflections on Bodily Life Support," *Journal of Religious Ethics* 16, no. 2 (1988): 273–305.

to give bodily life support by attempting to demonstrate that there is no general positive duty to give assistance to others and hence no specific duty to offer bodily life support.[1] I intend to clarify the "special nature" of bodily life support by explaining its immunity from what I regard as the legitimate general requirements of both social justice and beneficence.

Minimal Assistance Ought to Be Required by Law

The obligation to assist others has roots in both justice and beneficence. The obligation to give assistance to another can be derived from two very different conceptions of justice. On the one hand, it can spring from a reciprocal theory of justice. Minimal assistance is required because all persons have received and continue to expect to receive such "mutual aid" from others. On the other hand, it can be argued that there are certain primary goods—like self-preservation, health maintenance and procreation—toward which human communities are naturally inclined, and therefore justice required *prima facie* that all persons pursue these communal goods.

Each theory, *albeit* in very different manners, helps illumine the moral intuition that a starving "thief" can have a right to or can legitimately claim the "stolen" bread. To the degree that an agent is responsible for his or her neighbor's "need"—that is, has profited in some fashion from the exploitation which produced and sustains it—to that same degree, he or she is required by justice to go beyond this minimal level of assistance. In some cases then, the starving "thief" may be said to have a right to *this* "donor's" bread.

However, no single "donor" can be justly required to carry a genuinely communal burden. It is not always the case that the starving "thief" has a right to *this* "donor's" bread. For these reasons the tradition has rooted the general obligation to give assistance in beneficence as well as justice. Charity is possible for three reasons: (i) not all persons carry their fair share of social burdens; (ii) some communal responsibilities cannot be fairly distributed, but rather fall by virtue of the natural and/or historical lottery on the shoulders of single individuals or institutions; (iii) persons can voluntarily give up their fair share of social benefits.

What has all this to do with bodily life support, especially with child-bearing and organ donation? First, it establishes that (nonbodily) life support can be required by the demands of justice of both individuals and communities. However, it also establishes that such life support can sometimes be at least in part a matter of charity. Why? Because for a variety of reasons, single individuals are asked to shoulder a burden, the responsibility for which is not theirs alone. It is important to understand that *both* organ donation and childbearing are always in part (if not largely) acts of charity.

This has been clearly recognized in regard to organ donation and is expressed well in the gift ethos which illumines that activity.

. . .

Likewise, childbearing is always in part (if not largely) an act of charity. This, however, has not been widely understood nor is it reflected in the traditional ethos surrounding abortion. The life support of children is a *joint* parental responsibility as well as a communal one. Yet during the gestation period this burden cannot be equitably distributed even in theory. Mothers alone carry children to term. The fact that *every* pregnant woman carries far more than her fair share of this responsibility is simply vividly dramatized when pregnancy results from rape or the failure of contraceptive measures, when it threatens the mother's life, or when it is accompanied by total paternal or social abandonment.

However, simply because both organ donation and childbearing are acts (at least in part) of charity does not automatically mean they ought not be required. Because justice cannot always enjoin this "donor" to give his or her loaf of bread to the starving "thief" does not mean that such a gift is purely discretionary.

. . .

Bodily Life Support is a Gift

. . .

The giving of bread to the starving thief is only minimally discretionary because the bread belongs to the donor only in a minimal way. Even if one assumes on a penultimate level, as did Thomas Aquinas, that the notion of private property best serves communal needs and responsibilities, vis-a-vis the goods of the earth, it does not follow that one can ultimately possess or own wealth or property, etc. One is finally only a steward over such goods. The saving of the drowning child is more discretionary than the giving of the bread because an agent's actions, labor, skills, etc., belong more to him or her—are more personal—than property. Hence, they are more of a gift.

. . .

What is the extent of the discretionary nature of bodily life support? Can it ever be said that a needy "thief" has a right to this "donor's" blood, bone marrow, or womb, etc.? What kind of gift is this? Is the giving of such assistance through organ donation or pregnancy ever obligatory? If persons have a general obligation to assist others based on the demands of both justice and beneficence, may this not include bodily forms of life support? If not, why not? Persons do not have a duty to give bodily life support to others. Nobody, simply as a human being in need, has a claim to the use of another's body.

. . .

I would argue that "man's 'sovereignty over himself' to use Kierkegaard 's phrase, is fundamental to any serious moral view of life" (Gustafson, 1968:112). Bodily integrity is viewed descriptively as a foundation of agency or condition necessary for human action. In the work of Alan Donagan, *The Theory of Morality* (1979), such a condition becomes the basis for a normative judgment. In order for a person to act morally, his or her bodily integrity must be respected by others. (Indeed, we do not hold persons accountable for choices made under undue duress or coercion.) Therefore the agent must respect these same features of agency in others.

. . .

In summary, one may wish to argue that beneficence may legitimately require of all persons the giving of certain kinds of "gifts," particularly of objectifiable possessions. Nevertheless, the more personal the gift, the more "gifty" and discretionary it becomes. I can think of no more personal and intimate type of gift than the gift of one's bodily self-whether given sexually, in pregnancy, through various forms of organ donation, or as sacrificed for another. The more a gift belongs to, indeed is, another, the more truly it is a gift.

. . .

The ethos of gift-giving that currently pervades the practice of organ transplantation is the only ethos appropriate to the "special nature" of all forms of bodily life support. This ethos should be extended to our moral understanding of both pregnancy and abortion. Health care professionals (and I would add moral theologians) are appropriately described by Fox and Swazey (1974) as "keepers of the gates," that is, as agents who facilitate gift-giving and who guard against the theft or confiscation of what by its very nature can only be freely given. In her discussion of the wider moral framework of abortion. Beverly Wildung Harrison in *Our Right to Choose* makes the following assertion:

> We need also to acknowledge the bodily integrity of any moral agent as a foundational condition of human well-being and dignity. Freedom from bodily invasion . . . is no minor or marginal issue morally; rather, it is central to our conception of the dignity of the person. (Harrison 1983: 196)

My purpose in this section has been to explain and justify the axiom. The conclusion that neither pregnancy nor organ donation should be mandatory does not imply that all or even most refusals to offer bodily life support (through organ donations or childbearing) can be morally justified. Bodily integrity is a necessary but not self-evidently sufficient condition of morality.

Bodily Life Support: A Christian Feminist Assessment of Its Meanings

The overarching purpose of this section of my essay is to assess the gift ethos in light of the feminist suspicion of any moral framework that might call for the self-sacrifice of women. Though I have explained why I believe bodily life support should not be mandated of any person, I have yet to examine what it might mean for a Christian to give or refuse to give such gifts either through organ donation or childbearing.[2] Clearly "ought" in this instance does not mean required. Furthermore, as the proposed analogy reveals, the decision to bear a child, like that to donate organs, is a complex decision through which the gift-giver attempts to serve and balance a number of competing values.

Though they may be obvious, a brief rehearsal of some of these competing responsibilities is in order insofar as it will establish the context for my analysis of self-sacrifice and its refusal. Let us begin by listing some of the factors that might enter into a decision for or against donating an organ. The donor's general physical and emotional health and life-situation, the value of and likely impact of donation upon his or her life-plan (including present as well as future career considerations and family and social life ramifications), the extent to which the community (family, church, and townspeople) will support (both financially and emotionally) the donor and his or her dependents, the value of the recipient's life as well as the recipient's best interests (which are not in all cases *obviously* served by extending that person's life), and any special responsibilities of a contractual origin that the donor may have to either the recipient or others-all of these factors are normally considered relevant to a decision regarding organ donation.[3] Obviously, there is considerable room for conflict among these goods, and it is not always possible to balance them. In some circumstances, they may be mutually exclusive, that is, sometimes morally legitimate concerns must be sacrificed for the sake of other concerns.

Decisions regarding childbearing are analogous. *All* of the factors identified above are likewise morally relevant to a woman's decision to abort or bear a child.

. . .

Abortion is never a "simple" choice based on a single factor, such as the value of fetal life or maternal health. Pregnancies become problematic when no way of balancing the various responsibilities outlined above can be found. Whether terminated *or not,* these pregnancies never have morally "happy" endings. At best in such tragic circumstances, one aims to follow the least evil course of action. As Whitbeck demonstrates, women do not ever "want" abortions. Medea is a false image of women; it is the product of misogyny. Those who take women's experiences seriously could never describe an abortion, whether spontaneous or induced, as "a matter of little consequence." Further, women ought not be deceived about or veiled from the developmental reality of aborted fetal lives. Paternalism, however beneficent in origin, robs women of the opportunity to face their situation and their decision truthfully, with integrity, courage, and self-respect. Within this wider understanding of the problem, let us first unravel and then critically assess the traditional claim that Christians ought to give bodily life support, even when this entails self-sacrifice.

. . .

Traditional Christian Faith Presumptions

As Hauerwas notes, "the Christian respect for life is first of all a statement, not about life, but about God" (1981:226). Indeed, in the first instance it is a statement about God's ultimate sovereignty over all of life. A voluntarist commitment to or love of the potential recipient is not the necessary moral precondition for the giving of bodily life support. On the contrary, such bearing of the other is the condition for the understanding of what love is in a world where God, not humankind, is in ultimate control.

Before God humans stand in radical poverty, their life and value hang, as it were, by a providential thread. From this perspective, human existence and worth come as a gift from God. Apart from this presumption of nakedness, any human activity—including the giving of bodily life support—will become a form of idolatrous, self-aggrandizement. Thus, for the Christian to offer bodily life support is to convict oneself to a life of radical poverty in a world where God is sovereign.

Implicit in such an adoption of the other is a latent valuation. It is a sign of the ultimate trustworthiness of life. It is also a symbol of hope, for the world provides little objective evidence that such confidence is justified. Presuming that life is a gracious gift from God does not entail being deceived about the frailty and faultedness of human existence. Like the presumption of a person's innocence, this belief is indefeasible. While it readily admits the existence of counterexamples (like guilty persons), they do not undermine the presumption itself. It is for Christians a faith claim made from under the shadow of the Cross. For example, it is not to assert that objectively renal failure or fetal deformations are gracious gifts. Rather it is to assert that the lives of those who suffer from such evils, despite their costly and burdensome features, remain gracious gifts. It is to consent to one's own frail and faulted life as gracious gift. It is not to seek or to yield passively to suffering, but rather when unavoidable, to adopt it.

The Moral Implications of the Traditional View

Furthermore, the faithful agent is one whose particular responses to others and whose life as a whole is characterized by these presumptions. The Christian not only comes to perceive life as gracious gift but becomes a gift-giver, extends favors, mercy, etc., to others. To see faithfully one's life as graced is, in a word, to live graciously. In his Biblical theology, *Sharing Possessions,* Luke T. Johnson (1981:108) concludes that "the mandate of faith in God is clear: we must, in some fashion, share that which has been given to us by God as a gift." To grasp, hoard, or hold on to the world's goods, including ourselves, is not a proper thanksgiving. As Johnson (1981:99) notes in his exegesis of Sirach, "it is not enough to keep from oppression and injustice; covenant with God demands that we deliver the oppressed."

. . .

Thus sharing the gift of life seems to be a consequence of accepting the cosmology of Christian faith. Monika K. Hellwig writes of this dominical calling,

> In a wide sense we are all called to be parents to one another, to bestow on others the life and blessing with which we have been blessed, that is, to bless others with the substance of our own lives. (Hellwig, 1976:44)

This leads to at least one other kind of reason Christians may offer for such self-giving. This latter reason focuses not so much on what Christians are called to do, but rather on who they are called to be.

Christians are called to be images of God in the world. The paradigmatic example of such an image is the Kenotic Christ (Phil. 2:5-8), whose outpouring is celebrated in the Eucharist. For Christians the death of Jesus is *not* adequately portrayed as the surrogate sacrifice of the perfect scapegoat, the merits from which they passively profit. Instead the death of Jesus is seen as foundational to a covenant community in which Christians are active participants.

. . .

In her reflections on the meaning of the Eucharistic claim that one person can be the bread of another, Hellwig writes:

> Literally and physically this is always true of the mother of the unborn or unweaned child, and it is not accidental that the Bible uses the image of mother to describe God's nurturing. . . . Nor is it accidental or unduly fanciful that mystics have spoken of Jesus and his relationship to the Church in terms of motherhood. (Hellwig, 1976:27)

My purpose here has been three-fold. First, I wished to give some indication of how central self-giving, indeed sacrifice, is to Christian faith and to the sacramental expressions which constitute the Church. Second, I sought to highlight the explicit connection that has been made in the tradition between childbearing and God's own self-giving. Far from being owed anyone or a right, childbearing is most appropriately viewed as a gracious gift, not unlike God's own gratuitous Presence. Third, I have suggested that organ donation can be rendered intelligible and meaningful within this same vision of life.

Notes

1. Within the Anglo-Saxon legal tradition, strangers are usually not required to aid or rescue one another. Indeed, when it reviewed the old common-law crime of "misprision of a felony," the US Supreme Court of 1822 ruled that strangers were not required even to report crimes to legitimate authorities.
2. My attention to the distinctively Christian rationales behind the gift ethos should not be interpreted as a claim that *only* Christians can intelligibly engage in bodily life support. There are lots of non-Christian frameworks which can render gift-giving meaningful.
3. This is clearly not meant to be a comprehensive list. It is, however, a representative sample of the variety of factors relevant to such decision-making.

References

[Fox, Renee C. and Judith P. Swazey, 1974. *The Courage to Fail*. Chicago: University of Chicago Press, 1974.]

Gustafson, James M. 1968 *Christ and the Moral Life*. New York: Harper and Row, Publishers.

Harrison, Beverly Wildung 1983 *Our Right to Choose: Toward a New Ethic of Abortion*. Boston: Beacon Press.

Hauerwas, Stanley 1981 *A Community of Character*. Notre Dame, IN: University of Notre Dame.

Hellwig, Monika K. 1976 *The Eucharist and the Hunger of the World*. New York: Paulist Press.

Johnson, Luke T. 1981 *Sharing Possessions*. Philadelphia: Fortress Press, 1981.

Whitbeck, Caroline 1983 "The Moral Implications of Regarding Women as People: New Perspectives on Pregnancy and Personhood," *Abortion and the Status of the Fetus*, edited by William B. Bondeson et al. Dordrecht, Holland: D. Reidel Publishing Company, 247–272.

35

Motherhood as Moral Choice

Rebecca Todd Peters

Rebecca Todd Peters is a feminist social ethicist and professor of religion at Elon University. She received her PhD from Union Theological Seminary in New York, is ordained in the Presbyterian Church (USA), and serves on the Planned Parenthood Clergy Advocacy Board. She is the author or editor of eight books. In this excerpt, Peters argues for a new understanding of parenting as a sacred trust that reflects the covenant bonds forged between parent and child. From this standpoint, motherhood is not an inevitable consequence of heterosexual activity but a moral choice that women make in response to a calling to motherhood.

The idea of motherhood as a moral choice is a positive Christian ethic of abortion rooted in a sexual ethic of responsibility that promotes sex within healthy and stable relationships, advocates the use of birth control, and recognizes that the primary purpose of sex is not procreation. In fact, many Christians already hold such a view. Within such an ethic, individual women and couples must recognize the possibility of pregnancy and be prepared to act responsibly if a pregnancy occurs. When we reframe the social problem as "how do we respond to an unplanned pregnancy?" we ask different moral questions. These questions don't presuppose a right and wrong answer but instead require us to think about how the whole context of a woman's life is part of the discernment process.

After all, the profoundly moral decision to have a baby will, at minimum, require significant alteration of a woman's daily life for the next nine months. The physical toll that pregnancy takes on a woman's body is remarkable. It

Source: Rebecca Todd Peters, *Trust Women: A Progressive Christian Argument for Reproductive Justice* (Boston: Beacon, 2018).

includes fatigue, nausea, indigestion, cravings, back pain, sleeplessness, weight gain, not to mention labor and delivery or a C-section, or any of the pregnancy-induced conditions that can threaten a woman's life. And yet the decision to parent a child is an even more demanding and long-term moral decision than the decision to give birth. Given that less than 1 percent of women will choose adoption for their children, the majority of women who decide to accept and embrace an unplanned pregnancy are making the significant moral decision to welcome a child into their life.[1] While placing a child for adoption can be an admirable moral decision, qualitative research indicates that most women who do so are not choosing between adoption and abortion but are choosing between adoption and parenting.[2]

. . .

This reality is further confirmed by a recent study known as the Turnaway Study, which followed women who sought abortions but were turned away because they were past the gestational limit of the clinic. Researchers found that even though their study was composed exclusively of women who actively tried to terminate their pregnancies, only 9 percent of the women in that study placed their children for adoption.[3] The evidence indicates that when women decide to continue an unplanned pregnancy, the overwhelming majority are making a lifelong commitment to love, care for, and raise that child. Unwanted pregnancies can become wanted pregnancies, and most women who carry a pregnancy to term do develop an obligation toward their prenate* —an obligation that translates into a desire to keep and raise their child. The Turnaway Study also found that although both women who received abortions and those who were turned away were in comparable economic positions when they were pregnant, one year later, 76 percent of the turnaways (86 percent of whom were living with their babies) were receiving federal assistance compared with 44 percent of the women who had received abortions.[4] In highlighting the economic struggles that some women seeking abortions face, the Turnaway Study shows that women's decisions are influenced by their very real concerns about their ability to financially care for potential children.

For many Christians, the question of whether to have a child is deeply theological. Theologian Kendra Hotz describes parenthood as a calling that not everyone is called to fulfill. She challenges us to think beyond the personal joy and gratification that raising children may bring and to think

---

*Eds.: The term "prenate" refers to the developing products of conception as long as they remain inside the body or uterus.

more deeply about whether the choice to have children is also "a faithful expression of what God is doing—through our lives—in the world." She argues that "the choice for parenthood is bigger than what pleases me; it is also about God's reconciliation of all things."[5]

In the Protestant tradition, individual well-being is intimately linked to vocational calling. The idea that there is deep and abiding value in the work of our lives and that we have a responsibility to discern our calling—vocationally and relationally—in communion with God reflects the importance Christians place on discernment. While discernment often includes consulting with one's community, discerning who God is calling you to be is ultimately a process between an individual and God. A willingness to accept one's calling is an expression of honoring God and respecting the holiness of life that is at the heart of living life as a Christian. Christians regard parenting as a sacred trust in which parents enter a covenant relationship to care for, nurture, and bring up a child to love and know God. It is not a responsibility to be taken lightly but one that requires full knowledge of the commitment and the sacrifices required. If a person is to honor God and the covenant, then any covenant commitment to parenting must be entered into willingly.

When we frame parenthood as a covenant relationship that parents establish with their children, we recognize the powerful social force that human relationships have in shaping personhood. Feminist social ethicist Beverly Harrison explains that personhood, as a reflection of the power of love in community, helps build up individuals by deepening relationships that bring forth genuine community. Her description of love as "the power to act-each-other-into-well-being"... aptly depicts the loving act of a woman who embraces her pregnancy and assents to love her prenate into well-being with her very body and lifeblood.[6] We bring one another into being through our love, support, and care and we cannot survive outside of community.

In recognizing the importance of relationships and love in shaping personhood and human community, and the unique role that birth mothers play in calling their prenates into personhood, we need to reconfigure our understanding of the moral relationship between the prenate and the woman. Only then can we develop a new moral understanding of both pregnancy and abortion. According to this new view, the woman must *assent to* the relationship after recognizing her pregnancy. A woman's acceptance of a pregnancy and her willingness to enter into a relationship with the prenate signals the beginning of her moral obligation to carry that particular pregnancy to term. Still, in a reproductive justice framework, this moral obligation is not absolute. Although childbearing is a calling and a covenant relationship to which a women must assent, conditions in her life may change during the pregnancy such that she may feel the need to withdraw her assent and end the pregnancy. As a liminal category, pregnancy is inherently changing and often unstable. Because the process of becoming requires a pregnant woman's whole body and much more, her willing participation is a prerequisite for pregnancy to be understood as a moral act. Coerced pregnancy under any circumstances, for any reason, is a fundamentally immoral act that violates bodily integrity, respect for individual persons, and the human rights of individuals to choose to procreate or not to procreate.

To honor women's moral wisdom to discern God's calling, we must view a woman's moral obligation to a prenate as a covenant commitment that requires her assent. Actively embracing pregnancy as a covenant responsibility also reflects the moral conditions necessary for such a serious decision. With pregnancy, a woman is obligated to care for herself in particular ways and is later morally and materially obligated to the baby after it is born (either to raise the child or to entrust its care to an adoptive family).

Thinking about the moral status of the prenate as contingent on a woman's acceptance of her pregnancy is a more nuanced way of considering the question of the moral status of the prenate. It is also consistent with a Christian ethical approach to abortion, which focuses on a woman's assent to pregnancy as a necessary component. This approach reflects a Christian theological anthropology centered on relationship and interdependence. Christians believe that we were created to live together in communities of love and support. From this theological perspective, life is not simply about being born, but also about being named, claimed, and welcomed into community and nurtured into being. These characteristics of human dependence and interdependence are in stark contrast with a world that celebrates individuality and independence. They are also morally significant as we contemplate questions of pregnancy, reproduction, and parenting.

When women make decisions about their capacity to carry and bear children, they are also realistically assessing their own capacity to do what is necessary to nurture and care for a pregnant body and the developing prenate. Although the decision to accept a pregnancy and to protect and care for that prenate is an altruistic decision, the opposite decision—to terminate a pregnancy for which one is not ready or able to commit to—is also a responsible choice on the part of the pregnant woman. The decision to abort is often a reflection of self-care. The self-care may be motivated by a wide variety of circumstances. It might reflect a woman's desire to finish school so that she can get a decent job and care for herself and her family. It might reflect an attempt to protect herself in the midst of an abusive relationship. It might reflect her constrained economic reality and the difficulty she has in caring for existing children. It might reflect an acceptance of personal limitations in caring for a baby or another baby at that moment in her life. It might reflect the dissolution or fragility of her relationship with her partner. It might reflect a thousand and more different realities that represent the very real life circumstances out of which women daily make the decision to end a pregnancy so that they can tend to themselves and their current life circumstances. Self-care is not the same thing as selfishness. Until we recognize the difference, we will continue to misinterpret women's actions in misogynist and damning ways that shame women or that attempt to control their behavior.

The completely unfounded perception that women seek abortions casually or without completely understanding the ramifications of their decision can be traced back to those dominant cultural assumptions about woman's nature as the weaker sex, about women's social position as submissive to men, and about God creating women as helpers for men. The subtle (or not-so-subtle) message here is that women can't be trusted to make important life-altering decisions for themselves and that such decisions must be made by male authorities (doctors, the state, judges, priests) who are better able to assess what is in a woman's best interest.

. . .

Respecting Women's Moral Decision Making

We have seen that the failure to trust women to make decisions about their reproduction is rooted in misogyny and sexism. But prejudice based on gender is complicated and intensified when it intersects with racial stereotypes about the sexuality and family values of black and brown women as well as class-based stereotypes about poor women. In her book, *Killing the Black Body*, legal scholar Dorothy Roberts carefully outlines how "derogatory icons of Black women—Jezebel, Mammy, Tragic Mulatto, Aunt Jemima, Sapphire, Matriarch, and Welfare Queen" not only stereotype, demean, and oppress black women, but also undermine black women's access to reproductive justice.[7] These various mythologies weave an intersecting racist web that attacks black women from every possible angle—portraying them as paradoxically both domineering and lazy, wily and stupid, hypersexualized and asexual, as well as genetically deficient, hyperfertile and a host of other derogatory characteristics. This racist mythology laid the groundwork for legislation that incarcerates pregnant women for negligence, for sterilizing women of color without their informed consent, and for treating pregnant women who want abortions like children. Concerns that women make abortion decisions casually arise largely from middle-class, white ideas about what "proper" families should look like as well as moral assumptions about "proper" sexual behavior. Many white, middle-class Americans regard abortion regulations that reflect these middle-class, white assumptions as reasonable.

A Christian ethic of abortion rooted in reproductive justice begins with affirming that abortion is a decision with moral implications while also rejecting the narrow moralistic values that seek to police women's sexual behavior. A responsible ethical response to an unplanned pregnancy includes asking the very serious question of whether one is able to welcome a child into the world and to make a covenant with that child to be a loving and caring parent. When women ask themselves if they can accept an unplanned pregnancy, they are asking a serious moral question without exerting bias that there is a right and wrong moral response. A pregnant woman and her partner who are thinking carefully, morally, and responsibly about their situation, their existing moral obligations, and their capacity to embrace the joys and challenges of either parenting or placing a child for adoption are engaging in meaningful moral discernment. To say that abortion is a moral action is not a Christian argument but rather a moral one consistent with Christian teaching. Many of the actions related to our sexual behavior are moral actions: whether and when to have sex and with whom; whether to use birth control; whether to have children; and, of course, how to respond to a particular pregnancy. These actions have associated moral questions related to how we embody and express our sexuality. These are moral questions because they relate to two of the most fundamental and intimate aspects of our personhood and our identity—our sexuality and our bodies.

The ability to discern good from evil and to act for the good is what we call *moral agency*. It is this ability that Genesis 3 tells us makes humankind "like God." When we recognize that one of the most fundamental aspects of our humanity, our moral agency, is the result of Eve's actions—we can read this story in entirely new ways. Genesis is not a historical record; rather it is full of stories known as *etiologies*, which are stories that people tell to explain or understand themselves and the world in which they live. As an etiology, the story of the Fall explained to our ancestors the physical dangers and realities of childbirth as well as why growing food was so toilsome. The millennia that separates our world from the world of our biblical ancestors means that we no longer read the Bible for scientific explanations. Instead, people of faith read it to seek its moral wisdom. Even as an etiology, the story of Eve seeks to explain why humanity can distinguish right from wrong; it marks our moral agency as part of what it means to be made "in God's image." Reinterpreting Eve's actions as the origin of one of humankind's deepest connections with the divine offers a new warrant for respecting the moral agency of women.

The assumption that just because you get pregnant means you should have a baby not only is outdated, but also reflects biased and demeaning assumptions about women, motherhood, pregnancy, and children. Whether it is an unplanned and unwanted pregnancy — or a wanted pregnancy in which the circumstances of the pregnant woman or the prenate have changed—women actively seek abortions as moral agents taking active steps to shape their future. In women's moral decision about unplanned pregnancies, we see much of what psychologist Carol Gilligan found more than thirty years ago.[8] Gilligan notes that women base much of their moral reasoning on their existing moral relationships and obligations and that they evaluate the possibility of future moral obligations in light of their capacity to act responsibly in an imagined potential relationship. When women evaluate these possibilities, they consider many factors, including their financial ability to care for a child or another child, their ability to provide a safe and loving home for a child, and their ability to honor their own health and well-being, including their career and vocational plans.

Cultural expectations that women should welcome pregnancy and children are rooted in patriarchal expectations about what women should want and how women should respond to motherhood or potential motherhood. They are also rooted in middle-class, white assumptions about two-parent households where men make money to take care of their families. Romanticized expectations about how families ought to be ordered and what roles men and women play in these families continue to underlie cultural expectations about pregnancy and parenting. When women do not fit this mold, empathy and sympathy are often withheld from them and they are instead judged for their perceived moral laxity. This moral laxity is often associated with sexual activity: having sex outside marriage, having sex without the willingness to welcome a child, or having sex without contraception.

Women are not supposed to enjoy sex, desire it, or have sex unless they are willing to "suffer the consequences" or "accept their responsibility" or any other of the familiar cultural tropes that are used to portray expectations about how women should behave in light of an unplanned and unwanted pregnancy. Most women like sex as much as men do. Women's desire to have sex for pleasure and/or as part of their intimate relationships is normal and can be a healthy part of women's well-being. For many women, having an abortion *is* "accepting their responsibility" in a situation where having a child or another child would be an irresponsible decision.

. . .

When we shift from judgment to justice, we become the kind of community that helps women solve problems and live healthy and safe lives rather than blaming and shaming them for decisions they make in good faith about their future and their families. This reimagined vision of childbearing is the foundation of an ethic of reproductive justice.

Notes

1. J. Jones, *Adoption Experiences [of Women and Men and Demand for Children to Adopt by Women 18-44 Years of Age in the United States, 2002* Vital and Health Statistics series 23, no. 27 (Washington, DC: US Department of Health and Human Services, Centers for Disease Control and Prevention, 2008): 1-36]; Diana Greene Foster, Heather Gould, Jessica Taylor, and Tracy A. Weitz, "Attitudes and Decision Making Among Women Seeking Abortions at One U.S. Clinic," *Perspectives on Sexual and Reproductive Health* 44, no. 2 (June 1, 2012): 117–24.
2. Gretchen Sisson, "'Choosing Life': Birth Mothers on Abortion and Reproductive Choice," *Women's Health Issues* 25, no. 4 (July 2015): 349–54.
3. Gretchen Sisson, Lauren Ralph, Heather Gould, and Diana Greene Foster, "Adoption Decision Making among Women Seeking Abortion," *Women's Health Issues* 27, no. 2 (March 1, 2017): 136–44.
4. [Diana Greene] Foster, "Socioeconomic Consequences of Abortion Compared to Unwanted Birth" [presented at the American Public Health Association, San Francisco, October 30, 2012].
5. Kendra G. Hotz, "Happily Ever After: Christians without Children," in *Encountering the Sacred: Feminist Reflections on Women's Lives*, ed.

Rebecca Todd Peters and Grace Yia-Hei Kao, eds., London: T&T Clark, [2018]).

6. Beverly Harrison, "The Power of Anger in the Work of Love," in *Making the Connections: Essays in Feminist Social Ethics* (Boston: Beacon, 1985), [11].

7. [Dorothy] Roberts, *Killing the Black Body* [*Race, Reproduction, and the Meaning of Liberty* (First Vintage Books edition, 1997; repr., New York: Vintage, 1999)], Introduction.

8. Carol Gilligan, *In a Different Voice: Psychological Theory and Women's Development* (Cambridge, MA: Harvard University Press, 1982).

36

Contesting Abortion as Sin

Margaret D. Kamitsuka

Margaret Kamitsuka is Professor Emeritus of Religion at Oberlin College, Ohio. This excerpt makes the theological case for why abortion should not be labeled as sin. This discussion constitutes part of Kamitsuka's larger argument for a Christian theological position that grants the value of fetal life, while also upholding the pregnant person's moral agency for reproductive self-determination.

In some way, shape, or form, pro-life proponents see abortion as sinful. At the most compassionate side, if one can call it that, there is a discourse about "abortive moms" as sinners, but partially victimized ones[1]—coerced into abortion by selfish partners or angry parents, manipulated by unscrupulous abortion providers, and then traumatized by regret. There are a number of pro-life writers who promote these views, such as self-described psychologist David Reardon and Eastern Orthodox writer Frederica Mathewes-Green, who focus on issues such as the psychological and spiritual trauma that "post-abortive women" experience. On the latter point, Reardon writes: "One could argue that the harm that the woman suffers is greater since her soul is damaged by abortion, while the child only suffers physical death and remains spiritually untouched."[2] Mathewes-Green has been a strong advocate of showing compassion to these post-abortive women because doing so, she believes, will produce genuine repentance that will prevent any future abortions. By interviewing women recruited from pro-life postabortion counseling groups (which is not a random sampling), Mathewes-Green finds data in support of this compassion-oriented approach. As one woman said,

Source: Margaret D. Kamitsuka, *Abortion and the Christian Tradition: A Pro-choice Theological Ethic* (Louisville: Westminster John Knox, 2019).

speaking retrospectively about her abortion, "I also realized that, even though I did this terrible thing, God loves me; he loved me even before I said, 'I'm sorry, it was wrong.'"[3] This type of pro-life advocacy supports organizations that have ministries to serve women with counseling and retreats where they can repent of the wrong they have done and ask forgiveness from God and from their aborted fetus.

At the other end of the pro-life spectrum are those voices criticizing the trope of the victimized postabortion woman who needs compassion. One sees these arguments from scholars such as Francis Beckwith, who criticizes the pro-life strategy of "appealing to the pregnant woman's self-interest to persuade her not to have an abortion." Beckwith argues that this so-called softball strategy "may result in nurturing . . . a philosophical mindset that is consistent with abortion's moral permissibility,"[4] because it does not insist on calling abortion "unjustified homicide."[5] More politically extreme versions of Beckwith's rigorist call-a-sin-a-sin viewpoint can be found in the writings of militant anti-abortion activists. Some radical anti-abortion proponents claim that women who abort are guilty of "premeditated murder."[6] Extremist anti-abortion groups support penalizing women who abort and even using violence against abortion clinics and abortion providers. One ultra-right-wing Christian website states more baldly what Beckwith says indirectly: "The 'pro-life movement' in this nation has made the woman into a victim. That's right—they actually want us to believe that the woman who hires a paid assassin to murder her own child is in fact a victim herself."[7] There are a number of assumptions grounding this kind of rhetoric, whether scholarly or extremist: the two central ones are the claim that the fetus is a person, not just analogous to a born child but actually substantially equivalent to a born child; and the claim that the fetus needs to be protected (via strict abortion bans) from its gestating mother. . . .

Pro-choice proponents reject calling abortion sin—mostly invoking the notion of tragedy. There is a realistic basis for this viewpoint, if one thinks about the human condition—its brutishness and precariousness, especially for vulnerable classes of people—and the fact that, short of the eschaton, the believer has only partial knowledge of God's ways and sees only as if "through a glass, darkly" (1 Cor. 13:12 KJV). When human finitude combines with the inability to see how to move forward with an unintended pregnancy, one has the recipe for a tragic choice. That said, I disagree with Daniel Maguire's claim that "abortion is always tragic."[8] Calling all abortions tragic could imply that gestating fetal life is a pregnant woman's intrinsic and not overly onerous moral obligation, but life circumstances tragically make it impossible for her to follow through. . . . I insist on recognizing pregnancy as a risky and significant demand. . . . If a woman decides not to continue her pregnancy because she has already committed herself to other obligations, that decision, should not be spoken of as tragic, any more than one would call tragic a person's decision not to be a live organ donor. No physician would ever say to the potential donor, "You must avert the tragedy of my patient dying and give him your kidney" or "It's a tragedy that you are not opting to be a kidney donor." Some women's abortions are felt by them as tragic since they wish they could have had more options to be able to do otherwise, but not all abortions should be categorized as such.

Pro-choice scholars invoke the notion of tragedy, in part, to garner sympathy for women with unwanted pregnancies, and I agree that sympathy is in order; however, the category of tragedy can inadvertently mask the fact that abortion is a decision—to my mind, a maternal decision—that a gestating women has the responsibility and the authority to make. . . . I [have] insisted on the necessity of seeing abortion as a woman's morally serious maternal decision that there be no child born to whom she would have further mothering obligations. If one takes the position that abortion is a woman's decision, and not just a calamity that befalls her, then one has to face head on, theologically, the pro-life charge that abortion is an intentional sin.

There are at least four reasons why a choice for abortion should not be seen as ipso facto intentional sin. First, there is no clear theological basis for declaring that abortion is a sin of murder, because that judgment can only be made within a mind-set that has already predetermined that abortion is the intentional and unwarranted killing of a person. . . . Historically, deeming abortion to be homicide was largely a canon law development linked to the criminalization of abortion in the Middle Ages; even then, the crime did not apply to the unformed fetus but only to the ensouled, formed fetus—that is, a legal person.[9] Pro-life proponents today reject the unformed/formed conceptuality but try to sustain the charge of homicide with a variety of biblical, theological, and philosophical arguments. [Elsewhere,] I have shown the instability and confusion of pro-life claims to fetal personhood from conception (based on genetics, the *imago Dei*, biblical descriptions of life in the womb, probabalism, and so on). . . . I suggested that the term "person"— whose commonplace meaning is an embodied, born individual— cannot be said to apply unambiguously to a human being existing contingently and contiguously to its mother's body. A fetus, thus understood, is neither innocent nor an aggressor, neither mere human tissue nor preborn baby. Its death, by miscarriage or abortion, is not negligible, as women's own words attest. One cannot say that a fetus is a nonperson. Neither can one say that abortion of a still-developing fetus is the murder of a person in any commonplace meaning of the word. Abortion is undeniably the demise of a developing human being, but because pregnancy is a sui generis type of human experience, abortion death is a sui generis type of death. Abortion is the only situation in which one human agent causes the death of a human being developing within her own body. It is death that is not accidental, but it is death without malice. The one who dies is not a nonperson but not a person either. Hence, abortion cannot be said to constitute the sin of murder.

Second, even if someone concedes that "murder" is not an appropriate word for abortion, the argument could still be made that the destruction of uterine life constitutes a sinful denial of its value. I agree with the premise about uterine life having value but disagree that its destruction should be necessarily seen as denying its value, no matter how paradoxical that sounds. I have argued for seeing value as inhering at every emergent stage of a human organism for multiple reasons: it is genetically human, developing toward personhood, and intimately existing contingently and contiguously to its gestating mother.[10] If the discourse of women who abort is any indication, a pregnant woman's "no" to further gestation is rarely a denial of the value of life in her womb; indeed, many women speak of aborting their "baby." Even feminist philosophers invoke Emmanuel Levinas's notions of the ethical demand of the "face" of the Other, including the fetal Other.[11] A woman's "no" to gestational hospitality may be expressed as an immediate desire simply not to be pregnant anymore, and that desire is valid, in and of itself, for all the reasons I have given about the burdens and risks of pregnancy. In addition, abortion decisions can be seen as an acknowledgment that the woman feels unable to take on the caring relationship of nurturing, birthing, and being the mother of this baby—whether she uses those words or not. . . . Pro-life accusations that women who abort are callous and, hence, sinful do not even cohere with their own research data, which documents some women as admitting anguish over their abortion.[12] To pro-life proponents, women's admission of anguish is proof of sin; I take it as proof of a moral conscience and, hence, a tacit acknowledgment of fetal value. As such, abortion cannot be said to be an ipso facto sin of denying fetal value.

Third, even if one accepts that abortion is not a sin against a fetal person and not a denial of fetal value, it could still be a sin against God. Most theologians would agree that sin is a relational category including so-called horizontal relationships among humans in the world and the vertical God-human relationship. A pro-choice theologian cannot rule out that a woman may be sinning against God, in some way, in her act of abortion, if one accepts the aptness of the biblical assertion "all have sinned and fall short of the glory of God" (Rom. 3:23). However, this biblical assertion about sin cuts both ways: if a woman might sin in her abortion, so might pro-life protesters in their self-righteous and judgmental attitudes. . . . If, when, and the degree to which any abortion (or any judgment about that abortion) involves alienation from God—that can only be determined by the individual's own conscience, *coram Deo*, since God alone will "test the mind and search the heart" (Jer. 17:10). There is no objective way to know if, or the extent to which, a particular act of abortion death has damaged a woman's relationship with God, and thus there is no justifiable theological reason for assuming that a woman's act of abortion has automatically alienated her from God.

Abortion cannot be judged, from the outside, to be a sin against God simply because a death has occurred. Theologically, if God is acknowledged as the "maker of all things both seen and unseen" (Nicene Creed), then to destroy any part of God's creation—including fetal life, however one views it—could be a sin against the Creator. However, God has chosen to wrap uterine life in a veil of obscurity: "Just as you do not know how the breath comes to the bones in the mother's womb, so you do not know the work of God, who makes everything" (Eccl. 11:5). There is no definitive theological or biblical teaching, or even a preponderance thereof, to establish that every fetus is ordained by God for life on earth. Impregnation should not be taken as an indubitable sign of God's providential will that a child should be gestated and born. . . . For this reason, a woman's decision not to continue to gestate her fetus until birth cannot be deemed ipso facto sin against God. On the other hand, compelling a woman to gestate a fetus against her will strikes me as a callous act and an act of hubris, even if done with the best intentions toward the fetus.

A fourth reason for why one should not call abortion a sin is supplemented by feminist analyses about women surviving under conditions of patriarchy and other oppressions. It is not a sin to survive. As Asian American feminist theologian Rita Nakashima Brock has so perceptively explained, women, who for so long were praised for being obedient and passive, must learn another mode of existing in order to survive and build a decent future for themselves and their families. Brock, who has worked to bring the issue of domestic violence and sexual abuse into the sphere of theological reflection, argues that one of the most destructive aspects of the Christian tradition is its privileging of notions such as Christ's purity and obedience unto death.

For those people who experience various forms of abuse, and the resulting internalized shame, these ideals of obedience and purity are devastating. Brock suggests that marginalized groups, such as Asian American women like herself, struggle analogously from the exploitation that falls upon them as a result of "seeking to be good or clinging to trust in the power of others." To all these marginalized survivors, Brock says: "We must lose innocence in order to gain hope." Instead of innocence, Brock prefers the category of wisdom, which she associates with being "strong, strategically smart, skeptical, cunning, caring, . . . politically savvy"—attributes that she believes fit Jesus of the Gospel narratives.[13] Those who abandon romantic notions of purity may be labeled as sinners, in part because taking the path of wise survival may involve acts of moral ambiguity.

I find Brock's category of being wise, rather than obedient, as aptly applicable to many women who face difficult reproductive decisions. This category further shows that it may not be appropriate to call every abortion a tragedy. It is not a tragedy for a woman to survive. To put this idea into a biblical key, we might say that [Mary's] *fiat mihi* [("be it unto me," Luke 1:38 KJV)] may be an obedient, trusting response to an unplanned pregnancy but may not always be the wise and feasible response. In some situations, what a woman deems as necessary for her survival (whether physical, economic, emotional, or something else) may mean she loses her so-called innocence in lieu of a wise course of action. This kind of survival cannot be appropriately labeled sin.

Notes

1. Frederica Mathewes-Green, *Real Choices: Offering Practical Life-Affirming Alternatives to Abortion* (Sisters, OR: Multnomah Books, 1994), 124.
2. David C. Reardon, "A Defense of the Neglected Rhetorical Strategy (NRS)," *Ethics & Medicine* 18, no. 2 (2002): 25.
3. Mathewes-Green, *Real Choices*, 125.
4. Francis J. Beckwith, "Taking Abortion Seriously: A Philosophical Critique of the New Anti-Abortion Rhetorical Shift," *Ethics & Medicine* 17, no. 3 (2001): 161.
5. Beckwith, "Taking Abortion Seriously," 162. . . .
6. Michael Bray, *A Time to Kill: A Study concerning the Use of Force and Abortion* (Portland, OR: Advocates for Life, 1994), 21.

7. Matthew Trewhella, "Should Women Be Punished for Murdering Their Own Son or Daughter by Abortion?" *Army of God* (n.d.), https://www .armyofgod.com/MatthewTrewhella WomenPunishedAbortion.html. For more on this group, see Jennifer Jefferis, *Armed for Life: The Army of God and Anti-Abortion Terror in the United States* (Santa Barbara, CA: Praeger, 2011). . . .

8. Daniel C. Maguire, "Abortion: A Question of Catholic Honesty," *Christian Century* 100, no. 26 (1983): 805.

9. See [Margaret D. Kamitsuka, *Abortion and the Christian Tradition: A Pro-choice Theological Ethic* (Louisville: Westminster John Knox, 2019),] chap. 1 . . .

10. See [ibid.,] chap. 5. . . .

11. For my discussion of this Levinasian point, see [ibid., 186–7]. . . .

12. See David C. Reardon, "Women Who Abort: Their Reflections on Abortion," *Post-Abortion Review* 4, no. 1 (1996). . . . I have criticized Reardon's research and credentials elsewhere. See Margaret D. Kamitsuka, "Feminist Scholarship and Its Relevance for Political Engagement: The Test Case of Abortion in the U.S.," *Religion and Gender* 1, no. 1 (2011): 26.

13. Rita Nakashima Brock, "Losing Your Innocence but Not Your Hope," in *Reconstructing the Christ Symbol: Essays in Feminist Christology*, ed. Maryanne Stevens (Mahwah, NJ: Paulist, 1993), 40, 42–3.

37

A Womanist Theo-Ethic of Reproductive Justice

Toni M. Bond

One of the founders of the reproductive justice (RJ) movement, Toni Bond has worked in the reproductive health, rights, and justice movement for over twenty-five years. A self-described "fierce womanist and RJ activist," Bond connects theological reflections with the grassroots voices and lives of women of color. This excerpt, adapted from her doctoral dissertation at Claremont School of Theology in California is an original contribution to this volume. In it she offers insights into how a womanist commitment to the dignity of African American women and to the principles of RJ contribute to what she calls a "theology of sexual autonomy."

The parameters of reproductive justice (RJ) begin with recognizing Black women as moral agents with the ability to act independently. Recognizing Black women as moral agents includes valuing their inherent dignity and self-worth. Reproductive justice theory not only affirms Black women as human beings with agency, it counters the notion that Black women are inferior and incapable of thinking for themselves. It is because Black women have practical reasoning capabilities that they can make decisions about their reproductive and sexual lives. Intricately tied to agency is autonomy. Reproductive justice theory holds that Black women must have the agency to make autonomous decisions about whether to carry a pregnancy to term or to have an abortion or even to be sexually active or to practice abstinence. Finally, valuing Black women's agency includes acknowledging the value and authority of individual narratives about their reproductive and sexual lives.

Source: Toni M. Bond, "Faithful Voices: Creating a Womanist Theo-ethic of Reproductive Justice," PhD. Diss. (Claremont School of Theology, 2020).

I have constructed a womanist theo-ethic of reproductive justice that expands the reproductive justice theory and framework by naming and assigning ethical value to Black women's agency, resistance, and resiliency in their reproductive and sexual lives. The first key virtue of reproductive justice is practical wisdom. Reproductive justice values the practical wisdom Black women exercise to make prudent decisions about their reproductive and sexual health. It further recognizes that Black women utilize their practical wisdom to discern what is right for them at a particular moment in time, with consideration for what will be in their own best interest, is beneficial to their families, and takes into account available support systems within their communities.

The second key virtue of reproductive justice is resistance. Resistance represents Black women's embodied activism and determination to push against patriarchy, chauvinism, forms of religion that try to colonize Black people's bodies, and white supremacy. Black women engage in acts of resistance when they refuse to adhere to patriarchal norms like refraining from premarital sex, which when targeted at Black sexuality, is rooted in a white supremacist ideology imposed upon them by family members, intimate partners, churches, and policy makers. Reproductive justice draws upon womanist theologian Kelly Brown Douglas's sexual discourse of resistance that calls upon the Black community to engage in a comprehensive form of discourse about Black sexuality.[1]

The final key virtue of RJ to which I assign value is resiliency. Resiliency as a virtue in reproductive justice theory speaks to Black women's capacity to not just endure, but to overcome and thrive against interlocking forms of oppression. Resiliency as a virtue is tied to fortitude in the midst of adversity. Black women demonstrate their resiliency when they transcend forms of reproductive and sexual oppression designed to control their procreative liberty, deny their moral authority to determine whether to bear children, and hinder their ability to have and maintain healthy families in healthy, vibrant communities.

A Theology of Sexual Autonomy

A theology of sexual autonomy disrupts the narrative that human sexuality is sinful or illicit if it is outside marriage, with more than one partner, or with an LBGTQIA partner. It supports autonomy of sexual preference and respects the autonomy of young people when they are mature enough to discern when it is the right time for them to engage in sexual activity and can provide informed consent, which I discuss further below. A theology of sexual autonomy teaches that sex is both sacred and beautifully gifted from God between two consenting individuals. Womanist theologian, Kelly Brown Douglas points out that,

> When sexuality is expressed in a way that provides for and nurtures harmonious relationships—that is, those that are loving, just, and equal—then it is sacred. Only when sexual expression is objectified and thus disconnected from harmonious relationships is it sinful. The measure of what is sinful has to do with whether or not it contributes to right/harmonious relationships with God, community, and others.[2]

A theology of sexual autonomy further identifies as sinful the shaming of individuals for having premarital sex, LBGTQ+ discrimination, and shaming and judging teenagers for becoming pregnant. Shame, judgment, and discrimination are acts that interfere with an individual's right to enjoy a harmonious relationship with God and the community.

In her discussion of evangelical sin and sexual purity, womanist ethicist Monique Moultrie observes that the sin is greater than just the woman's actions or 'going astray'. Instead, any sexual activity outside of the defined evangelical sexual boundaries of heterosexual, marital activity jeopardizes the salvation of the woman, her future children, and the greater Christian evangelical community who witness the woman's actions.[3] The very action of judgment that causes women and girls to feel shame and guilt and that alienates them from community must also be viewed as sinful because it is a defilement of their human psyche, an attack on their mental sense of self-worth. Womanist theologian, Delores S. Williams writes,

> Inasmuch as womanist theology takes the Bible seriously as a validating tool, a womanist notion of sin claims that defilement of black women's bodies and the resulting attack upon their spirits and self-esteem constitute the gravest kind of social sin of which American patriarchal and demonarchal society is guilty.[4]

As Williams notes, the defilement of Black women's bodies and attacks upon their individual spirit and self-esteem are particularly heinous forms of social sin because they leave lasting, residual scars that Black women internalize, which cause them to question their own value and self-worth. The judgment often meted out by the Black church upon women and girls for engaging in premarital sex, becoming pregnant as a teenager or as an unmarried adult, or for having an abortion disrupts the relationship Black women and girls have with God because it causes them to carry a burden of shame, which is counter-intuitive to God's love.

A theology of sexual autonomy also values the body and the ability to give consent. It necessarily recognizes the relationship between human embodiment, human identity, and human sexuality, and that all three are important within the context of humanity's relationship with God. Religious and theological anthropology scholar, Marc Cortez points out that sexuality is a core aspect of human existence and 'a natural and essential aspect of humanity'.[5] Sexual autonomy is vital to human embodiment and sexuality. Thus, a theology of sexual autonomy includes the right to be self-governing over one's body. Within that autonomy is the virtue of agency and the moral authority an individual has to be self-governing about with whom and when to have sex. God imbues us with free-will at birth, which once we are born connects with our ability to consent, for it is free-will that enables us to consent. Irenaeus of Lyons argued that God imbues humans with all that they are and all that they will become. He writes,

> For you did not make God, but God you. If, then, you are God's workmanship, await the hand of your Maker which creates everything in due time; in due time as far as you are concerned, whose creation is being carried out. . . . by preserving the framework you shall ascend to that which is perfect, for the moist clay which is in you is hidden [there] by the workmanship of God. His hand fashioned your substance.[6]

Therefore, any responsible doctrine of consent necessarily connects God's creation of humans imbued with free-will to their ability to consent.

Although we are born with the ability to consent, our reasoning capabilities must undergo a process of maturation before we can engage in a process of discernment to make decisions. Irenaeus believed that humans were born in a state of immaturity because they were created by God out of nothingness. From that state of immaturity, God continuously pours knowledge into humans bringing them to a state of maturity. In the case of providing consent around sexual autonomy, there are consensual age laws, which vary from state to state, to protect young people from sexual exploitation. Still, while those laws were designed to protect them from sexual predators, these same laws have also been used to deny young people their human right to make decisions to become sexually active, to obtain an abortion, and to carry pregnancies to term. Young people are capable of making important life decisions about their reproductive and sexual health. For example many young people, when confronted with unintended pregnancies engage in a discernment process around whether to carry a pregnancy to term and parent the child, place the child for adoption, or have an abortion, utilizing their reasoning capabilities to exercise their inherent free-will to consent to parent or not.

A theology of sexual autonomy also recognizes that just as young people have the moral capacity to exercise agency around their sexuality, teenage girls also have the capacity to parent a child if they are provided with the necessary social and economic supports. A theology of sexual autonomy counters the guilt that has been associated with premarital sex, teenage pregnancy, and teenage sexuality with sinlessness. It situates shame where it belongs, with oppressive theology. Guilt and shame are clarified in a theology of sexual autonomy as tools of oppression to keep sexual beings from being sexually liberated.

The reproductive justice virtue of resistance is also a part of a theology of sexual autonomy. Together with agency, resistance in a theology of sexual autonomy counters biblical interpretations that teach that the body is sinful and sex is taboo and engages with the biblical text through a womanist theological lens that is sex positive.[7] It further seeks to identify those places in the biblical text that speak of human sexuality as pleasurable, like the Song of Songs or 1 Corinthians 13 where love is referenced as patient and kind.

A theology of sexual autonomy is also a process-relational theology that speaks truth, life, and love into the life of the young teenager who is pregnant and acknowledges the virtue of resiliency and that young people do have the fortitude to raise healthy children when they are given adequate social and economic supports. Therefore, it is sinful when teenagers are not given the adequate social and economic supports to raise their children. Thus, the actual sin is not that the teenager has become pregnant, but that there are not enough economic and social programs supporting their development and creative transformation into a parent raising a healthy child. When the church chooses to shame and blame a teenage pregnancy, it is a sin against the young women because the church has chosen to ignore God's persuasive call to partner with God to positively influence the lives of a mother and her child.

Teenagers often do not feel comfortable talking to their parents about their decision to become sexually active and they fear talking to any of the leadership at their churches because they know they will more than likely be judged for desiring to become sexually active. But it begs the question of the difference it would make in the reproductive and sexual lives of young people if churches would create a welcoming atmosphere where the theology taught was about a God that partners with humans, that is continuously interacting with humans, transforming them and humans transforming God, and which teaches that the contours of human's lives are not fixed but ever-changing.

A theology of sexual autonomy stands in resistance to practices of calling teenage mothers or anyone else before church congregations to public repent for being sexual beings. A theology of sexual autonomy reconnects human sexuality with spirituality and affirms the agency and autonomy that comes directly from God.

A Theology of Reproductive Autonomy

Like sexual autonomy, a theology of reproductive autonomy also values the body and the ability to give consent. It recognizes the relationship between human embodiment, human identity, and procreative liberty. A woman's procreative liberty is primary in a theology of reproductive autonomy because the woman enters into a creative partnership with God to bring forth life. At the same time, it acknowledges that the ultimate decision of whether to bring forth a life rests with the woman because of the free-will imbued by God to consent.

A theology of reproductive autonomy is also interdependent. Decisions may be made independently, but they can have an impact that goes far beyond the individual, which is why it also values life. Valuing does not mean placing the life of the woman over the life of the fetus. Instead, it means valuing all life as sacred and, likewise, that the life of the woman and her capacity to discern whether it is an appropriate time to bring forth another human life is also sacred. This is especially important for Black women whose humanity has historically been denied and their ability to exercise procreative liberty, in creative partnership with God, around their pregnancies has been disrupted. Realizing the full humanity that God created Black women with recognizes that they are able to make decisions about their procreative liberty, free from human interferences that attempt to stand in the way of their reproductive autonomy.

Notes

1. Kelly Brown Douglas, *Sexuality and the Black Church: A Womanist Perspective* (Maryknoll: Orbis, 1999), 69.
2. Kelly Brown Douglas, *What's Faith Got to Do with It? Black Bodies/Christian Souls* (Maryknoll: Orbis, 2005), 215.
3. Monique Moultrie, *Passionate and Pious: Religious Media and Black Women's Sexuality* (Durham: Duke University Press, 2017), 23-4.
4. Delores S. Williams, 'A Womanist Perspective on Sin' in *A Troubling in My Soul* ed. Emilie M Townes (Maryknoll: Orbis, 1993), 144.
5. Marc Cortez, *Theological Anthropology: A Guide for the Perplexed* (New York: T&T Clark, 2010), 643.
6. Irenaeus of Lyons, *Against Heresies*, 4.39.2.
7. The International Society for Sexual Medicine defines sex positive as having positive attitudes about sex and feeling comfortable with one's own sexual identity and with the sexual behaviors of others. See "What Does 'Sex Positive' Mean?" *International Society for Sexual Medicine*.

Islam

38

Shiite Perspective on the Moral Status of the Early Human Embryo

Kiarash Aramesh

Kiarash Aramesh has his medical degree from Tehran University of Medical Sciences and his PhD in Healthcare Ethics from Duquesne University. His essay gives insight into Shiite perspectives on moral issues related to the embryo and early fetus. Shiism is the second largest branch of Islam (Sunni Islam being the largest), comprising approximately 10 percent of the global Muslim population. Iran functions as a center for Shiite theological and legal theory and rulings for Sharia law. Shiite Islam shares with Sunni Islam adherence to the Quran, but Shiites revere a different set of normative traditions (sunna) comprised of narratives (hadiths) about the Prophet Muhammad. Aramesh discusses the moral and legal implications of the issue of ensoulment and the embryo's implantation in the uterus.

Shiite Fiqh and the Early Human Life

Islamic *fiqh* (including its Sunni and Shiite branches), also referred as *Shari'a* law, has four main sources. The first and most important one is the Holy *Qur'an*, the primary source of Islamic law. The second source of Islamic law is the Tradition or *sunna*, which is what the prophet (and the innocent

Source: Kiarash Aramesh, "Shiite Perspective on the Moral Status of the Early Human Embryo: A Critical Review," *Journal of Religion and Health* 57, no. 6 (2018): 2182–92.

imams* in the Shiite school) said, did, or agreed to. The third source is *ijma*, which is the consensus of Islamic scholars (in Shiite jurisprudence, this source is used with limitations. Some authorities believe that only the cases of consensus that have been endorsed by an innocent Imam are valid). The fourth is reason (*aghl*) in the Shiite schools and analogy (*qiyas*) in the Sunni schools of jurisprudence (Motahari 2001, pp. 16–22; Fadel 2012).

In dealing with ethico-legal questions about the early human life, the most referred and cited resources are the Holy Qur'an and the *sunna*. However, Shiite jurists (like other scholars in other fields) have always read, understood, and interpreted these sources according to their scientific knowledge and understanding of human embryology. Therefore, studying the Shiite perspective on the ethical status of the early human life necessitates exploring the related parts in Qur'an and *sunna* and the way Shiite jurists understood and interpreted them and how their understanding has been evolved through history.

Qur'anic Embryology and the Meaning of *Nutfa*

The term *nutfa*, by which the semen and the early human embryo have been named in the most Islamic classical texts and scriptures, has been repeated 12 times in the Holy *Qur'an*. In some verses, the consecutive stages of embryonic and fetal development are described, for example:

> We created the human from an essence of clay. Then we made him, a drop (*nutfa*), in a secure receptacle (the womb). Then we created of the drop, a clot (of congealed blood) and we created the clot into bite size tissue, then we created the bite size tissue into bones, then we clothed the bones with flesh, and then produced it another creation. Blessed is Allah, the best of creators! (23:12–14)

. . .

Obviously, the term used for referring to the early human embryo in the Holy *Qur'an* and Islamic Holy Scripture is *nutfa*. Other terms, like *alaqa* (the clot) and *mudgha* (tissue) that represent the subsequent stages of fetal development, are not covered by this article (Sachedina 2009, pp. 131–134).

---

*Eds.: The Shiite tradition considers the valid successors to the mission of the Prophet Mohammed to be "innocent" or sinless imams.

According to the Holy Qur'an, *nutfa* is the very first stage of development of an embryo. Whether it is attributed to: (a) the sperm (male gamete) which continues to form an early embryo in the womb (the traditional understanding of embryonic development); or (b) just the result of conception which develops in the womb after fertilizing an egg by a sperm (the modern understanding of embryonic development), is not clear in the verses themselves (Ghaly 2014). However, the commentators and interpreters, based on their understanding of embryology, have read the text differently.

In some verses, the former interpretation is more obvious, for example:

> . . . was he not a drop of fluid which gushed forth? (75:37)

while, the proponents of the latter interpretation refer to the verses which denote a "mixed *nutfa*" as the very first stage of embryonic development, for example:

> Indeed, there came upon the human a period of time when he was an unremembered thing. We have created the human from a drop (*nutfa*), a mixture, testing him; we made him to hear and see. (76:1–2)

As seen above, the *Qur'an* describes the consecutive stages of embryonic growth and development, but does not provide any quantitative measures of the length of each stage. Muslim jurists have usually relied upon the *sunna* for determining the length of each stage and accordingly, estimating the time of the last development (*khalghan akhar*) that is supposed to bestow full ethical status to the human fetus. For this purpose, Shiite jurists appealed to the following quotations (*hadiths*) of the prophet and innocent Imams:

According to a *hadith* of the prophet Mohammad, narrated by and named after *Abdullah Ibn Masoud,* each of the developmental stages mentioned by *Qur'an*, *nutfa*, *alaqa*, and *mudgha*, lasts for 40 days. Therefore, the earliest possible time for ensoulment is 120 days after the formation of *nutfa*. This *hadith* is narrated by Sunni sources; however, some Shiite authorities also appealed to this *hadith* for this purpose (Fadel 2012; Muhaqiq Karaki 1993, p. 406; Shahid Thani 1993, p. 195). In Shiite sources, there are also other *hadiths* from the Shiite innocent Imams denoting the same or other descriptions for the Qur'anic stages of embryonic development (Ibn Babvaiy 2009, p. 311; Koleini 2009, p. 347; Sachedina 2009, pp. 132–133).

As a matter of fact, in describing natural issues—from the human body to astronomic facts—the *Qur'an* never obviously contradicts the knowledge of the era in which the Prophet lived. Therefore, the commentators and interpreters of the *Qur'an*, before the modern era, had never understood the

Qur'anic verses describing the growth and development of fetus in contradiction with Aristotle's or Galen's descriptions of the early human life. Accordingly, they did not consider any difference between semen and the early human embryo (before 40th day) (Ghaly 2014).

Even now, some commentators and jurists utilize this word with ambiguity. Some others, however, clearly recognize the findings of modern science, which show the very difference between sperm (the male gamete) and early embryo (the result of conception in which a male and a female gamete are combined to form a zygote and then the zygote multiplies to form the embryo) (Tabatabayi 1987, p. 209).

It seems that some interpretations with regard to the moral status of the human embryo in Islamic revelations have been based upon the traditional understandings of human embryology, rooted in the ancient Greek and Medieval Islamic medical sciences (Ghaly 2014). On the other hand, the permitted extent of relying on the modern scientific findings in ethical conclusions is not agreed upon among Islamic schools of thought. Therefore, some interpreters and jurists rely on the traditional understandings that equate *nutfa* to the semen and the first stages of embryonic development in the womb and others see the fundamental differences between the sperm and the early embryo and consider *nutfa* as equal to only the early human embryo. This ambiguity in the adopted embryologic account (traditional or modern) has resulted in some degrees of discrepancy and contradiction among their ethical viewpoints (Alai and Rezai 2009).

The Importance of Implantation

In their assessment of the tort committed against the fetus, jurists have regarded the implantation of the *nutfa* in the uterus as the beginning point of the sacred embryonic life beyond which any infliction of harm to it necessitates a compensation (*diya*) (Najafi 1981, pp. 373–389). Before implantation, destroying the *nutfa*, without any justifiable reason, is considered morally disliked but, according to the majority of Shiite scholars, no monetary compensation has been considered for it (Esfandyari 2013). The monetary compensation gets higher with the growth of the embryo and fetus and reaches its maximum level after 120 days, which is the very point of ensoulment (Aramesh 2009a, b).

. . .

Blood Money for Pre-implantation Embryo

Bearing in mind that no monetary compensation (*diya*) is considered for destroying pre-implantation embryo, it seems that there is no ethical relevance and worth for such embryos. Some contraceptive methods like intrauterine device (IUD), which prevents implantation thus destroys the early embryo, have been approved by religious authorities and used widely in contraception clinics in Iran. Most Shiite scholars, however, consider this stage of embryonic life as respectful, which means that it should not be wasted or destroyed without having a justifying reason. Medical research and health-related interventions such as contraception or infertility treatment are among such reasons.

Ensoulment and Its Implications

As mentioned above, the later phases of fetal development, including the one in which ensoulment takes place, are beyond the scope of this article. However, because of the important implications of this event on the ethical and legal status of the human fetus, it is worth mentioning, albeit briefly. According to Muslim jurists, including the Shiite ones, ensoulment, which is the breathing of divine soul into the human body, takes place after 120 days of embryonic life after conception. This belief is derived from the embryologic information provided by the *Qu'ran* and the *sunna* as described above in this paper. It does not mean that this is the exact time of ensoulment, but it means that ensoulment never takes place before 120 days after conception.

After the very point of ensoulment, the human fetus is considered a human person entitled to all moral and legal advantages attached to personhood. Before this point, however, the human embryo or fetus (including the early human embryo) is not considered a human person entitled to all legal and ethical rights. Accordingly, killing the human embryo or fetus before ensoulment is forbidden but is permissible under certain circumstances. After ensoulment, however, the fetus is considered an inviolable human person (Larijani and Zahedi 2006a, b).

References

Alai, H., & Rezai, H. (2009). *Examining the contradictions between Qur'anic verses and biomedical science.* (in Persian).

Aramesh, K. (2009a). A closer look at the abortion debate in Iran. *American Journal of Bioethics, 9*(8), 57–58.

Aramesh, K. (2009b). Iran's experience on religious bioethics: An overview. *Asian Bioethics Review, 1*(4), 318–328.

Esfandyari, A. (2013). *How Much is Diya for Abortion?* (in Persian).

Fadel, H. E. (2012). Developments in stem cell research and therapeutic cloning: Islamic ethical positions, a review. *Bioethics, 26*(3), 128–135.

Ghaly, M. (2014). Pre-modern Islamic medical ethics and Graeco–Islamic–Jewish embryology. *Bioethics, 28*(2), 49–58.

Ibn Babvaiy, A. (2009). *Fiq-o-rreza.* Qom: Nashroleslami (in Arabic).

Koleini, M. (2009). *Alkafi* (Vol. 7). Qom: Dar-al-Hadith. (In Arabic).

Larijani, B., & Zahedi, F. (2006a). Changing parameters of Abortion in Iran. *Indian Journal of Medical Ethics, 3*, 130–131.

Larijani, B., & Zahedi, F. (2006b). Health promotion, Islamic ethics and law in Iran. *DARU Journal of Pharmaceutical Sciences, 14*(Suppl. 1), 7–9.

Motahari, M. (2001). *Osul e Fiqh-Fiqh.* Tehran: Sadra (in Persian).

Muhaqiq Karaki, S. N. (1993). *Jami' Almaaqasid fi Shar' o Alhavaid* (Vol. 1). Qom: Al Albeit (in Arabic).

Najafi, M. (1981). *Javahir A-lKala, Fi Sharaye' Al-Islam* (Vol. 43). Beirut: Dar ul Ihya' (in Arabic).

Sachedina, A. (2009). *Islamic biomedical ethics.* New York: Oxford University Press.

Shahid Thani, Z. A. (1993). *Masalik ol Afham fi Sharh Shara'i al Islam* (Vol. 9). Qom: Mu'ssesa AlMa'arif AlIslami (in Arabic).

Tabatabayi, M. (1987). *Almizan Fi Tafsir Qur'an* (N. Hamediani, Trans. Vol. 20). Qom: Allame Foundation (in Persian).

39

Controversies and Considerations Regarding the Termination of Pregnancy for Foetal Anomalies in Islam

Abdulrahman Al-Matary and Jaffar Ali

Abdulrahman Al-Matary is a physician at the Department of Neonatology, King Fahad Medical City Riyadh, Saudi Arabia. Jaffar Ali taught for many years at the University of Malaya, Kuala Lumpur, Malaysia. Their article notes how Islam tends to be liberal regarding the legality of abortion but only prior to when ensoulment is said to occur on day 120 of pregnancy. The authors urge lawmakers in Muslim majority countries for more accommodations regarding the permissibility of abortion after ensoulment in cases where a TOP (termination of pregnancy) is warranted because of a severe fetal abnormality.

Healthcare providers are oftentimes confronted with ethical issues regarding peoples of different cultures, the resolution of which differs from that of their own [1-3].

The inability of service providers to effectively handle sensitive issues such as the termination of pregnancy (TOP) can result in enormous prolonged suffering for both the parents and the affected children. It is therefore crucial for healthcare workers to be sensitive to the norms of

Source: Abdulrahman Al-Matary and Jaffar Ali, "Controversies and Considerations Regarding the Termination of Pregnancy for Foetal Anomalies in Islam," *BMC Medical Ethics* 15, no. 1 (2014): 1–10.

different cultures to be able to deal effectively with specific ethical issues. In particular, it is crucial to be adequately acquainted with the norms of the major faiths of the world, especially when dealing with matters of a sensitive nature such as TOP. Islam allows TOP under certain conditions if the pregnancy has not progressed beyond the 120th day of pregnancy, which is also referred to as the day of ensoulment. This is crucial because if a diagnosis is delayed for any reason, then TOP will become illegal if attempted past the 120th day. Delays in diagnosis have contributed to considerable suffering for both parents and the affected children. Both speed and a timely intervention are critical in the management of foetal anomalies in the Muslim patient.

There is now a large volume of compelling empirical evidence [1-28] indicating that considerable pain and suffering is experienced by the mothers of anomalous foetuses because they did not undergo TOP due to cultural reasons or because they were delayed and could not perform a TOP before the 120th day of pregnancy. A review of the literature and anecdotal evidence suggest this predicament to be due to (i) a lack of knowledge on the part of parents, which is compounded by guilty consciousness; (ii) a delay in the early and rapid diagnosis of foetal anomalies due to a flawed or inefficient referral system; and (iii) the lack of expert clerical opinions.

. . .

Ethics: The Islamic Viewpoint

Islamic law is derived from (i) the Qur'an; (ii) the recorded authentic sayings and precedents set by the Prophet (*Sunnah*) and the prophetic decrees (the compilation or the records of the *Sunnah* are called *Hadith*); and (iii) the *ijtihād*. The ijithad can be defined as the rulings deduced from the Islamic principles based on the Qur'an and *Hadiths* by learned scholars who arrive at religious edicts or *Fatwas* to address a particular situation [2,11].

When Does Life Begin?

All Abrahamic religions and indeed all religions forbid the taking of a life [29-31]. In Islam, in the context of the embryo, the question arises whether it is a living entity? Logically a lifeless entity feels no pain nor is it sensitive to its environment, and therefore, the ethics of its externally engineered demise is less debatable and therefore less questionable and more permissible than if the entity is a living individual and the need to abort is a necessity. In all Abrahamic religions and in most religions, the question of the soul is paramount [32]. A living individual not only has a physical body but also has a soul. Therefore, it follows that an embryo is not an individual until it has a soul. This, in Islam, is generally believed to take place at approximately 120 days after fertilisation [2,14,32,33] although some schools of thought may argue that life begins the moment the sperm fertilises the egg. On the basis of the *Hadith,* Muslims assume the former to be correct. It is noteworthy that one school of Islamic thought allows embryo research up to 14 days post fertilisation for the benefit of the advancement of science [18].

An embryo becomes an individual with the full rights of a living person only after it is bestowed a soul, prior to which, it is just an entity, soulless and hence, lifeless as it were, to most Islamic scholars; therefore, it has limited rights but is not devoid of rights. In consideration of these points, the general belief in Islam is that the embryo begins life following ensoulment at day 120 after fertilisation [2,14,32,33]. It is noteworthy that the embryological development of humans is described in detail in the Glorious Qur'an. A detailed description concerning the embryo and foetal development in the Glorious Qur'an appears to have some parallel with current scientific knowledge [34].

Views of the Four *Sunni Madhabs* (Schools of Thought)

Sunni Muslims belong to one of the four major schools of thought, which are called *Madhhabs,* viz: *Hanafi; Shafi'i; Maliki;* and *Hanbali.* The *Madhabs* are neither clans nor sects but only schools of thought. These four schools of *Sunni* thought derive their Islamic rules from the Qur'an, the *Hadith* and new rules based on the *Ijtihad.* The generally accepted belief is that abortion is forbidden at any stage of a pregnancy on the basis of the following verses from the Qur'an.

> ". . . . And do not kill the soul which God has forbidden except for the requirements of justice . . . . . ." [Glorious Qur'an, Al- An'am 8: 151].

Thus, the termination of a pregnancy, even at the earliest possible stage, without medical justification is not allowed (even for social or economic reasons), as stated in the Glorious Qur'an:

> ". . . do not Kill your children for fear of want: We shall provide sustenance for them as well as for you. Verily the killing of them is a great sin." [Glorious Qur'an, Al- Esraa' 15: 31].

Religious Edicts and the Law

The *Hanafi'* and many of the *Shafi'i* schools state that abortion is permissible until the end of four months, only if one has legitimate grounds for abortion (Table 1). While the *Maliki* and *Hanbali* schools state that abortion is permissible at the request of both the parents for up to 40 days with a legitimate cause, this is principally prohibited from day 40 onwards [35,36].

. . .

The International Islamic *Fiqh* (Islamic Jurisprudence) Council

The International Islamic *Fiqh* Council (IIFC; Academy) is an Islamic *Sunni* institution of the World Muslim League that is based in Mecca, Saudi Arabia. Its members are representatives of individual countries where Islam is the predominant religion. They are chosen by their respective governments as

Table 1 Views of Muslim Sunni Legal Schools of Thought and Shi'ite Sect on Termination of Pregnancy

Sects/Schools	Sunni Maliki	Sunni Hanbali	Sunni Hanafi	Sunni Shafiie	Shi'ite
Abortion permissible?	No	No	No	No	No
If legitimate when abortion is permissible?	≤40 days	≤40 days	≤120 days	≤120 days	≤120 days

the senior-most Islamic scholars of their respective countries. Their main task is to meet on a regular basis to discuss current debatable issues affecting Muslims and to formulate rulings for resolving such issues.

The IIFC has ruled the following:

If proven by a committee of at least two competent and trustworthy medical experts on the basis of medical examinations with the use of appropriate equipment and laboratory findings before 120 days of pregnancy that the foetus has serious anomalies that will be present at birth, only then is it permissible to abort after the request of the parents.

When the pregnancy reaches or is beyond the 120th day, abortion becomes totally forbidden and is deemed a form of murder that will result in prosecution [35,36,37] unless the continuation of the pregnancy to full term poses a risk to the mother's life; abortion shall then be considered permissible. This decision must be based on the opinions of at least two competent and trustworthy medical experts in the field.

This ruling was based on revelations derived from Glorious Qur'an:

". . . No soul shall have imposed upon it a duty but to the extent of its capacity; neither shall a mother be made to suffer harm on account of her child. . . ." [Glorious Qur'an, Al- Baqara 2:233].

. . .

The Current Ruling in Saudi Arabia on Abortion

. . . In early 2011, the SC* of Saudi Arabia issued an edict (Fatwa no. 240 dated 16 January 2011) [38] legalising abortion in certain circumstances.

. . .

1. Abortion of a malformed foetus after 120 days of conception or 19 weeks of gestation following ensoulment is permissible if the pregnancy is certain to cause the death of the mother.
2. Abortion of a malformed foetus before 120 days or prior to ensoulment is permissible if it is certain that the foetus will die following birth or if it has severe incurable disabilities.

---

*Eds.: The Standing Committee for Scientific Research and for Issuing Edicts, Preaching and Guidance

3. Abortion of the foetus at any stage of pregnancy is permissible if intrauterine death was confirmed.

4. Abortion shall not be permissible under any circumstance without a medical report from a specialised and trustworthy committee composed of at least three competent physicians following written informed consent of both parents or the mother alone if the pregnancy and its continuance was affecting or will affect her health. The consent can be provided by persons delegated by the parents if the parents are not able to provide the same for any valid reason. The signed consent must be retained in the medical records of the mother [38].

. . .

Rule number two above states that abortion is permissible prior to ensoulment if the malformed or defective condition of the foetus is incurable. A large number of foetal anomalies are considered incurable and thus may be amenable to therapeutic abortion. More importantly, under this edict the mothers are empowered to decide on their own whether to proceed with TOP, which provides significant freedom to the mother to safeguard her well-being irrespective of external influences.

. . .

The issue of the termination of a pregnancy past 120 days of pregnancy due to severe foetal anomalies in Islam lies somewhere between the *permissible* and *forbidden*. In other words, it is a "grey area" in the interpretation of the Islamic literature that very few scholars venture into or will be led to discuss. Due to the enormous amount of pain and suffering that the mothers of affected foetuses endure, the authors implore scholars to re-visit and debate the issue further for pregnancies beyond the 120th day. The authors urge Muslim law makers to deliberate and consider abortion past the 120th day of fertilisation to avoid substantial hardship to mothers and family members if it is certain that the severely anomalous foetus will decease after birth or will be severely malformed and physically and mentally incapacitated after birth.

References

1. Shaw A: "They say Islam has a solution for everything, so why are there no guidelines for this?" Ethical dilemmas associated with the births and deaths of infants with fatal abnormalities from a small sample of Pakistani Muslim couples in Britain. *Bioethics* 2012, 26(9):485–92.

2. Gatrad AR, Sheikh A: Medical ethics and Islam: principles and practice. *Arch Dis Child* 2001, 84:72–75.

3. Der Wal JT G-v, Manniën J, Ghaly MM, Verhoeven PS, Hutton EK, Reinders HS: The role of religion in decision-making on antenatal screening of congenital anomalies: a qualitative study amongst Muslim Turkish origin immigrants. *Midwifery* 2013, 29:S0266–6138(13)00106-X.

4. Agay-Shay K, Friger M, Linn S, Peled A, Amitai Y, Peretz C: Periodicity and time trends in the prevalence of total births and conceptions with congenital malformations among Jews and Muslims in Israel, 1999–2006: a time series study of 823,966 births. *Birth Defects Res A Clin Mol Teratol* 2012, 94(6):438–448.

5. Al-Alaiyan S, Alfaleh KM: Aborting a malformed fetus: A debatable issue in Saudi Arabia. *J Clin Neonatol* 2012, 1(1):6–11.

6. Al Aqeel AI: Islamic ethical framework for research into and prevention of genetic diseases. *Nat Genet* 2007, 39(11):1293–1298.

7. Aramesh K: A closer look at the abortion debate in Iran. *Am J Bioeth* 2009, 9(8):57–58.

8. Bryant LD, Ahmed S, Ahmed M, Jafri H, Raashid Y: 'All is done by Allah'. Understandings of Down syndrome and prenatal testing in Pakistan. *Soc Sci Med* 2011, 72(8):1393–1399.

9. Bundey S, Alam H, Kaur A, Mir S, Lancashire RJ: Race, consanguinity and social features in Birmingham babies: a basis for prospective study. *J Epidemiol Community Health* 1990, 44:130–135.

10. Chaabouni H, Chaabouni M, Maazoul F, M'Rad R, Jemaa LB, Smaoui N, Terras K, Kammoun H, Belghith N, Ridene H, Oueslati B, Zouari F: Prenatal diagnosis of chromosome disorders in Tunisian population. *Ann Genet* 2001, 44(2):99–104.

11. Da Costa DE, Ghazal H, Al KS: Do not resuscitate orders and ethical decisions in a neonatal intensive care unit in a Muslim community. *Arch Dis Child Fetal Neonatal Ed* 2002, 86(2):F115–119.

12. Farag TI, Al-Awadi SA, Yassin S, El-Kassaby TA, Jaefary S, Usha R, Uma R, Mady SA, Fakhr M, Mannae M, *et al*: Anencephaly: a vanishing problem in Bedouins? *J Med Genet* 1989, 26(8):538–539.

13. Ngim CF, Lai NM, Ibrahim H, Ratnasingam V: Attitudes towards prenatal diagnosis and abortion in a multi-ethnic country: a survey among parents of children with thalassaemia major in Malaysia. *J Community Genet* 2013, 4(2):215–221.

14. Hedayat KM, Shooshtarizadeh P, Raza M: Therapeutic abortion in Islam: contemporary views of Muslim Shiite scholars and effect of recent Iranian legislation. *J Med Ethics* 2006, 32(11):652–657.

15. Husain F: Ethical dimensions of non-aggressive fetal management: a Muslim perspective. *Semin Fetal Neonatal Med* 2008, 13(5):323–324.

16. Jafri H, Ahmed S, Ahmed M, Hewison J, Raashid Y, Sheridan E: Islam and termination of pregnancy for genetic conditions in Pakistan: implications for Pakistani health care providers. *Prenat Diagn* 2012, 32(12):1218–1220.

17. Sasongko TH, Salmi AR, Zilfalil BA, Albar MA, Mohd Hussin ZA: Permissibility of prenatal diagnosis and abortion for fetuses with severe genetic disorder: type 1 spinal muscular atrophy. *Ann Saudi Med* 2010, 30(6):427–431.

18. Serour GI: Islamic perspectives in human reproduction. *Reprod Biomed Online* 2008, 17(Suppl 3):34–38.

19. Sharony R, Kidron D, Amiel A, Fejgin M, Borochowitz ZU: Familial lethal skeletal dysplasia withcloverleaf skull and multiple anomalies of brain, eye, face and heart: a new autosomal recessive multiple congenital anomalies syndrome. *Clin Genet* 2002, 61:369–374.

20. Sher C, Romano-Zelekha O, Green MS, Shohat T: Utilization of prenatal genetic testing by Israeli Moslem women: a national survey. *Clin Genet* 2004, 65(4):278–283.

21. Teebi AS: Autosomal recessive disorders among Arabs: an overview from Kuwait. *J Med Genet* 1994, 31(3):224–233.

22. Zlotogora J, Haklai Z, Rotem N, Georgi M, Rubin L: The impact of prenatal diagnosis and termination of pregnancy on the relative incidence of malformations at birth among Jews and Muslim Arabs in Israel. *Isr Med Assoc J* 2010, 12(9):539–542.

23. Zlotogora J: The molecular basis of autosomal recessive diseases among the Arabs and Druze in Israel. *Hum Genet* 2010, 128(5):473–479.

24. Zlotogora J, Haklai Z, Leventhal A: Utilization of prenatal diagnosis and termination of pregnancies for the prevention of Down syndrome in Israel. *Isr Med Assoc J* 2007, 9(8):600–602.

25. Zlotogora J, Hujerat Y, Barges S, Shalev SA, Chakravarti A: The fate of 12 recessive mutations in a single village. *Ann Hum Genet* 2007,71(Pt 2):202–208.

26. Zlotogora J: Is there an increased birth defect risk to children born to offspring of first cousin parents? *Am J Med Genet A* 2005, 1(3):137A–342.

27. Zlotogora J, Haklai Z, Rotem N, Georgi M, Berlovitz I, Leventhal A, Amitai Y: Relative prevalence of malformations at birth among different religious communities in Israel. *Am J Med Genet A* 2003, 15(1):59–62.

28. Zlotogora J, Leventhal A, Amitai Y: The impact of congenital malformations and Mendelian diseases on infant mortality in Israel. *Isr Med Assoc J* 2003, 5(6):416–418.

29. Lewis JA: Jewish perspectives on pregnancy and child bearing. *Matern Child Nurs* 2003, 28:306–12.

30. Markwell HJ, Brown BF: Bioethics for clinicians: 27. Catholic bioethics. *Can Med Assoc J* 2001, 165:189–92.
31. Pauls M, Hutchinson RC: Bioethics for clinicians: 28. Protestant bioethics. *Can Med Assoc J* 2002, 166:339–343.
32. BBC: *Religion & Ethics - When is the foetus 'alive': The stages of fetal development.* 2011.
33. Alamri YA: Islam and abortion. *J. Islamic Med Assoc North Am* 2011, 43(1):39–40.
34. Moore KL: A Scientist's interpretation of references to embryology in the Qur'an. *J. Islamic Med Assoc North Am* 1986, 18(1):15–17.
35. Al-Maqdesse AAMM, Al-Maqdesse AAMM, Shams A-D: *Cairo (Egypt): Aalam Al-Kotob.* 1985:281.
36. Al-Mardawi AAAS: *Alensaf fi ma'refat alrajeh men alkhelaf. Vol.1.* Beirut. Lebanon: Dar El Fikr; 1956:386.
37. Council of the World Muslim League: *Proceedings of Conference of The Fiqh (Islamic Jurisprudence).* 1990.
38. Preaching and Guidance in Saudi Arabia: *Proceedings of the Standing Committee for Scientific Research and Issuing Edicts.* 2011.

40

Sufi Ethics: Legal Rulings in Religious Context

Marion Holmes Katz

An expert in Islamic law and gender, Marion Holmes Katz teaches at New York University. Her essay offers an extensive discussion of Sunni theological and legal writings on abortion that is highly recommended for anyone pursuing research in this area. We have excerpted the portion of Katz's discussion of the twelfth-century philosopher and theologian Abu Hamid al-Ghazali. Already an eminent Muslim scholar, al-Ghazali left his teaching post mid-career to live for a period with a Sufi community, imbibing their more mystical beliefs and practices. He eventually produced a synthesis of Sufi-influenced Islamic teaching on many topics, including abortion. Al-Ghazali probed the spiritual intentions regarding contraception and abortion, finding the former mostly permissible and the latter mostly not, although he seemed to imply that some early abortions may constitute a less serious moral transgression.

At least since the thirteenth century, Sufism has been an influential supplementary (and sometimes competing) frame of ethical and spiritual reference for many—or even most—Muslims. The nature of the sources makes it more difficult to address specific, concrete ethical issues through a

Source: Marion Holmes Katz, "The Problem of Abortion in Classical Sunni Fiqh," in *Islamic Ethics of Life: Abortion, War, and Euthanasia*, ed. Jonathan E. Brockopp (Columbia: University of South Carolina Press, 2003), 23–50.

Sufi lens than through that of *fiqh*.* While *fiqh* works tend to deal with such issues as reproductive behavior in fairly exhaustive detail, works dealing with Sufi *akhlāq** frequently treat the issue of moral self-improvement in broad and general terms. Thus, it is relatively difficult to find explicit discussions of an issue such as abortion. At this point, however, it may be useful to examine one very widely respected example of the synthesis of Islamic law and Sufi self-improvement. This may give a more comprehensive sense of the religious world within which Sunni Muslims have made decisions about ethical issues such as abortion.

An interesting example of the interaction between the two discourses (*fiqh* and Sufism) is provided by one of the most influential Islamic scholars of the Middle Ages, the author of one of the most widely read and deeply cherished syntheses of Islamic teachings in the history of the tradition. This is Abu Hamid al-Ghazali (d. 1111 C.E.), whose magnum opus *Ihyā' 'ulūm al-dīn* ("The Revivification of the Religious Sciences") is until today both ubiquitous and revered in most parts of the Sunni Muslim world. Al-Ghazali's religious life, touchingly described in his autobiographical work *al-Munqidh min al-dalāl* ("The Deliverer from Error"), was marked by religious upheaval. After a crisis of faith in which he became unable to teach Islamic law, al-Ghazali left his prestigious academic post in the imperial capital of Baghdad to spend years in searching and meditation. His survey of the various paths to faith available in his time (law, theology, philosophy, Shi'ism, and Sufism) led him to a synthesis in which adherence to the normative discourses of law and theology was informed by an experiential conviction nurtured by Sufi practice. For the mature al-Ghazali, Islamic law and Sufi ethics were complementary. Crucially, he believed that *fiqh* applied exclusively to externals, while Sufism addressed the conditions of the heart.[1] Thus, for al-Ghazali *fiqh* is essentially a branch of politics, a discipline devoted to regulating the this-worldly affairs of human beings so that they can pursue their final rewards in peace. The heart of the spiritual struggle, meanwhile, goes on in a subjective realm inaccessible to the discourse of *fiqh*.

. . .

However, precisely because al-Ghazali's Sufi ethics *(al-akhlāq al-ṣūfiya)* deal with the subjective states of human hearts, they do not deal primarily

---

*Eds.: *Fiqh,* legal theory.
*Eds.: *Akhlāq,* the practice or study of virtue.

with ethical problems as understood in the modern west. Sufi ethics, for al-Ghazali, is not ultimately concerned with actions at all. "How many a lower soul (*nafs*)," he reflects in the *Iḥyā'*, "is receptive to acts, but not to moral characteristics!"[2] Thus, the same act can have very different ethical evaluations depending on the subjective spiritual state of the actor. A Sufi's refusal to accept charity, for instance, can be good or bad depending on the state of the *nafs*.[3]

How would a schema such as al-Ghazali's, in which *fiqh* regulated external human affairs and sufi ethics disciplined individual hearts, apply to an issue such as abortion? As it happens, we need not speculate; al-Ghazali provides one of the most detailed and thoughtful medieval discussions of the issue of abortion in his *Iḥyā'*. Based on this passage, al-Ghazali is sometimes cited by modern authors as an example of the absolute prohibition of abortion;[4] however, on closer examination his discussion is as ambiguous as it is rich.

The idea that al-Ghazali was a firm opponent of abortion seems to be based on two analogical arguments that he makes, one negative and the other positive. Firstly, al-Ghazali states that neither infanticide (*wa'd*, or the burying of unwanted offspring) nor abortion (*al-ijhāḍ*) is to be equated with *coitus interruptus*, because both involve the destruction of an already extant being (*mawjūd ḥāṣil*). Secondly, he compares conception (in his medical terminology, the mixture of the male and female "semen," *mā'*, or the male semen and the woman's menstrual blood) to the "offer" and "acceptance" that constitute a legal contract. Withdrawal differs from abortion in that the man's semen in itself cannot form a child, just as an offer in and of itself does not create a contract. "After the offer and the acceptance [have occurred]," however, "reneging constitutes cancellation, nullification, and rupture [of the contract]."[5]

Al-Ghazali's argument does differ from those of some other authors in that he emphasizes the moment of conception (i.e., the mixing of the sexual fluids of the man and the woman) as a decisive dividing point in the creation of the child. Before conception, al-Ghazali argues, any steps taken to prevent conception (ranging from the refusal to marry, through refraining from sexual intercourse with the spouse, to *coitus interruptus*) simply represent failures to realize a potential good. Thus, such actions are not forbidden; they are, rather, instances of falling short of the ideal (*tark al-afḍal*). Abortion and infanticide are qualitatively different from contraception in that they involve an offense (*jināya*) against an extant being; they represent the infliction of a positive wrong rather than the negation of a potential right.[6]

However, it is not necessarily the case that al-Ghazali's argument that both infanticide and abortion constitute a *jināya* implies an equal and absolute prohibition of both actions. Islamic law, which represents a fully synthesized combination of law (in the sense of judicially enforceable norms) and ethics (in the sense of moral standards providing voluntary orientation for the actions of individuals), has diverse and ambiguous ways of identifying and treating "bad" actions. In this case, al-Ghazali places abortion and infanticide on a continuum of moral odium:

> [The destruction of the fetus] also has different degrees. The first degree of existence is when the semen falls into the womb, mixes with the woman's semen and becomes ready to receive life; spoiling this is an offense *(jināya)*. When it becomes a clump and a blood clot . . ., the offense is more serious . . . When the spirit is breathed into [the fetus] and the form is completed . . ., the offense becomes even more serious. The utmost degree of seriousness in the offense is after the child is born alive.[7]

Thus, it is not entirely clear how serious an offense early abortion would be in al-Ghazali's schema. It certainly falls short of murder, which presumably would be the final degree in his progression. Interestingly, al-Ghazali is also credited with the opinion that it is permissible to abort a drop of semen or a blood clot but forbidden to abort a clump of flesh.[8] Samira Bayyumi explains the rationale for this position as follows:

> This [opinion] is based on the Shafiʿi teaching that the drop of semen and the blood clot do not have the subtle form of the fetus *(sūrat al-janīn al-khafīya)* that the midwives, who are the experts [in this area], know; thus, they [i.e., the Shafiʿis] require the *ghurra** for a clump of flesh but not for a drop of semen or a blood clot.[9]

The apparent conflict between the sliding scale of moral turpitude described in *Iḥyā' 'ulūm al-dīn* and this second opinion attributed to al-Ghazali may be a function of the dual application of the *fiqh* to ethical evaluation of one's own actions before the fact and to the definition of civil and criminal offenses to be demonstrated and punished after the fact. Following al-Ghazali's schema as a moral guide for one's own actions, one would ideally choose not to abort a developing fetus at any point after conception, although the lesser seriousness of the transgression might justify doing so early in the pregnancy under some conditions. Using his schema as a guideline for identifying and

---

*Eds.: *Ghurra,* payment or fine.

penalizing transgressions after the fact, however, one would need to introduce another factor: the necessity for some kind of proof that a pregnancy had existed in the first place. From this point of view, only at the point when medical personnel (in this case, midwives) could discern the emerging form of the fetus could an offense be demonstrated to have occurred. At this point, however, there is a disjunction between the two forms of *shar'ī* discourse, the normative and the legal. It is resolved by making an analogy from the case of legal investigation (primarily, the demand for compensation for a fetus miscarried as a result of assault) to the case of personal moral action. Thus, the moral odium of abortion is incurred only if a pregnancy can be proven to have existed.

Al-Ghazali also provides an interesting examination of the possible motives for contraception, motives that might also be considered with respect to abortion. He enquires into this matter because, while he considers contraception to be permissible, he allows that the motivating intention *(al-niyya al-bā'itha)* may in itself be morally reprehensible. He lists five possible motives, only two of which he considers illegitimate. The first applies to slave women; the owner may want to avoid conception so that a slave woman could not gain a claim to emancipation by bearing his child. The second is the preservation of the beauty and health of the woman. The third is the fear of hardship resulting from excessive offspring. Al-Ghazali endorses all of these motives as permissible, although the third represents a failure to achieve the ideal state of *tawakkul,* or reliance on Divine Providence. The only motives he brands as sinful are the fear of conceiving daughters rather than sons, and a woman's excessive fear of the pollution resulting from childbirth, an obsession with ritual purity that al-Ghazali associates with the Kharijite heresy.

. . .

Al-Ghazali's emphasis on the importance of procreation is firmly rooted in his understanding of the nature of the human person and its realization in married life. Like other Islamic jurists (and unlike many Christian thinkers), al-Ghazali does not consider procreation to be the sole rationale for the sexual tie of marriage. The satisfaction of sexual urges which might otherwise lead to corruption and sin and the spiritually restorative enjoyment of intimacy and companionship are both independent, although subordinate, objectives of marriage. The legitimacy of marital intercourse is in no way contingent upon the possibility of conception. However, al-Ghazali places sexual satisfaction and personal companionship second and third in his list of the benefits of marriage (the fourth and fifth are the time saved by delegating household responsibilities to one's wife and the moral fortitude gained by patient endurance of her bad behavior). The first and most important benefit of marriage, in al-Ghazali's view, is procreation. Al-Ghazali considers procreation to be a fundamental objective of human nature as created by God (the *fiṭra;* see Qur'an 30:30).[10]

Notes

1. Al-Ghazālī, *Iḥyā' 'ulūm al-dīn* (Beirut: Dār al-Fikr, 1414 A.H./1994 A.D.), 1:28-9.
2. Al-Ghazālī, *Iḥyā'*, 5:176.
3. Al-Ghazālī, *Iḥyā'*, 5:129-31.
4. See [Umm Kulthūm Yaḥyā Muṣṭafā al-Khaṭīb, *Qaḍīyat tahdīd al-nasl* (Jidda: al-Dār al-Su'ūdīyah li'l-nashr wa'l-tawzī', 1982),] 152.
5. Al-Ghazālī, *Iḥyā'*, 2:58.
6. Ibid.
7. Al-Ghazālī, *Iḥyā'*, 2:65.
8. [Samīra Sayyid Sulaymān Bayyūmī, *al-Ijhāḍ wa-āthāruhu f'i'l-sharia'a al-islāmīya* (Cairo: Dār al-Ṭabā'a al-Muḥammadīya bi'l-Azhar, 1989)], 19.
9. Ibid., 23.
10. Al-Ghazālī, *Iḥyā'*, 1:28.

41

Family Planning, Contraception, and Abortion in Islam

Sa'diyya Shaikh

Sa'diyya Shaikh received her PhD in religion from Temple University and is professor of religion at the University of Cape Town, South Africa. She researches the intersection of Islamic studies and gender studies and has written widely on gender justice issues affecting Muslim women. This essay offers a useful overview of the diversity of thought about abortion among different schools of thought within Islam. It also provides insight into a Muslim feminist perspective on contraception and abortion, which emphasizes theological principles of moral agency and discernment.

God and Humanity: *Tauhid, Fitrah,* and *Khilafah*

The belief in the oneness or unity of God, known to Muslims as the principle of Tauhid, is the center from which the rest of Islam radiates. It is a foundational ontological principle anchored within the deepest spiritual roots of the religion suffusing different areas of Islamic learning

Source: Sa'diyya Shaikh, "Family Planning, Contraception and Abortion in Islam: Undertaking Khilafah," in *Sacred Rights: The Case for Contraception and Abortion in World Religions*, ed. Daniel Maguire (New York: Oxford University Press, 2003), 105–19.

that includes theology, mysticism, law, and ethics in varying ways. While transience, finitude, and dependence define everything else, God is the only independent source of being.[1] As such, God is primary to our understandings of the very meaning of reality and is constitutive of the ultimate integrity of human beings.[2]

According to the Qur'an, human beings are uniquely imbued with the spirit of God and in their created nature have been granted privileged knowledge and understanding of reality.[3] Human weakness, on the other hand, is presented primarily as the tendency to be heedless and forgetful of these realities. God's revelations through the various prophets in history are an additional mercy intended to remind one about what is already ingrained at the deepest level of one's humanity. Mediating between faith and heedlessness is the human capacity for volition and freedom of choice. This uniquely endowed human constitution with an inborn capacity for discernment is called the *fitrah*.

Within Islam, therefore, while humanity is primed for goodness, our moral agency is bound to the freedom of choice and the active assumption of responsibilities that ensue from such agency. This understanding of human purpose and potential is reflected in a pervasive Qur'anic concept called *khilafah* that can be translated as trusteeship, moral agency, or vicegerency, where the subject of this activity, the human being, is referred to as the *khalifah*, that is, the trustee, the moral agent, or the vicegerent. This core Qur'anic concept provides the spiritual basis for understanding ethical action in Islam. Within this framework, each individual, as well as every community, is responsible for the realization of a just and moral social order in harmony with God's will.[4] In Islam, enacting one's moral agency is intrinsic to a right relationship with God.

. . .

Sexism and Gender Justice

Another pivotal area of concern relates to Islamic perspectives on gender relations and marriage, and their implications for family planning. The notion that God's unity is reflected in the equality and unity of humankind provides a basis for a strong critique of sexism and gender hierarchy. The Qur'an explicitly asserts the fundamental equal worth of male and female believers, as well as the fact that gender relations are intended to be cooperative and mutually enriching.[5] This ethos of reciprocity between women and men is further reinforced in the Islamic understanding of marital relationships.

The Qur'an presents marriage and children as a gift from God to be cherished and enjoyed.[6] As such, marriage is valued and encouraged in most Muslim cultures. Despite this incentive to have a family, neither marriage nor children are considered obligatory in the life of a Muslim man or woman.

. . .

Contraception

Contraception has a long history in Islam that needs to be situated in relation to the broader Islamic ethos of marriage and sexuality. In Islam if one chooses to marry, this is not automatically linked to procreation. Within the Islamic view of marriage, an individual has the right to sexual pleasure within marriage, which is independent of one's choice to have children.[7] This type of approach to sexuality is compatible with a more tolerant approach to contraception and family planning.

Historically, the various Islamic legal schools with an overwhelming majority have permitted coitus interruptus, called *azl*, as a method of contraception.[8] This was a contraceptive technique practiced by pre-Islamic Arabs and continued to be used during the time of the Prophet with his knowledge and without his prohibition.[9] The only condition the Prophet attached to acceptability of this practice, which was reiterated by Muslim jurists, was that the husband was to secure the permission of the wife before practicing withdrawal. Since the male sexual partner initiates this technique, there needs to be consensual agreement about its use by both partners for two primary reasons. First, the wife is entitled to full sexual pleasure and coitus interruptus may diminish her pleasure. Second, she has the right to offspring if she so desires.[10] These requirements speak to the priority given in Islam to mutual sexual fulfillment as well as consultative decision making between a married couple in terms of family planning.

As early as the ninth century female contraceptive techniques such as intravaginal suppositories and tampons were also a part of both medical and judicial discussions in Islam.[11] While medical manuals listed the different female contraceptive options and their relative effectiveness, legal positions differed around whether the consent of the husband was necessary or not with the use of female contraceptives. In classical Islamic law, which informs contemporary Islamic jurisprudence law, the majority position in eight out of the nine legal schools permits contraception.[12]

. . .

Abortion

In Islamic scholarship the positions on abortion are more varied and less consensual than the approaches to contraception. Historically, the Muslim legal positions range from unqualified permissibility of an abortion before 120 days into the pregnancy, on the one hand, to categorical prohibition of abortion altogether, on the other. Even within a single legal school the majority position was often accompanied by dissenting minority positions.[13]

Some of the key ethical and legal considerations in addressing the abortion question relate to understanding the nature of the fetus, the process of fetal development, and the point at which the fetus is considered a human being. While scientific inquiry has illuminated the process of fetal development with progressively more clarity, the question of when a fetus is considered a human being is open to varying interpretations. The following Qur'anic verses are central to understanding some of the ways in which Muslim thinkers approach these issues.

> He creates you in the wombs of your mothers
> In stages, one after another
> In three veils of darkness
> Such is Allah, your Lord and Cherisher. (Q 39:6)

> We created the human being from a quintessence of clay
> Then we placed him as semen in a firm receptacle
> Then we formed the semen into a blood-like clot
> Then we formed the clot into a lump of flesh
> Then we made out of that lump, bones
> And clothed the bones with flesh
> Then we developed out of it another creation
> So Blessed is Allah the Best Creator. (Q 23:12-13)

Given these scriptural teachings, Muslim scholars have understood that the fetus undergoes a series of transformations beginning as an organism and becoming a human being. An authenticated prophetic tradition provides a more detailed time frame for understanding the pace of fetal development: "Each of you is constituted in your mother's womb for 40 days as a *nutfa* (semen), then it becomes an *alaqa* (dot) for an equal period, then a *mudgha* (lump of flesh) for another equal period, then the angel is sent and he breathes the *ruh*, (spirit) into it."[14]

Together the Qur'anic verses and the prophetic tradition have been understood to describe a sequential process where the fetus undergoes a series of changes and finally culminates in becoming a full human being when it is "ensouled."[15] According to the Qur'an, this culmination point denotes a significant shift since the fetal organism is transformed into something substantively different from its previous state as is reflected in the verse "then we developed out of it another creation" (i.e., a human being). In the prophetic tradition this same point of transition into a human being is described as the point at which the angel breathes the spirit into the fetus at 120 days.

Medieval Islamic scholars also found support for the Qur'anic position and the prophetic teachings from Greek medicine, which had a corresponding understanding of the stages of fetal development.[16] Contemporary medical technology has developed such that we are able now able to detect vital signs of a fetus like brainwaves and heartbeat. While these advances in medical knowledge are informative and help to illuminate decisions, they still do not provide us with definitive criteria for determining when a fetus becomes fully "another creature," that is, a human person. While science can contribute to a description of the fetal development, it is outside of scientific method to determine the point of spiritual transition into the full human essence. For human beings, any designation of when a fetus constitutes a full human life can be contested since we are unable to know this unambiguously. Thus, revelation and prophetic inspiration remain a crucial way of understanding this issue from an Islamic perspective.

The narratives from the primary Islamic sources provide Muslim thinkers with a way to generate an estimated criterion for establishing personhood during the process of fetal development. This in turn has direct implications for the ethical and legal approaches to the question of abortion in Islam.

The view that the fetus is ensouled at 120 days, thereby becoming a human person and thus a legal personality, was integrated into Islamic jurisprudence.[17] Hence, for example, if someone injures a pregnant woman, causing her to miscarry the fetus, the amount of compensation due to her is based on the stage of fetal development. Causing the miscarriage of an ensouled or what is called a "formed" fetus is considered a criminal and religious offense and the mother needs to be compensated for the full blood money (*diya*) as though it were a case of a child already born.[18] A lesser remuneration is due if the fetus was considered "unformed." According to Islamic law only a formed fetus that is miscarried or accidentally aborted has the right to inheritance (to pass on to relatives), to be named, and to have a ritual burial.

From this perspective, the abortion of a formed fetus, that is, after 120 days, is considered a criminal offense and prohibited by all Islamic legal schools. Exceptions to this prohibition, however, include situations where the mother's life is in danger, where the pregnancy is harming an already suckling child, or where the fetus is expected to be deformed.[19] Relating to an abortion prior to the 120-day period, there are four different positions in classical Islamic, which have been summarized in the following way by Shaykh Jad al-Haq:[20]

1. Unconditional permission to terminate a pregnancy without a justification or fetal defect. This view is adopted by the Zaydi school, and some Hanafi and Shafi'i scholars. The Hanbali school allows abortion through the use of oral abortifacients within 40 days of conception.
2. Conditional permission to abort because of an acceptable justification. If there is an abortion without a valid reason in this period it is considered to be disapproved (*makruh*) but not forbidden (*haram*). This is the opinion of the majority of Hanafi and Shafi'i scholars.
3. Abortion is strongly disapproved (*makruh*). This is the view held by some Maliki jurists.
4. Abortion is unconditionally prohibited (*haram*). This reflects the other Maliki view, as well as the Zahiri, Ibadiyya, and Imamiyya legal schools.[21]

Such diversity in perspectives characterizes the Islamic legal canon, which contains contrary positions where both permissibility and prohibition of abortion are considered legitimate. This range of positions suggests a flexibility to the way in which Muslim societies have historically approached the issue of abortion. Moreover, the extensive discussions of specific types of abortifacients in medical manuals of the classical Islamic world reflect that it was a part of the social reality.

. . .

It is not surprising that despite the diversity characterizing Islamic legal perspectives on abortion, which even include views of its permissibility, the realities of many contemporary Muslim societies reflect a tendency to adopt a more rigid approach. Part of this motivation, rightfully, is to ensure that people do not adopt an uncritical acceptance of easy abortions since the decision to terminate a potential realization of a human life is a grave decision not be taken lightly or without circumspection. Indeed, the gravity of this whole enterprise bolsters the case for a responsible approach to family planning including reliable contraceptive usage, which would, for the most part, preempt the need for abortion.

. . .

For those that oppose abortion, a compassionate and merciful attitude would include focusing on transforming social structures so that having children does not create hardships for the mother, the family, and the society. This would be a more socially constructive use of energy than the crusade against abortion. A concern for the welfare of the fetus without a concern for its continuing welfare as a human being reflects a limited, if not hypocritical approach.

In Islam, if an individual or a couple are considering the possibility of an abortion it is imperative that they do so with a full awareness of the gravity of such a decision. In this situation, I would present that being a *khilafah*, or moral agent, requires a careful consideration of all the factors, weighing up the different demands and needs of the specific situation, and like in all things, intentionally keeping one's sense of *taqwa*, or God-consciousness, at the forefront. Islamically, the freedom to act as the *khalifah* is intrinsically accompanied by accountability and responsibilities at the personal, social, and religious levels. Often the specifics of a given context determine what the most responsible alternative is. Given these considerations, from within the Islamic perspective there is room for a pro-choice perspective where the individual *khalifah* engages all sources of Islamic guidance—the Qur'an, the prophetic traditions, and the legal positions, as well as his or her own intellectual, moral, and ethical capacities—to inform a decision about abortion.

Notes

1. Qur'an 55:26-27.
2. Qur'an 59:19.

3. Qur'an 15:29.
4. See Fazlur Rahman, *Major Themes of the Quran* (Minneapolis: Bibliotheca Islamica, 1980), p. 18.
5. Qur'an 33:35; 16:97; 9:71.
6. Qur'an 16:72; 25:74.
7. Islam also recognizes the spiritual dimensions of sexuality as explored by medieval mystical philosopher Ibn Arabi, who stated that in accordance with the spiritual state of the partners, the act of sexual union has the possibilities for unparalleled mystical unveilings and experiences of the divine. See Ibn Al-Arabi, *Bezels of Wisdom*, trans. R. W. J. Austin (Mahwah, N.J.: Paulist Press, 1980), p. 274.
8. See *Islam's Attitude Towards Family Planning* (Cairo: Ministry of Waqfs and Ministry of Information, 1994), pp. 27–34, and Abdel Rahim Omran, *Family Planning in the Legacy of Islam* (London: Routledge, 1992),] pp. 145–182.
9. Omran provides an extensive discussion on the *al-azl* tradition in *Family Planning*, pp. 115–142.
10. [Basim Musallam, *Sex and Society in Islam* (Cambridge: Cambridge University Press, 1983)], pp. 31–36.
11. Ibid., pp. 77–88, 37–38.
12. Omran, *Family Planning*, pp. 145–167.
13. Musallam, *Sex and Society*, pp. 57–59.
14. Muslim, *Book of Qadr*, hadith no. 4781.
15. Ibn Qayyim al-Jawziyya, *Al-Tibyanfi aqsam al-Qur'an* (Cairo, 1933), pp. 374–375.
16. Musallam, *Sex and Society*, p. 54.
17. For detailed legal implications of the religious view of fetal development, see Muhammad Salaam Madkur's *Al-Janin wa Ahkam al-muta'alliqa bihi Ji al-fiqh* (Cairo, 1969).
18. Musallam, *Sex and Society*, p. 57.
19. Omran, *Family Planning*, p. 192.
20. Jad al-Haq Ali Had al-Haq, *al-Fatawa al Islamiyya min Dar al-lfta al-Misriyya* (Cairo: Wazara al-Awqaf/ al Majlis al-A'la Ii al Shu'un al-Islamiyya, 1983), vol. 9, pp. 3093–3109.
21. The Zahiri, Ibadiyya, and Imammiyya schools all have a limited following.

Part 5

Abortion and Religion in Public Life

Introduction to Part 5

Religion is a central aspect of human culture, and its presence and influence are evident in aspects of what religious studies scholars term "material religion," such as legal codes, religious buildings, and shrines as well as in more intangible things like beliefs and attitudes about diet and dress, marriage, and sex, for example. Religion is never separate from culture, and religious adherents live out their faith engaging in the same kinds of activities as their nonreligious counterparts such as voting, saying the pledge of allegiance, and paying taxes. Some of the fiercest clashes that mark our public life occur when believers bring their religious commitments to bear on issues that affect us all. We are familiar with some of these historical instances, such as the 1925 Scopes trial where the teaching of new evolutionary theories became a controversy affecting school board decisions. The controversial nature of our public discussion of abortion reflects one space where religion continues to play a prominent role in the public square.

While some people hold that abortion and religion should be relegated to the private sphere, this is neither desirable nor possible. People, including religious people, exist whole and complete in both private and public spaces, and public institutions and entities like healthcare facilities and government interact with and care for people who are religious. While the distinction between public and private spaces in society is reasonable, people do not divide themselves so easily. Additionally, international religious institutions like the Vatican continue to hold considerable political power in the world. In often less overt ways, religious people who also happen to be doctors, counselors, elected officials, teachers, judges, police officers, and so on hold various forms of political and social power. Their actions and behavior as public figures are often informed by their private and personal beliefs. In short, religion is present in public life whether we like it or not.

In this final section, we turn to representative examples of the ways that religious views and practices regarding reproductive realities have had an influence in the public sphere from the late twentieth century to today. We highlight, in particular, how religion engages institutions, communal practices, and public media where abortion issues are adjudicated, regulated, and debated. Proponents on both sides of the abortion issue press their case at the hospitals where they work or are treated, at convention centers where they hold religious gatherings, in legal documents they submit to courts, and in religious views they publicize from pulpits, on billboards, and through the internet.

We begin Part 5 with the account from the Dirks and Relf book of how an activist wing of the religious prochoice movement mobilized Protestant clergy and rabbis across the country in the late 1960s to form the Clergy Consultation Service, which helped thousands of women access abortion services prior to *Roe*. Religious abortion rights activism before the legalization of abortion in 1973 consisted of mostly small groups of mainline Protestant and progressive Jewish men and women who lobbied in support of the liberalization of abortion laws, as Rachel Kranson's essay about the Women's League for Conservative Judaism documents. Meanwhile, the Catholic Church hierarchy in the 1960s was actively mobilizing its prolife platform that went into high gear after 1973 with pastoral and legislative plans, while prochoice Catholics raised their (albeit less powerful) voices in dissent, as Patricia Miller's essay shows.

The *Roe v. Wade* decision was a turning point for reproductive realities in the United States. As Stacy Scaldo shows, the US Supreme Court, despite maintaining the appearance of being immune to religious influence, accepted and engaged with *amicus* briefs from denominations and religious groups. *Roe* also proved to be a lightning rod for the prolife movement. Brian Massingale takes issue with the prolife attempt to compare *Roe* to the infamous nineteenth-century *Dred Scott* decision denying citizenship to Black people. Some Christian extremists have eschewed legal debates, the pulpit, and peaceful prolife demonstrations. Aaron Winter details how a number of committed white Christian militant groups have engaged in direct violent acts of domestic terrorism against abortion healthcare clinics and providers.

Crisis pregnancy centers, which constitute a massive public prolife presence in the United States, is the topic of Ziad Munson's article. These centers are often well-funded and well-resourced clinic-like settings, equipped with ultrasound machines and staffed by committed Christians, who believe they are the ones offering pregnant women real choices. Meanwhile at Catholic-run medical centers, staff are required to follow Vatican-approved ethics guidelines, which can create dilemmas for physicians treating a pregnant patient facing a medical crisis, as recounted in the essay by Freedman et al. Sometimes, people who are pregnant have unexpected medical conditions that require emergency terminations, which are largely prohibited in Catholic hospitals. Bernard Prusak discusses how Catholic moral teachings have real ramifications for pregnant patients and hospital staff in his case study analysis of an emergency abortion that was authorized at a Catholic hospital in Phoenix, Arizona.

Conservative prolife African American activists, ranging from leaders in the Nation of Islam to Alveda King, have preached that abortion is not just murder but racial genocide—a message that Shyrissa Dobbins-Harris associates with the concept of "misogynoir." Monique Moultrie shows how some progressive Black Christians reject any attempt to coopt the Black Lives Matter theme into an antiabortion campaign for "Black Babies Matter." Many devout Muslims who do not yet wish to have children turn to religious authorities for guidance about contraception and other matters of sexual practice. L. L. Wynn and Angel Foster study how Muslims living in the United States seek out online *fatwas* in English or Arabic on these issues.

We noted in the introduction to this volume that the task of social ethics is to help people engage in deep and considered examination of contemporary social problems in ways that contribute to thoughtful analysis and understanding with the goal of developing robust ways to address those problems. New questions and controversies related to abortion and religion will continue to arise in the public sphere. The chapters in this section offer a range of ways in which religious people have endeavored to address abortion in the public square from the late 1960s through today. It is important to examine and evaluate the actions, strategies, and motivations of the people and groups represented in these chapters—and the consequences (intended or not) of their positions and actions. Doing so can generate insights and learnings that are transferable to other problems and issues not covered in this volume. We hope that critical engagement with the topics, perspectives, strategies, and experiences presented here will help prepare you to participate in more robust, nuanced, and productive conversations about abortion and religion in public life.

As you read the essays in this section, we encourage you to consider the following:

1. Pay attention to the theme of "religious freedom" as you read these articles. Where does it show up? How are authors invoking this principle? How would you describe the issue of religious freedom in relation to the question of legal access to abortion?

2. Try to identify the various modes and methods used by religious adherents (prolife or prochoice; authoritative leaders or lay people) to bring their religious views into the public square regarding abortion. What are constructive and democratic ways that religion can play a meaningful role in the public sphere?

3. Identify the various ways these articles analyze how rhetoric and argument reflect religious ideas and values. How do these analyses help you think about the conversation in our pluralistic democratic society in new or different ways?

4. Where and how do different forms of religious power and authority emerge in the public sphere? How is this power and authority used? Are there criteria you can identify that would help evaluate the appropriateness of religious action in the public sphere?

42

A History of the Clergy Consultation Service on Abortion:

The Counselors

Doris Andrea Dirks and Patricia A. Relf

D. A. Dirks earned a PhD in educational leadership from Western Michigan University and teaches at Mount Royal University, Canada. Patricia A. Relf is a freelance writer based in the Cleveland area and has served on the board of a Michigan affiliate of Planned Parenthood. Their book provides a detailed history of how pastors and rabbis mobilized in the late 1960s to develop a counseling and referral service to help women at a time when abortion was either illegal or highly restricted in every US state. Two key figures in the Clergy Consultation Service mentioned in this excerpt are the Reverend Howard Moody of Judson Memorial Church in New York City and American Baptist minister Spencer Parsons, who was dean of Rockefeller Chapel at the University of Chicago.

The 1960s gave rise to many radical movements and many feminist groups. The Clergy Consultation Service on Abortion was unique. It was overwhelmingly a white, male, middle- and upper-class, middle-aged group of mainline Protestant and Jewish clergy. Yet it really was a radical, feminist, populist group: radical in that it sought an overthrow (not just amendment)

Source: Doris Andrea Dirks and Patricia Relf, *To Offer Compassion: A History of the Clergy Consultation Service on Abortion* (Madison: University of Wisconsin Press, 2017).

of existing abortion laws; feminist in that it worked to return to women power over their reproductive choices; populist in that it strived to serve women of every socio-economic status, race, and religion. They saw their clerical status as useful to women's fight for abortion rights even if most of them were men, just as many of the same clergy had found their status useful in the civil rights struggle even if they were white.

In 1972, the national office estimated the total number of CCS members at 3,000.[1] ... A majority of CCS clergy whose affiliations we know came from mainline denominations: Presbyterian, Methodist, Baptist, Episcopalian, UCC or Congregational, Unitarian, and Lutheran roughly in that order. Jewish clergy were less well represented, and nearly all were from the Reform tradition, with just a few Conservative rabbis. There were also clergy from the Disciples of Christ, Church of the Brethren, Reformed Church, and five listed as Roman Catholic. We found one or two representatives from each of the Friends (Quaker), Associate Reformed Presbyterian, Ethical Culture, Christian Methodist Episcopal, and Swedenborgian Church.

. . .

Theology of Protestant Counselors

Of course religion was not just a protection and status enhancement for the CCS. The members felt genuinely called to act on their beliefs. [Rev. Howard] Moody felt keenly that organized religion as well as the law had oppressed women, and he wrote an essay in 1967 called "Man's Vengeance on Woman: Some Reflections on Abortion Laws as Religious Retribution and Legal Punishment of the Feminine Species."[2] He laid primary responsibility for punitive antiabortion laws at the feet of Protestants, not Roman Catholics. He wrote, "If the Catholics seemed to be unnaturally obsessed with the future salvation of an unbaptized fetal soul, the Protestants were preoccupied with removing the visual product of woman's immorality and sin. . . . Protestants do not share with our Catholic brothers any belief in the instant animation of the fetus, so the only reasonable justification that we can give for the present abortion law is some innocuous defense of the 'sanctity of life.'" Moody went on to condemn the law as forcing women to seek dangerous illegal abortions. "It is hard to draw any other conclusion from the background and history of the present law than that it is directly calculated, whether conscious or unconscious, to be an excessive and self-righteous punishment, physically and psychologically, of women. . . ." Moody called on Protestants, as the most responsible for the law, to take up the fight to repeal it. "The time is long overdue for a crusade by the Christian church against the outrageous injustice of the present laws. Our silence and timidity have been to condone the law and acquiesce in the suffering."[3]

. . .

Theologically, Moody argued that free choice is essential to being human. He wrote in his memoir, "My understanding of free choice is that the right to choose is a God-given right with which persons are endowed. Without choice, life becomes a meaningless routine and humans become robots. Freedom of choice is what makes us *human* and *responsible*. And for women, the preeminent freedom is the choice to control her reproductive process." He viewed "the deification of the *conceptus*" as heretical, saying that in his theology, being born is not a right but a gift of God and a woman. "*Rights* begin with birth—they are a birthday present—hence *birthright*. Now we are born and have rights, but even then the rights are not absolute or indisputable. Even after birth our rights are fought for, denied and balanced against those who are already here and whose own rights limit and confine our own."[4]

. . .

Many of the pastors we interviewed expressed the opinion that their pastoral counseling necessitated a commitment to compassionate care for women with unwanted pregnancies—their CCS work was simply part of their job as ministers. As we have noted, they were also involved with the social movements of the day, particularly in civil rights and antiwar organizing, and women's rights seemed a natural part of that work.

. . .

The Rabbis

The CCS rabbis we interviewed, and those who wrote on the subject, believed that Jewish teaching permits abortion: the living person (the mother) takes precedence over the potential person (the fetus). A founding member of the CCS, Reform Rabbi Israel Margolies of Beth Am Congregation in New York, speaking at an Association for the Study of Abortion conference in 1968 said, "Until a child is actually born into this world, it is literally part of its mother's body, and belongs only to her and her mate. It does not belong to society at all, nor has it been accepted into any faith. Its existence is entirely and exclusively the business and concern of its parents, whether they are married or not. It is men and women who alone must decide whether or not they wish their union to lead to the birth of a child, not the synagogue or church, and certainly not the state."[5] Rabbi Morton Bauman, a member of the Los Angeles CCS, told the Los Angeles *Herald-Examiner* much the same thing, adding, "I think it's criminal for any child to enter this world unwanted. Having a child doesn't teach a lesson or solve a problem. Religion, not the state, is the institution which teaches ethics and morality, therefore each individual should abide by the teachings of his church and not call upon the state to impose those teachings on others."[6]

Reform Rabbi Balfour Brickner strongly criticized any Bible-based argument that the fetus be considered a full person, saying Exodus 21:22-55 addresses the issue directly. He said,

> Two people are fighting, and a woman is standing by. In the middle of the fight, she is wounded. The ax head falls off, or a rock hits her, and it hits her in her belly, and she's pregnant, and she miscarries. Or she loses the fetus. So the question is raised and answered: Are the people involved in the fight guilty of murder? And the answer is, of course, no. And the reason they're not guilty of murder is because the fetus is only a fetus, and not a living person. . . .[7]

He wrote elsewhere, "According to Jewish law, a child is considered a 'person' only when it has 'come into the world.' The fetus in the womb is not a person until it is born. The Rabbinical principle is *lav nefesh hu*—'It is not a living soul.'"[8] In general, Brickner told us, Jews were very willing to be involved with Planned Parenthood and family planning. "Jewish women were the best practitioners of birth control in the world—still are. I remember I once had a conversation with my then-mother-in-law, who was at that time in her late seventies or eighties, and I once said to her, 'Ethel, what did you folks do when you got pregnant?' And she laughed at me, and she said, 'Why do you ask such a dumb question? Everybody had a doctor'—and she was a New Yorker—'everybody had a doctor in Brooklyn.' Which was to say there wasn't a time when abortion and abortion services were not considered as a viable option and used and practiced as a viable option, certainly among lots and lots of Jewish women."[9]

. . .

Black Clergy

Loretta Ross writes that the majority of abortions available to black women in the 1950s and the early 1960s were provided by doctors and midwives operating illegally. Black midwives provided most of the abortion and contraception services for black women in the deep South. Ross says that in the 1960s "underground abortions were facilitated by churches and community-based referral services" but does not mention the CCS by name.[10]

Relatively few black clergy joined the CCS, and probably for different reasons than the rabbis. Many in black communities were suspicious of the white medical establishment, especially regarding reproductive health, for good reasons going back to such horrors as Dr. James Marion Sims's experimentation on enslaved women and children. The eugenics movement in the early twentieth century openly advocated advancing "superior" (white) genes and repressing those of "inferior" races, and Margaret Sanger, the founder of Planned Parenthood, at least for a time used the scientific-sounding language of the eugenics movement to promote women's right to contraception.[11] She argued that the use of birth control was both moral and eugenically beneficial. Legal scholar Mary Ziegler writes that to win support for Sanger's version of eugenics, between 1920 and 1928 the *Birth Control Review* (established and edited by Sanger) featured "racialist and anti-immigration" articles. Though she was never a proponent of abortion, Sanger wrote that birth control and "its general, though prudent, practice must lead to a higher individuality and ultimately a cleaner race."[12] In the United States, the racist eugenic legacy played itself out in the Tuskegee experiments that began in 1932, in which black men suffering from syphilis believed they were in a treatment program but in fact had treatment withheld (finally ending in 1972). Additionally, black women were far more likely to undergo forced sterilization than were white women; in fact, in the South especially, black women sometimes went to the hospital to give birth and were sterilized after the delivery. Hospital abortion committees imposed sterilization as a condition of providing an abortion more often for black women than for whites. In the 1960s, as the civil rights movement grew, this history of abuse by white medical providers became more public, causing some black leaders—mostly young men—to conclude that the white-controlled political system had a stake in suppressing and oppressing the black population.[13]

The Black Panther Party was the only nationalist group to support free abortions and contraception, although not without controversy within its own ranks. In 1967, the Black Power Conference held in Newark, New Jersey, resolved that birth control was a form of "black genocide."[14] Nkenge Toure and Angela Davis both made comments about women in the party wanting access to birth control and abortion, but noted that some men tried to shut down family planning clinics in New Orleans and Pittsburgh.[15] Black congresswoman Shirley Chisholm wrote in 1970, after she became honorary president of NARAL, that "there is a deep and angry suspicion among many blacks that even birth control clinics are a plot by the white power structure to keep down the numbers of blacks, and this opinion is even more strongly held by some in regard to legalizing abortions. But I do not know any black or Puerto Rican *women* who feel that way. To label family planning and legal abortion programs 'genocide' is male rhetoric, for male ears. It falls flat to female listeners, and to thoughtful male ones."[16] Many other women of color also fought for contraception and abortion rights, often combining the fight with that against sterilization abuse to complete their contention that they should have full reproductive control of their own bodies—to reproduce as well as not to.[17] Of course, some of the women who sought abortions through the CCS were black.

. . .

The Catholic Church and the CCS

. . .

The CCS clergy had contacts among priests and nuns who were sympathetic. Most did not appear on public lists of CCS members. One who participated openly was Sister Barbara Voltz of the Catholic Newman Center at University of Wisconsin-Milwaukee. She spoke publicly in 1972 as a representative of the Milwaukee Area CCS. Although she regarded herself as a nun, she had resigned from her order, the School Sisters of Notre Dame, and became a member of the noncanonical organization Sisters for Christian Community.[18] [Rev. Spencer] Parsons said that at least one Roman Catholic priest who later left the priesthood and two nuns, one the prominent feminist theologian Anne E. Carr, were members of the Chicago CCS, and although they did not make referrals, they met with Catholic women who wanted further counseling following their abortions. "When [women] felt very badly about being Roman Catholic and having had an abortion, she was very helpful. And I had priests in Chicago who did the same thing. They said, 'Don't send me anybody initially to counsel, because this would be very awkward for me. But if you have anybody who needs to reflect on this and think about it, I'd be glad to be of help,'" Parsons recalled. Carr also attended counselor training sessions to educate the Protestant and Jewish clergy about Catholic beliefs and explain some of the struggles that Catholic women would be going through when they came for counseling.[19]

Moody said that he had referred Catholic women who had doubts to a priest from the Newman Center at New York University. "A lot of Catholic women, there was an ambivalence. They knew that they'd be excommunicated, they knew—they loved the church, they went to church, they did—but they couldn't do this. They couldn't have the child. But when there was an ambivalence, I knew that I could refer to him, and that he would be as gentle as he could be. I knew how he'd handle it," Moody said.[20]

. . .

CCS members counseled many Catholic women, generally in proportion to the number of Catholics in the general population. Reports from CCS chapters in 1969 said that in Cleveland, 40 percent of CCS counselees were Roman Catholic; New Jersey CCS reported that slightly under half were Catholic.[21] . . .

Congregations and the CCS

Few of the clergy we spoke with suffered negative repercussions from their congregations or denominations at least for their abortion counseling. Of the Protestant or Jewish denominations represented among the CCS clergy, none had official proscriptions against abortion. The U.S. Episcopal Church was supportive of abortion law reform and the CCS, although the international Anglican Communion had declared an "abhorrence of the sinful practice of abortion" in 1930. Some individual evangelical Protestant ministers had opposed abortion in the 1930s and 1940s; it is safe to say that there weren't many fundamentalists among the CCS clergy. In 1961, the National Council of Churches declared general opposition to abortion except in case of danger to a woman's life or health.[22] Beginning in 1963, the Unitarian Universalist Association of Congregations passed a series of resolutions supporting "the right to choose contraception and abortion as a legitimate expression of our constitutional rights."[23] In 1968, Moody and Parsons both spoke at the American Baptist Convention in favor of a resolution stating that "abortion should be a matter of responsible, personal decision," and that legislation should permit termination of pregnancies before the twelfth week. That resolution—though it was not official church policy and was not binding on any member or congregation—was adopted.[24] . . . Many other denominations issued statements supporting changes in abortion laws, including the Greek Orthodox Archdiocese of North and South America (1966), the Episcopal Church (1967), the Union of American Hebrew Congregations (1967; now known as the Union for Reform Judaism), the United Church of Christ (1970), the United Methodist Church (1970), and the Moravian Church of America (1970).[25] Even the Southern Baptist Convention, representing one of the more conservative of the mainline denominations, approved a national resolution in 1971 accepting in principle the reforms of the ALI [American Law Institute]* model; after the *Roe v. Wade* decision, the Southern Baptist news service viewed the decision as one that advanced "the cause of religious liberty, human equality, and justice."[26]

Notes

1. This number was reported in "Legal Abortion: How Safe? How Available? How Costly?" *Consumer Reports* 37, no. 7 (July 1972),470, and in CCS internal correspondence from the same period, Judson Archive, NYU. . . .
2. Howard Moody, "Man's Vengeance on Woman: Some Reflections on Abortion Laws as Religious Retribution and Legal Punishment of the Feminine Species," *Renewal* (February 1967).
3. Ibid.
4. [Howard Moody, A Voice in the Village: A Journey of a Pastor and a People (N.p.:Xlibris, 2009)], 331-332.
5. Israel R. Margolies, "A Reform Rabbi's View," in Robert E. Hall (ed.), *Abortion in a Changing World: The Proceedings of an International Conference Convened in Hot Springs, Virginia, November 17-20, 1968, by the Association for the Study of Abortion* (New York: Columbia University Press, 1970), vol. 1, 33.
6. Kit Snedaker, "Abortion," California Living, *Los Angeles Herald-Examiner*, January 18, 1970, 15-25.
7. Balfour Brickner, interview by the authors, June 12, 2003, New York.
8. Balfour Brickner in Angela Bonavoglia (ed.), *The Choices We Made: Twenty-five Women and Men Speak Out about Abortion* (New York: Four Walls Eight Windows, 2001), 192.

---

*Eds.: The American Law Institute drafted model legislation to reform abortion law.

9. Brickner interview.

10. Loretta J. Ross, "African-American Women and Abortion: A Neglected History," *Journal of Health Care for the Poor and Underserved* 3, no. 2 (1992), 279-281.

11. Ross, "African-American Women and Abortion," 171. . . .

12. Mary Ziegler, "Eugenic Feminism: Mental Hygiene, the Women's Movement, and the Campaign for Eugenic Legal Reform, 1900-1930," *Harvard Journal of Law & Gender* 31 (2008), 111.

13. Martha C. Ward, *Poor Women, Powerful Men: America's Great Experiment in Family Planning* (Boulder, CO: Westview Press, 1986), 92.

14. Harriet A. Washington, *Medical Apartheid: The Dark History of Medical Experimentation on Black Americans from Colonial Times to the Present* (New York: Harlem Moon, 2006), 2 (Sims), 158 (Tuskegee), 192-193 (eugenics), 196-199 (Sanger, Black Power Conference).

15. Ross, "African-American Women and Abortion," 282.

16. Shirley Chisholm, *Unbought and Unbossed*, 40th anniversary ed. (Washington, DC: Take Root Media, 2010), 130.

17. Amy Kesselman notes that other black women activists also spoke out on behalf of abortion at the time, including Frances Beale, Patricia Robinson, Florynce Kennedy ("Women versus Connecticut: Conducting a Statewide Hearing on Abortion," in Rickie Solinger [ed.], *Abortion Wars: A Half Century of Struggle, 1950-2000* [Berkeley: University of California Press, 1998], 66n36), and Dr. Dorothy Brown, a Tennessee state legislator (Ross, "African-American Women and Abortion," 183; Jael Silliman, Marlene Gerber Fried, Loretta Ross, and Elena R. Gutiérrez, *Undivided Rights: Women of Color Organize for Reproductive Justice* [Cambridge, MA: South End Press, 2004], 55). The authors note that the Young Lords, a Puerto Rican nationalist organization, supported abortion rights as the Black Panthers did, but a similar Chicano organization in Los Angeles, the Brown Berets, saw birth control and abortion as genocide (223-224).

18. Keith Spore, "Abortion Hearing Bares Emotions, *Milwaukee Sentinel*, April 14, 1972; Dorothy Austin, "A New Kind of Nun in a New Kind of Ministry," *Milwaukee Sentinel*, April 21, 1972.

19. Parsons interview.

20. Moody interview.

21. Report to the Chicago CCS on the meeting of the National CCS in New York, NY, on May 28, 1969, folder 5, box 1, Chicago CCS Records, UIC.

22. Daniel K. Williams, *Defenders of the Unborn: The Pro-Life Movement before Roe v. Wade* (New York: Oxford University Press, 2016), 28, 41; Lambeth Conference, Resolution 16, "The Life and Witness of the Christian Community—Marriage and Sex" (1930).

23. Pew Research Center, "Religious Groups' Official Positions on Abortion," January 16, 2013.

24. *Year Book of the American Baptist Convention 1968-1969* (Valley Forge: American Baptist Board of Education and Publication), 52-53, 125.

25. Rosemary Nossiff, *Before* Roe: *Abortion Policy in the States* (Philadelphia: Temple University Press, 2001), 54-55n84; Linda Greenhouse and Reva B. Siegel, *Before* Roe v. Wade: *Voices That Shaped the Abortion Debate before the Supreme Court's Ruling* (New York: Kaplan, 2010), 69-70.

26. Gorney, *Articles of Faith*, 188. The Southern Baptist Convention did not rescind its approval of moderate abortion law reform until 1980, according to Williams, *Defenders of the Unborn*, 237.

43

The Battle over Abortion in the Catholic Church

Patricia Miller

Patricia Miller, a Washington DC–based freelance journalist, writes widely on the intersections of public policy, sexuality, and the Catholic Church. Her award-winning book *Good Catholics* tells how Catholic authorities mobilized a prolife advocacy movement. In this excerpt, we see how the anticontraception work of the Catholic Church in the early 1900s morphed into antiabortion work during the 1960s, leading up to the *Roe* Supreme Court decision. At the same time, Miller recounts, the organization Roman Catholics for the Right to Choose was constituted. Readers may be interested to read further in Miller's book regarding how that organization later became Catholics for a Free Choice (CFFC) and finally the current Catholics for Choice (CFC).

The Catholic bishops of the United States have been organized as a national entity since 1919, when the National Catholic Welfare Conference was established to advocate for Catholic interests in a country that was often hostile to Catholics. Since their large-scale arrival in America in the 1800s, Catholics had been viewed with suspicion because their primary allegiance was believed to be to the Vatican in Rome, not to the United States. Many also worried that the Catholic bishops would try to influence civil law to reflect Catholic doctrine. Throughout the nineteenth and the first half of the twentieth centuries, anti-Catholic discrimination was widespread. Few Catholics could be found in boardrooms, elite schools, or country clubs. Catholics largely lived apart from mainstream Protestant society, with their

Source: Patricia Miller, *Good Catholics: The Battle over Abortion in the Catholic Church* (Berkeley: University of California Press, 2014).

own working-class neighborhoods and schools organized around parish life. Local bishops were powerful figures whose authority over the faithful was unquestioned, and the hierarchy worked to emphasize the patriotism of their flock and protect them from discrimination.

The post–World War II era brought widespread change to this parochial world. Catholics assimilated into the mainstream, leaving their urban neighborhoods for the suburbs and gaining entry to institutions once reserved for WASPs, including the ultimate pinnacle of American achievement, the presidency itself, with the election of John F. Kennedy. The power of the bishops and the church began to decline, as did the need for them to protect Catholics from the outside world. The church convened the Second Vatican Council from 1962 to 1965 to discuss how it should respond to these changes and how it should relate to the modern world.

. . .

The social issues that Vatican II urged the bishops to focus on were economic development, the fostering of peace in an age of nuclear weapons, and, most significant for the history of the church and the United States, abortion.[1] No issue would capture the attention of the Catholic hierarchy quite like abortion. The movement to legalize abortion challenged not just the hierarchy's prohibition against abortion as an "unspeakable crime," but also its belief that sex needed to be linked to procreation to preserve the sanctity of marriage. The bishops had long seen the maintenance of conventional sexual morality—even for non-Catholics—as their special purview. In 1921, as birth control was gaining widespread acceptance, New York Archbishop Patrick Hayes got the police to shut down a public discussion of contraception sponsored by the Voluntary Parenthood League. He defended his action as a "public duty" carried out not in a "sectarian spirit," but in the broad interest of protecting society from the pernicious effects of family limitation.[2]

They may have lost the battle over birth control, but the bishops had a new, even more consequential fight on their hands. From the mid-1960s onward, members of the Catholic hierarchy turned much of their attention to preventing the further legalization of abortion. As abortion reform gained momentum in California in the mid-1960s, the Diocese of Los Angeles hired Spencer-Roberts Associates, the political consulting firm that managed Ronald Reagan's successful gubernatorial campaign, to lobby against the measure. It organized the first "Right to Life" League, which was named by a local bishop based on wording from the Declaration of

Independence, consisting of Catholic clergy and a handful of local anti-abortion activists. The idea was to create the appearance of widespread Catholic grassroots opposition to abortion reform so that it didn't look like Catholic opposition was a top-down effort, which might have reawakened fears about the Catholic hierarchy trying to impose its values in a pluralistic society.

When the abortion reform measure was reintroduced in the California Legislature 1967, these anti-abortion activists were flown by Spencer-Roberts to Sacramento to testify against the bill.[3] The abortion reform bill passed anyway and was signed by Governor Reagan, but the "Right to Life" movement had been concocted just as the fight over abortion reform was heating up. . . .

That same year the Catholic hierarchy began to construct a national grassroots network to oppose liberalization of abortion laws. . . . The NCCB also encouraged individual bishops to develop right-to-life groups. The bishops provided local groups, which were often just one or two activists, with places to meet, administrative support, free publicity in church bulletins and, perhaps most invaluably, exhortations from the pulpit for Catholics to work to oppose abortion.[4]

. . .

In 1968, the bishops' Family Life Bureau created the National Right to Life Committee (NRLC) as a formal structure to coordinate the activities of local right-to-life groups and to give the fledgling prolife movement a national presence. It would become the single most powerful anti-abortion group nationally and was wholly a creation of the Catholic bishops.

. . .

Despite opposition from the Catholic bishops, a tide of abortion reform swept the nation between 1967 and 1970, as twelve states—mainly those without a strong Catholic Conference—reformed their abortion laws.[5] Most of these early abortion reform efforts were championed by men who were interested in making abortion more "humane" by broadening the circumstances under which doctors could legally perform the procedure. But the late 1960s brought a new constituency interested in changing abortion law: women. . . . [I]ncreasingly women realized that personal issues like abortion were as important to women's rights as workplace equality. On a practical level, the ability to control their fertility was essential to women's ability to access the higher education and workforce opportunities that had been reserved for men. On an emotional level, women began to acknowledge that they were angry that they were the ones who had to pay such a high price for an unwanted pregnancy.

It's hard to conceive of what a starkly different world it was for women in terms of sexuality and reproduction in the mid-1960s. The Pill had been introduced only in 1960, and although it was already rewriting the rules of sexual behavior, it still had its limitations. Early oral contraceptives had very high doses of estrogen, which caused side effects for many women and led them to discontinue use. Access to birth control also was limited by law. As late as 1965, twenty-nine states had laws limiting access to contraceptives. Some banned birth control from being advertised or information about birth control being distributed. Others allowed only doctors or pharmacists to distribute contraceptives and banned drug stores from selling condoms. Many states banned minors from buying contraceptives. Social convention also played a role. Many doctors would not prescribe contraceptives to unmarried women because they were afraid of promoting promiscuity, and many pharmacists kept condoms behind the counter for the same reason.[6]

A handful of Catholic states like Connecticut and Massachusetts still banned birth control even for married couples. The right of married couples to use contraception was not officially sanctioned until 1965 in the *Griswold v. Connecticut* Supreme Court decision, which recognized the right of privacy within marriage. Unmarried couples would have to wait until 1972's *Eisenstadt v. Baird* to be granted the same right. It was a society in flux. The old strictures were gradually falling away as the sexual revolution gained steam, but women did not yet necessarily have the tools to take advantage of the newfound sexual liberation that was being espoused.

. . .

Speaking at the First National Conference on Abortion Laws in 1969, which led to the establishment of the National Association for Repeal of Abortion Laws (NARAL), the first national abortion rights organization, Betty Friedan spoke the words that would become a rallying cry for a generation when she asserted that "there are certain rights that have never been defined as rights, that are essential to equality for women. . . . The right of women to control her reproductive process must be established as a basic and valuable human civil right." Like her feminist colleagues, she dismissed the idea of abortion reform: "Don't talk to me about reform—reform is still the same—women, passive object. Reform is something dreamed up by men."[7]

. . .

Repeal also found support from another, more surprising quarter. Influential Jesuit law professor Robert Drinan created a stir when he said that from the perspective of Catholic moral teaching it would be better for all abortion laws to be repealed than for the government to be in the business of deciding who should and should not be born, as it would be forced to do under reform measures. He advocated the complete repeal of laws prohibiting abortion in the first twenty-six weeks of pregnancy, with abortion treated as homicide thereafter.[8]

With support for repeal growing, Friedan and the New York chapter of NOW decided the time was ripe to push for repeal in New York State. It was a long shot. In a state that was 40 percent Catholic, the Catholic Church had used its clout in the legislature to turn back abortion reform efforts in 1967 and 1968.

. . .

Despite ferocious lobbying from the Catholic hierarchy and after a dramatic last-minute vote switch by a legislator in a conservative, heavily Catholic district, who stood to gravely acknowledge that he was signing his political death warrant but said in good conscience he could not be the person to let the bill fail, the New York Legislature passed the law on April 9, 1970. Governor Nelson Rockefeller signed the bill in spite of a last-minute plea from New York Cardinal Terence Cooke.[9]

The New York bill was essentially a compromise between the repeal and reform positions. It became the model for broad-based abortion legalization when it was in effect codified by the U.S. Supreme Court in *Roe v. Wade*.

. . .

The near-death experience of the New York State abortion law was a wake-up call to abortion rights activists. . . . By 1970 there was a right-to-life committee in just about every state. Between 1970 and 1973, after a string of successes, abortion reform efforts failed in state after state, most of them heavily Catholic. "If it weren't for the Catholic Church, the law would have been changed years ago," groused one legislator after three failed attempts to liberalize abortion law in Ohio.[10]

Supporters of legal abortion had good reason to fear the power of the Catholic Church. The hierarchy had been the most formidable opponent of the legalization of birth control. Once contraception gained acceptance in the 1930s, the bishops couldn't do much about middle-class women who received birth control through private physicians for "health" reasons, which the courts declared legal. They did, however, prevent the opening of public birth control clinics in northeastern cities that served largely immigrant and poor populations, blocked state legislatures from legalizing birth control, and turned back efforts to provide federal funding for family planning programs for the poor.[11]

. . .

Although the abortion liberalization movement had been worried about the Catholic Church for some time, most activists were reluctant to attack the church directly for fear it would allow the bishops to hide behind charges of anti-Catholicism. But there was a way to rebut the bishops on abortion without running the danger of being called anti-Catholic: have other Catholics do it.[12]

. . .

In September 1971, an organization calling itself Roman Catholics for the Right to Choose announced its support for the repeal measures before the state assembly. Mary Robison, the group's chair, said, "It appears . . . at least in the public mind—that opponents of abortion law repeal are Roman Catholics. Many undoubtedly are. But many Roman Catholics do not agree with the stand taken by our church in this regard."[13]

Roman Catholics for the Right to Choose was the first explicitly Catholic abortion rights organization and marked a new chapter in the evolving effort to legalize abortion, as Catholics for the first time went public with their support of abortion rights. The organization sent the assembly a petition in favor of repeal with the names of 500 Catholics. It said that while not all the signers found abortion "personally acceptable," they were in agreement "in our belief that our Church should not attempt to use civil law to impose its moral philosophy upon our non-Catholic neighbors."[14]

Notes

1. See *Gaudium et Spes*, Dec. 7, 1965, which called abortion and infanticide "unspeakable crimes."
2. "Hayes Denounces Birth Control Aim," *NYT*, Nov. 21, 1921.
3. Keith Monroe, "How California's Abortion Law Isn't Working," *NYT*, Dec. 29, 1968; [Connie Paige, *The Right to Lifers: Who They Are, How They Operate, Where They Get Their Money* (New York: Summit, 1983)], 56.
4. [James Risen and Judy Thomas, *Wrath of Angels: The American Abortion War* (New York: Basic, 1998)], 19.

5. These states were Colorado, Arkansas, California, Delaware, Georgia, Kansas, Maryland, New Mexico, North Carolina, Oregon, South Carolina, and Virginia. [Leslie J. Reagan, *When Abortion Was a Crime: Women, Medicine, and the Law in the United States, 1867-1973* (Berkeley: University of California Press, 1997)], 331.

6. Peter Kihss, "Bill for Liberalizing New York Statue Goes to State Senate," *NYT*, June 8, 1965.

7. [Linda Greenhouse and Reva Siegel, *Before Roe v. Wade: Voices That Shaped the Abortion Debate before the Supreme Court's Ruling* (New York: Kaplan, 2010)], 39.

8. Fred Graham, "A Priest Links Easing of Abortions with Racism," *NYT*, Sept. 8, 1967.

9. Bill Kovach, "Final Approval of Abortion Bill Voted in Albany," *NYT*, April 11, 1970.

10. In 1972, reform efforts failed in George, Indiana, Rhode Island, Colorado, Delaware, Maine, Kansas, Iowa, Illinois, Michigan, Pennsylvania, Massachusetts, and Connecticut. Jurate Kazickas, "Counterattack on Abortion Gains Ground," *NYT*, Aug. 14, 1972.

11. See [David J. Garrow, *Liberty and Sexuality: The Right to Privacy and the Making of* Roe v. Wade (New York: Macmillan, 1994)]; and [Donald T. Critchlow, *Intended Consequences: Birth Control, Abortion, and the Federal Government in Modern America* (New York: Oxford University Press, 1999)], for a history of the bishops' efforts to suppress state and federal funding for birth control.

12. Ti-Grace Atkinson, president of the New York chapter of NOW, criticized the organization for not taking on the church directly, which was one reason she left to join a more radical group of feminists. "If you've got a position on abortion, you've got one on the church," she said. See [Judith Hole and Ellen Levine, *Rebirth of Feminism* (New York: Quadrangle, 1971)], 90.

13. "Catholics Ask for Free Choice in Abortions," *Pittsburgh Post-Gazette*, Sept. 25, 1971.

14. Letter to the Members of the Commonwealth of Pennsylvania General Assembly, from Mary S. Robison, Roman Catholics for the Right to Choose, Sept. 1971, Pennsylvania State Archives, Harrisburg, PA, Pennsylvania Historical and Museum Commission.

44

Roe v. Wade:
Setting the Stage
for Pro-Choice
Religion-Based Holdings

Stacy A. Scaldo

In this excerpt, law professor Stacy Scaldo analyzes how religion-based arguments, represented in *amicus* briefs, played a significant role in the *Roe v. Wade* decision. Despite the Court's ostensible efforts to avoid including religious reasons as a basis of the decisions, Scaldo finds that aspects of the prochoice religious groups' reasoning in their brief can be found in the Court's "holding" or determination in refusing to rule on prolife claims regarding fetal personhood. She also notes that the *Roe* ruling acknowledged both that religious beliefs are deeply tied to the debate about abortion and that there is no agreement among religions on the question of when life begins. Those interested in knowing how these dynamics are found in subsequent Supreme Court decisions on abortion can read Scaldo's entire essay.

In *Roe*, the Court was tasked with deciding whether the Constitution supported a woman's right to choose to terminate her pregnancy through abortion.[1] The Texas law prohibiting abortion except when necessary to save the life of the pregnant woman was challenged by Roe, whose desire to abort

Source: Stacy A. Scaldo, "Life, Death & the God Complex: The Effectiveness of Incorporating Religion-Based Arguments into the Pro-Choice Perspective on Abortion," *Northern Kentucky Law Review* 39 (2012): 421–66.

was not connected to any life threatening condition.[2] The Court held 7-2 that the Constitutional right to privacy, as recognized in *Griswold v. Connecticut*,[3] included the right to terminate a pregnancy by abortion.[4] The Court set up a three stage analysis and determined that the state's levels of interest in a pregnancy vary depending upon the trimester:

   a. For the stage prior to approximately the end of the first trimester, the abortion decision and its effectuation must be left to the medical judgment of the pregnant woman's attending physician.
   b. For the stage subsequent to approximately the end of the first trimester, the State, in promoting its interest in the health of the mother, may, if it chooses, regulate the abortion procedure in ways that are reasonably related to maternal health.
   c. For the stage subsequent to viability, the State in promoting its interest in the potentiality of human life may, if it chooses, regulate, and even proscribe, abortion except where it is necessary, in appropriate medical judgment, for the preservation of the life or health of the mother.[5]

In purpose and effect, the court created a sliding scale of autonomy based upon this trimester framework, acknowledging a women's complete autonomy over the pregnancy during the first trimester and providing varying levels of acceptable state interference as the pregnancy continued into the second and third trimesters.[6]

1. The Briefs

Only two amicus curiae briefs on behalf of religiously affiliated groups were filed in the *Roe* case—one in favor of the pro-choice argument and the other in favor of the pro-life argument. The brief in favor of the pro-choice argument was filed on behalf of the following churches or organizations: the American Ethical Union, the American Friends Service Committee, the American Humanist Association, the American Jewish Congress, the Episcopal Diocese of New York, the New York State Council of Churches, the Union of American Hebrew Congregations, the Unitarian Universalist Association, the United Church of Christ and the Board of Christian Social Concerns of the United Methodist Church.[7] The brief presented two main arguments in favor of finding the statutes at issue unconstitutional: (1) that the abortion laws at issue invaded the right to privacy[8]; and (2) that they were an invalid exercise of police power.[9]

The facially religious argument is contained within the broader argument as to the improper use of police power.[10] The section's title presumes that the belief that "the product of every conception is sacred" is a religious view.[11] Based upon this viewpoint, the pro-choice amici argued mainly that protecting fetal life based upon the premise that the product of every conception is sacred (a religious view) violates the Establishment Clause of the First Amendment.[12] Amici noted that the interest in the fetus stems, in its essence, from a misplaced "'moral' concern for the 'potential of independent human existence.'"[13] They argued that this moral concern is misplaced if it outweighs a "greater moral outrage: the deep human suffering of adults and children alike, that results from compelling one to continue an unwanted pregnancy, to give birth to an unwanted child, and to assume the burdens of unwanted parenthood."[14] Therefore, because not all people, and not all religions, regard the product of every conception as sacred, a law that prohibits abortion based on the sacredness of the potential life, necessarily chooses and imposes upon its citizens one religion or one set of religious beliefs over another in violation of the Establishment Clause.

The brief in favor of the pro-life argument was filed on behalf of the Association of Texas Diocesan Attorneys.[15] The arguments made in this brief focused on the concept of personhood and the status of a fetus as a person.[16] In conformity with that argument, amici claimed:

> [N]o federal court can rationally dispose of the issues in this case without confronting and resolving the issue of whether an unborn child is a person under the constitutional concept of the person. It also tells that if the unborn child is a person within the meaning of the Constitution then a state has the right to enact a statute seeking to protect the constitutional right to life of the unborn child providing it has done so in a reasonable way.[17]

The concept of personhood would be the center of the debate in Roe. The Court's decision on the issue would set the stage for all future abortion regulation cases.

2. The Decision

As is evident from the opening paragraphs of the opinion, the Court in Roe did not expressly look to religion as the basis of the decision.[18] However, the introduction makes clear in both structure and content that religion and religious ideology were key components of the Court's reasoning.[19] Broken into three distinct but overlapping parts, the introduction sets the stage for the holding in *Roe* and its progeny.[20] First, the Court introduced the historical importance of the challenged legislation:

> The Texas Statutes under attack here are typical of those that have been in effect in many States for approximately a century. The Georgia statutes, in contrast, have a modern cast and are a legislative product that, to an extent at least, obviously reflects the influences of recent attitudinal change, of advancing medical knowledge and techniques, and of new thinking about an old issue.[21]

Next, the Court acknowledged the daunting task that lay ahead:

> We forthwith acknowledge our awareness of the sensitive and emotional nature of the abortion controversy, of the vigorous opposing views, even among physicians, and of the deep and seemingly absolute convictions that the subject inspires. One's philosophy, one's experiences, one's exposure to the raw edges of human existence, one's religious training, one's attitudes toward life and family and their values, and the moral standards one establishes and seeks to observe, are all likely to influence and to color one's thinking and conclusions about abortion.[22]

Finally, in an effort to demonstrate a principled detachment regarding a deeply morality-driven issue, the Court noted that its task was "to resolve the issue by Constitutional measurement, free from emotion and of predilection."[23]

The Court did not cite in pertinent part to either of the two amicus briefs filed by the religiously affiliated groups.[24] It also facially avoided any reliance on religion in setting forth the framework of the opinion in the introduction. It is clear, however, even from these initial paragraphs, that the pro-choice religious brief had a deep impact on the Court's ruling.

...

The purpose of the Court's foray into the historical practices and legal ramifications of abortion was to demonstrate that the laws at issue in the case were "of relatively recent vintage."[25] As the Court noted, these criminal abortion laws did not really begin to surface in mass until the late 19th century.[26] This is an important point from a religious perspective because it responded to a general societal belief that a pro-life stance had always been rooted in and connected to religious doctrine.[27] It also placed the pro-life stance in the context of belonging to the new fundamentalist-based Christian upstarts that had gained momentum in the previous half-century.[28] On several occasions throughout this analysis, the Court made a point of historical religious trends in support of and opposition to abortion.[29] It noted that "[a]ncient religion did not bar abortion,"[30] and that early Christian theology was inconsistent on the issue.[31]

After explaining why criminal abortion laws, in large part, did not exist until relatively recently, the Court examined three interests historically proffered by the state to justify its enactment and continued existence: (1) the discouragement of illicit sexual conduct; (2) the protection of the pregnant woman against an unsafe medical procedure; and (3) the protection of prenatal life.[32] The second state interest, that of protecting the pregnant woman against unsafe abortion procedures, was purely a medical interest, and the Court's determination as to the value of that interest was medical as well.[33] However, the first and third interests—discouraging illicit sexual conduct and protection of fetal life—included religious implications, both in the interest of the state and analysis by the Court.[34]

The Court acknowledged that the discouragement of illicit sexual conduct was neither an interest advanced by the state in the case nor was it suggested by amici.[35] The Court, however, determined it would be best to address as a first concern the occasional argument "that these laws were the byproduct of a Victorian social concern."[36] If not advanced by the state and not argued by amici, the reasonable assumption is that the Court was speaking to the public in anticipation of or in reaction to an ongoing argument based upon a particular set of religious and moral principles. This tends to fall in line with the Court's assessment of both late 19th century and current religious attitudes toward abortion.[37] The Court, in essence, was speaking directly to the pro-life religious sector of society and discounting any morally-based anti-abortion stance. The Court concluded, in line with the concessions of the pro-life argument, that the statutes at issue were overbroad in protecting the interest of discouraging illicit sexual conduct as "the law fail[ed] to distinguish between married and unwed mothers."[38]

The third interest of protecting prenatal life presented the Court with a different dilemma altogether. The parties to the case, amici, and in some way, the rest of society, were asking the Court to make a determination as to when life begins. The Court refused.[39] Although acknowledging that historical abortion statutes and cases "impliedly repudiate[d] the theory that life begins at conception,"[40] the Court carefully searched for middle ground. Instead of a finding on either side, it determined:

> [A] legitimate state interest in this area need not stand or fall on acceptance of the belief that life begins at conception or at some other point prior to life

[sic] birth. In assessing the State's interest, recognition may be given to the less rigid claim that as long as at least *potential* life is involved, the State may assert interests beyond the protection of the pregnant woman alone.[41]

With this one statement, the Court handed both the pro-life and pro-choice communities victory *and* defeat.

. . .

The Court's finding that the issue could be resolved without determining the status of a fetus beyond that of potential life would have equally far reaching implications. Facially, the Court took religion out of its reasoning.[42] But, in implicitly adopting the argument of the pro-choice religious amici, the Court: (1) determined that the right to privacy included a woman's right to choose to have an abortion;[43] (2) demonstrated that religion and how religious views affect the abortion debate were noteworthy considerations of its decision;[44] and (3) set the parameters for future religion-based arguments in Supreme Court abortion cases.[45]

First, the 'potential life' determination was essential to the Court's finding that the right to personal privacy includes the abortion decision. As stated above, if life begins at conception, the privacy right cannot extend to abortion as the life of the fetus is of equal status.[46] However, by calling the fetus 'potential life,' the Court was able to circumvent the issue of when life begins and expressly avoid the religious 'sanctity of life' argument. Because the potential life status impinges on the right to privacy an unqualified attribute, it "must be considered against important state interests in regulation."[47]

Second, in refusing to rule on the exact life status of the fetus·, the Court acknowledged how deeply religion and religious beliefs are tied to this debate.[48] In fact, the decision to avoid rendering life status to a fetus was based in part on the inconsistent religious theories:

> We need not resolve the difficult question of when life begins. When those trained in the respective disciplines of medicine, philosophy, and theology are unable to arrive at any consensus, the judiciary, at this point in the development of man's knowledge, is not in a position to speculate as to the answer.[49]

Further discussion of the differing views of religious groups continued with the Court noting that the predominant Jewish and Protestant positions held to the theory that life does not begin until live birth, that organized religious groups taking a position have regarded it as a matter for the conscience of the pregnant woman and her family, and that the Catholic pro-life stance was a relatively recent one.[50] As a consequence of these competing theories, the Court summed up its reasons for rejecting the sanctity of life argument by stating that it did "not agree that, by adopting one theory of life, Texas may override the rights of the pregnant woman that are at stake."[51] In making that determination, however, the Court did that very thing. By adopting one theory of life—that a fetus is only a potential life—the Court did not just override the rights of the fetus; it foreclosed the ability for the fetus to have any rights of equal measure that could validly compete with that of the pregnant woman at an early stage of pregnancy.[52] Instead the fetus only becomes important if the state can show an interest sufficiently compelling to vie for legitimate state regulation—a situation never present at the beginning stages of a pregnancy.[53] As future cases have noted, this state interest in fetal life is rarely sufficient to override the interests of the woman, even at the latest stage of a pregnancy.[54]

. . .

It is this potentiality of life, as opposed to the existence of it, which validates applying the right to privacy to the abortion decision. In essence, by refusing to determine when life begins and by referring to the fetus as "potential life," the Court did in fact answer the question of when life begins.[55] According to the Roe Court, life begins at live birth.[56]

With this framework in place, the Court set the parameters of the arguments by religious amici in future abortion cases.

Notes

1. *Roe v. Wade*, 410 U.S. 113 (1973) at 116.
2. *Id.* at 120. The companion case to *Roe, Doe v. Bolton* was filed by a married couple. *Id.* at 121; *Doe v. Bolton*, 410 U.S. 179 (1973). They claimed that the wife was suffering from a disorder that caused her physician to recommend that she not become pregnant. *Roe*, 410 U.S. at 121. The Does claimed that if she should become pregnant, they would wish to terminate the pregnancy. *Id.*
3. Griswold v. Connecticut, 381 U.S. 479 (1965).
4. *Roe,* 410 U.S. at 153.
5. *Id.* at 164-65.
6. *Id.* at 163-164.
7. Motion of Am. Ethical Union et al. as Amici Curiae in Support of Appellants' Position, with the Proposed Brief Attached, Roe v. Wade, 410 U.S. 113 (1973) (No. 70-18), 1971 WL 128051.

8. *Id.* at 14-20.
9. *Id.* at 20-34.
10. *Id.* at 31. (Subsection B.3.c. of the brief is titled: "The religious view that the product of every conception is sacred may not validly be urged by the States as a justification for limiting the exercise of constitutional liberties, for that would be an establishment of religion").
11. *Id.*
12. *Id.* at 31-32.
13. Motion of Am. Ethical Union et al., *supra* note 17, at 31-32 (quoting *Doe v. Bolton*, 319 F. Supp. 1048, 1055 (1970)).
14. Motion of Am. Ethical Union et al., *supra* note 17, at 31-32.
15. Brief Amicus on Behalf of Ass'n of Tex. Diocesan Attorneys, in Support of Appellee, *Roe v. Wade*, 410 U.S. 113 (1973) (No. 70-18), 1971 WL 134282.
16. *See id.*
17. *Id.* at 48-49.
18. *Roe*, 410 U.S. at 116-17.
19. *See generally id.*
20. *See generally id.*
21. *Roe*, 410 U.S. at 116.
22. *Id.*
23. *Id. . . .*
24. It did cite to the Brief of the Am. Ethical Union et al. in support of its statement that "organized groups that have taken a formal position on the abortion issue have generally regarded abortion as a matter for the conscience of the individual and her family." *See id.* at 160 and n. 58.
25. [*Roe*, 410 U.S.] at 129.
26. *Id.*
27. *Id.*
28. *Id.*
29. *See generally Roe*, 410 U.S. 113.
30. *Id.* at 130.
31. *Id.* at 134. Up until the 19th Century, Christian theology had come to accept the idea that the point of "mediate animation" occurred by the age of 40 days for males and 80 days for females. *Id.* According to the *Roe* Court, there was agreement that "prior to this point the fetus was to be regarded as part of the mother, and its destruction, therefore, was not homicide." *Id.* Due in large part to the lack of evidence to support the "40-80 day view," quickening became the critical point. *Id.*
32. *Id.* at 147-52.
33. *Id.* at 148-50 (noting that abortion prior to the end of the first trimester is relatively safe, mortality rates for abortion in the first trimester when performed in a legal environment are equivalent to or less than the rates

for normal childbirth, the risks to a woman increase as her pregnancy continues, and high mortality rates at illegal "abortion mills" strengthen the state's interest in protecting the woman's health later in the pregnancy).

34. *Id.* at 158, 150-152.

35. *Roe*, 410 U.S. at 148.

36. *Id.*

37. *See id.*

38. *Id.*

39. *Id.* at 159.

40. *Id.* at 151-52.

41. *Roe*, 410 U.S. at 150.

42. *See generally Id.* at 113.

43. *Infra* at 10-11.

44. *Infra* at 11.

45. *Infra* at 11-12.

46. Roe, 410 U.S. at 156-57.

47. *Id.* at 154-55 (noting that the right is "subject to some limitations; and that at some point the state interests as to the protection of health, medical standards, and prenatal life become dominant").

48. *Id.* at 159.

49. *Id.* at 159.

50. *Id.* at 160-61 (citing generally to the Motion of the Am. Ethical Union et al, *supra* note 17).

51. *Id.* at 162.

52. *Roe*, 410 U.S. at 163. (According to the Court, the compelling point for triggering the State's important and legitimate interest in protecting potential life was viability. The Court drew this line because "the fetus then presumably has the capability of meaningful life outside the mother's womb.")

53. *Id.*

54. *See generally Stenberg*, 530 U.S. 914; *Gonzales*, 550 U.S. 124.

55. [*Roe*, 410 U.S. at 164-5.]

56. *Id.*

45

The Women's League for Conservative Judaism and the Politics of Abortion, 1970–82

Rachel Kranson

A professor of religious studies, Rachel Kranson's scholarship focuses on post–Second World War Jewish life in America. Her essay on Jewish women's prochoice activism in the 1970s uncovers a story that has been overlooked in most accounts of secular prochoice and conservative Christian abortion battles. Kranson focuses on the Women's League, a national group representing women affiliated with the Conservative branch of Judaism in the United States. Noted for their promotion of Jewish culture among the network of Conservative synagogue "sisterhood" groups, they also spoke to political and societal issues. Kranson details how the Women's League developed a prochoice Jewish religious stance rooted in religious freedom rather than women's rights.

This essay traces the Women's League for Conservative Judaism's engagement in the issue of reproductive rights during the 1970s and early 1980s, as the hardened ideological positions that would later come to characterize the national debates over abortion were only just beginning to form. Members

Source: Rachel Kranson, "From Women's Rights to Religious Freedom: The Women's League for Conservative Judaism and the Politics of Abortion, 1970–1982," in *Devotions and Desires: Histories of Sexuality and Religion in the Twentieth-Century United States*, ed. Gillian A. Frank, Bethany Moreton, and Heather R. White (Chapel Hill: University of North Carolina Press, 2018), 170–92.

of Women's League first championed legal abortion in 1970, defending their position through expressly feminist arguments upholding reproductive autonomy as a woman's civil right. While they never backed down from their support for legal abortion, the political shifts of the late 1970s and early 1980s compelled them to develop a new language through which to discuss the issue. By 1982, they began to justify their stance on abortion through the principal of religious freedom rather than through an endorsement of women's rights.

Reframing access to abortion as a matter of religious freedom offered Women's League members a way to articulate their support for the procedure without publicly endorsing the notion of women's reproductive autonomy, an idea that had become increasingly controversial over the course of the 1970s. The late 1970s saw the "religious right," a coalition of socially conservative activists dominated by evangelical Protestants, emerge as the central religious voice in the national debates over reproductive rights. As much of the American public began to view a particularly right-wing, Christian opposition to abortion as a universal religious principle, the leaders of Women's League struggled to show that their backing of legal abortion did not conflict with their religious commitments. Reconfiguring access to abortion as a religious right enabled them to present their stance on abortion as a component of their spiritual worldview rather than as a capitulation to secular, feminist ideals.[1]

That an organization like Women's League, whose members overwhelmingly favored legal abortion and largely sympathized with the feminist movement, retreated from discussing abortion as a woman's right demonstrates the strong influence that the anti-abortion activism of the Christian right had on less conservative, even non-Christian, religious groups. The story of how this organization negotiated the issue of abortion, therefore, reveals the surprisingly broad impact of late twentieth-century religious conservatism.

. . .

In the late 1970s and early 1980s, these assumed linkages between religion and sexuality offered right-wing Christian leaders the chance to secure a powerful voice in American politics through their attempts to restrict sexual and reproductive behavior. This political climate forced representatives of American Judaism to consider carefully their statements on abortion. Because Jewish law does not support the idea of ensoulment at conception, nearly all Jewish legal authorities consider it necessary to terminate a pregnancy in some situations, most consistently in the case when a fetus endangers the life of the mother. On the other hand, few of the traditional Jewish authorities recognize a woman's right to choose an abortion independently, without first securing the permission of a rabbi. Since Jewish law neither prohibits abortion on principle nor allows women the right to curtail their pregnancies autonomously, the leaders of American Judaism have had license to participate in national debates over abortion in ways that reflect their complex political interests as much as their religious convictions. Tracing the ways that Jews discussed reproductive rights, therefore, affords us insight into the parameters of public religious discourse during the rise of the religious right. It offers a sense of the arguments that could, and could not, be made by the spokespeople of American Judaism if they expected their position to be taken seriously by politicians, the judiciary, the media, and the American public.[2]

. . .

Women's League passed its first resolution in support of abortion access at its 1970 biennial convention, during an especially dynamic social action plenary. The social action committee proposed resolutions on racial unrest, campus activism, the separation of church and state, and Soviet Jews. In spite of the increasing visibility of the feminist movement and the recent decriminalization of abortion in Hawaii and New York, however, they had not prepared a statement on the issue of reproductive rights.[3]

While reproductive rights may not yet have reached the political radar of the social action committee, these matters concerned Women's League members at the grassroots level. When the session moderator invited comments from the floor, delegates from the Midwest branch presented the women who attended the social action plenary with a resolution that they had prepared late the night before. This statement supported women's access to birth control and abortion, and the membership voted unanimously to adopt it.

. . .

This initial resolution on reproductive rights that Women's League passed unanimously in 1970 utilized the expressly feminist vocabulary of women's rights and women's choice to justify support for abortion and birth control. It proclaimed the "freedom of choice as to birth control and abortion" to be "inherent in the civil rights of women," adding that "all laws infringing on those rights should be repealed."[4]

With this statement, Women's League became the first branch of the Conservative movement to pass a national resolution on reproductive rights. Three years before *Roe v. Wade* made legal access to abortion the law of the land, five years before any other branch of the Conservative movement would declare support for legal abortion, and thirteen years before the Rabbinical Assembly would do so, the Women's League went on record declaring anti-abortion laws an infringement of women's civil rights. This language, in many ways, mirrored their previous resolutions supporting the civil rights of African Americans and religious minorities, but this signified the first time that either the Women's League or any national branch of the Conservative movement had treated women as a political entity with a distinct set of rights that ought to be secured.[5]

Significantly, and in spite of Women's League's identity as an expressly religious organization, this 1970 resolution did not refer to Jewish religious law or Jewish theology in its defense of reproductive rights. Indeed, neither the delegates at the convention nor the members of the social action committee deemed it necessary to consult with the rabbis of the Conservative movement—who, in these years before women's ordination, were by definition all men—before adopting this resolution. In 1970, during the heyday of the feminist movement and prior to the political ascendance of the religious right, Women's League members did not see a woman's legal right to abortion as being in conflict with a religious worldview. Rather, much like the members of the National Association for the Repeal of Abortion Laws, the National Organization for Women, and other advocates of liberal feminism, they conceived of reproductive rights as a cornerstone of women's political, social, and economic independence rather than a spiritual matter to be discussed with rabbinic authorities.

. . .

By the early 1980s, however, Women's League would overhaul its long-standing resolution on abortion in ways that reflected larger shifts in American politics that reframed abortion as a conservative issue associated with religious commitment. In the years before the *Roe* decision, Catholics led the political movement to limit abortion rights and the general public understood their opposition to abortion as a particularly Catholic issue. Anti-abortion sentiment gradually became ensconced in the mainstream of conservative politics over the course of the 1970s as Nixon courted the Catholic vote and sought to draw them into the Republican Party.

By the late 1970s, evangelical Protestants joined and then came to dominate the anti-abortion movement, working with Catholics and Mormons to oppose *Roe v. Wade.* By the 1980 election that pitted Jimmy Carter against Ronald Reagan, the influence of such politicized religious organizations as Jerry Falwell's Moral Majority and Beverly LaHaye's

Concerned Women for America, both established in 1979, deployed the religiously inflected language of "family values" against the vocabulary of "women's rights." Family values functioned as an ecumenical binding that held together the evangelical Protestants, Catholics, and Mormons who worked together for shared political goals despite their theological differences. Together, they sought to restrict access to abortion and contraception in addition to fighting against other proposals, such as state-sponsored childcare, that sought to help working mothers provide economically for their families. Their conception of these matters as assaults against what they saw as the God-given, traditional structure of the family, an institution they imagined as being led by a breadwinning father and nurtured by a full-time, procreative mother, struck a chord with many Americans. Moreover, their vision garnered a great deal of attention from Republican politicians who had been trying to bring these voters into their party for the better part of a decade.

Opposition to abortion emerged as a central component of this new political vision, achieving its primacy due to national anxieties over profound transformations to sexual and gender norms. From the late 1960s, arguments for abortion reform that sought to protect the health of (respectable, married) mothers competed with anti-abortion arguments that described the procedure as a means by which unmarried, sexually active women could escape the consequences of their promiscuity. As the ideas and rhetoric of the religious right gained currency, many politicians and much of the public began to view anti-abortion sentiment as a universal belief shared by all socially conservative people of faith and as a cultural litmus test for traditional religious leadership.[6]

Unsurprisingly, therefore, it was not until the late 1970s that prominent rabbis within the Conservative movement introduced Women's League members to new ways of thinking about the abortion issue that had little to do with women's autonomy. Robert Gordis, a renowned professor of biblical studies at the Conservative movement's Jewish Theological Seminary and a past president of the Rabbinical Assembly, challenged the way that Women's League members discussed reproductive rights. Gordis, by all accounts, was "very beloved" by the leaders of Women's League, who were grateful to him for consistently taking the time to speak at their national conventions. Women's League members, for their part, supported Gordis professionally and financially by regularly sponsoring and publicizing his scholarly work.[7]

Earlier, in the late 1960s, Gordis had become quite interested in the transformation of American sexual mores that occurred in the wake of improved birth control options, youth rebellion, and the feminist movement. He endeavored to write a Jewish response to this "sexual revolution," and the leaders of Women's League actively supported this project. In 1967, they funded the publication of Gordis's *Sex and the Family in the Jewish Tradition*, a thin volume that discussed Jewish texts and legal traditions concerning the sanctity of marriage, the positive value of licit, marital sex, and the permissibility of birth control. Though Gordis briefly mentioned the then-illegal abortion procedure as a tragic phenomenon signifying "danger and death for mothers and for offspring yet unborn," abortion did not appear as a major theme within this book. Nowhere in this volume did Gordis theologize abortion or delve into Jewish legal traditions concerning the procedure. While Gordis certainly did not endorse women's reproductive rights, he nonetheless painted abortion as a matter of social, rather than religious, concern.[8]

. . .

Though the Women's League continued to support legal abortion, its amended 1982 resolution justified this stance through the logic of religious freedom instead of through the principle of women's rights. In this formulation, proposed limits on abortion access did not place a woman's right to reproductive autonomy into jeopardy; rather, they threatened the right of Jews to free exercise of their religion. This resolution effectively erased women as a political entity with rights that ought to be secured and protected.

In addition to changing the central logic behind the organization's support for legal abortion, the amended statement also stressed that Jewish religious traditions did not support women's reproductive autonomy. It quoted Robert Gordis's claim that abortion needed to be "legally available but ethically restricted" and insisted that the members of Women's League deplored the "burgeoning casual use of abortion." With this language, the resolution echoed the Christian right's framing of abortion as a vehicle for sexual promiscuity and admonished the women who chose the procedure for their presumed moral deficiency. This revised resolution placed the issue of reproductive rights within a religious framework and painted women as a group whose sexuality and reproductive capacity needed to be monitored by moral, if not legal, arbiters.

Many of the delegates at the Women's League's biennial convention protested this revision to their abortion resolution and preferred to retain their original statement in support of women's reproductive autonomy. "Our members were very pro-choice," recalled Bernice Balter. "We really had to sell the halachic [Jewish legal] point of view. Some people found this point of view too restrictive . . . Whenever there was a complaint, I could always bring up the Torah as justification, which is what I did in this case." In spite of the objections, Women's League leaders moved forward with their revised statement on abortion that drew on the language of Jewish law, sexual conservatism, and religious freedom. The sexual politics of the early 1980s had made it unseemly, perhaps even untenable, for many religious organizations to continue to advance the principle of a woman's right to reproductive autonomy, even if they continued to support legal access to abortion.[9]

Notes

1. In this essay, I will be using the term "religious right" without quotes and treating it as if it were a singular and cohesive movement.
2. On the intricacies of Jewish law regarding abortion, see Rachel Biale, *Women and Jewish Law: An Exploration of Women's Issues in Halakhic Sources* (New York: Schocken Books, 1984); David Feldman, *Birth Control in Jewish Law: Marital Relations, Contraception, and Abortion as Set Forth in the Classic Texts of Jewish Law* (New York: New York University Press, 1968); and Daniel Schiff's *Abortion in Judaism* (Cambridge: Cambridge University Press, 2002), which brings a historical approach to rabbinic decisions regarding abortion and shows how the laws developed over time.
3. "Idea Exchange Sessions on Social Action," Convention Proceedings, National Women's League of the United Synagogue of America, Biennial Convention, November 15-19, 1970, 1970 Convention folder, 78-791 WLCJ Archives.
4. "Resolutions," Convention Proceedings, National Women's League of the United Synagogue of America, Biennial Convention, November 15-19, 1970, 1970 Convention folder, 126, WLCJ Archives.
5. While the United Synagogue did not pass a national resolution on abortion rights until 1975, its New York metropolitan region presented testimony in favor of abortion law reform before the New York State Legislature in 1967 during discussions over whether to liberalize state abortion laws. See "Abortion," *United Synagogue of America, Biennial Convention Proceedings* (New York: United Synagogue of America, November 16-20, 1975), 193-94.
6. Randall Balmer, *God in the White House: A History* (New York: Harper Collins, 2008), 93-105; Donald Critchlow, *Intended Consequences: Birth Control, Abortion, and the Federal Government in Modern America* (New

York: Oxford University Press, 1999), 208-10; Matthew Lassiter, "Inventing Family Values," in *Rightward Bound: Making America Conservative in the 1970s*, ed. Bruce Schulman and Julian Zelizer (Cambridge, Mass.: Harvard University Press, 2008), 13- 28; Daniel K. Williams, "The GOP's Abortion Strategy: Why Pro-choice Republicans Became Pro-life in the 1970s," *Journal of Policy History* 23, no. 4 (2011): 513-39; James P. McCartin, *Prayers of the Faithful: The Shifting Spiritual Life of American Catholics* (Cambridge, Mass.: Harvard University Press, 2010).

7. Seelig interview, May 14, 2014.

8. Robert Gordis, *Sex and the Family in the Jewish Tradition* (New York: Burning Book Press, 1967). Acknowledgment of the sponsorship of the Women's League appears on the copyright page. Brief mentions of abortion as a social phenomenon appear on pp. 12, 16, and 25-26.

9. Indeed, the internal dissension over amending this resolution was such that there is some discrepancy in the record over whether it actually passed. Balter, Seelig, and the Women's League record of resolutions indicate that the membership voted to pass the resolution, as did past president Audrey Citak in a 1992 article on reproductive rights. See Audrey Citak, "Tikkun Olam: Women's League's Mandate for Action," *Women's League Outlook* 62, no. 4 (June 30, 1992), 5; Balter interview, May 12, 2014; Seelig interview, May 14, 2014. On the other hand, a 1982 report in *Women's League Outlook* indicates that members voted against amending the resolution. See Norma Mann, "Very Much Part of the World," *Women's League Outlook* 53, no. 2 (Winter 1982): 18.

46

Mainstream, Militant, and Extremist Antiabortion Activism

Aaron Winter

Aaron Winter is Senior Lecturer in Criminology and Criminal Justice at the University of East London. He researches right-wing extremism, and in this article discusses how far-right Christian antiabortion groups in the United States are distinguished from more moderate ones. The objectives are the same, but Winter details how supposedly "godly" violence is a central tactic of extremist antiabortion Christian groups.

[T]he antiabortion movement can be divided up into three wings or sectors: mainstream, militant, and extremist. Yet the relationships and boundaries between these sectors and specific movements or organizations within them are blurry (both analytically and practically) and historically contingent, and they are explicitly contested within political debate, the media, movement propaganda, and scholarship. There is relative consensus on the fact that the distinctions and thus definitions of each wing are based on the distinction between ideology and tactics, and that while all oppose abortion and hold a great deal in common ideologically, they use different tactics to achieve their aim and assert that ideology, from the most mainstream and legitimate tactics to the most violent and extreme.

. . .

Source: Aaron Winter, "Anti-Abortion Extremism and Violence in the United States," in *Extremism in America*, ed. George Michael (Gainesville: University Press of Florida, 2013), 218–48.

The mainstream wing can be defined as that which pursues and advocates a prolife or antiabortion agenda targeting elected representatives, legislators, the medical profession, and abortion providers in order to affect opinion, changes in the law, restrictions on provision, rights and access (e.g., to late-term abortions), and, ultimately, the abolition of abortion. It is made up of mainstream conservative religious and political organizations such as the National Conference of Catholic Bishops' Committee for Pro-Life Activities and the National Right to Life Committee as well as members of the mainstream political parties, churches, religious groups, media outlets, and commentators. They pursue their agenda and objectives through legitimate, democratic, and nonviolent means such as lobbying, campaigning, supporting political campaigns or running for elected office, fundraising, public protest, advocacy, and propaganda. One example of this is the annual "March for Life" and another is the "Stop the Abortion Mandate," which was organized to protest Obama's health care reform through lobbying, attending town hall meetings, and writing a "Coalition Letter to Congress." The signatories to this letter included Priests for Life, Christian Medical Association, Focus on the Family Action, Christian Coalition of America, Americans United for Life, and many others.[1] Such organizations tend to reject violence.

The militant wing can be defined as those organizations and activists who seek to end abortion rights and provision not on a legal and political front, as the mainstream wing does, but on the front lines by targeting abortion providers (both clinics and doctors) and pro-choice rights and advocacy groups using direct-action tactics. These tactics include blocking clinic entrances by creating human blockades and locking themselves to clinic gates and doors, and harassment of providers and patients using both physical confrontation and propaganda in the form of visual images of abortions and aborted fetuses. The militant wing is made up of organizations such as Randall Terry's Operation Rescue, the Pro-life Action Network, Lambs of Christ, and Rescue America. Due to the confrontational nature of their rhetoric and tactics, the violence that has broken out at clinic protests and blockades or has been committed by individuals associated with these organizations through membership, possession of literature, or participation in the clinic protests, these militant organizations have often been implicated in violence, labeled extremists, and been the target of legislation to protect abortion providers.

The extremist wing is constituted by those antiabortion activists who advocate, threaten, or use violence against those who provide, receive, or support abortion. It is done with the intention of intimidating, injuring, or killing these targets in order to deter them or others, to exact retribution, to influence changes to the law, and to prevent or end the practice and availability of abortion. Such violence typically involves bombing, arson, assassination, assault, death threats, kidnapping, invasion, vandalism, and burglary.[2] There are a number of organizations associated with antiabortion violence, such as American Coalition of Life Activists and Missionaries to the Preborn, but typically violent attacks on abortion providers have been committed by lone individuals or lone wolves, those on the fringes of the movement or informal groups.[3] The most notable examples include Rev. Mike Bray, Rev. Paul Hill, John Salvi, Eric Rudolph, James Kopp, and Scott Roeder. Another significant "actor" in this wing of the movement is the Army of God. First appearing as a moniker used in a 1982 kidnapping and bombing, it has since appeared on death threats and claims of responsibility following numerous attacks. In its first decade, between its first appearance and 1994, the Army of God was linked to bombing and arson attacks on one hundred clinics.[4]

. . .

The sources of and justification for antiabortion extremism and violence are typically religious and primarily Christian, particularly fundamentalist Catholic, Protestant, and Mormon, thus overlapping with mainstream adherents, activists through religious identification, and theology if not tactics.[5] Yet there are also more extreme theologies, such as Christian Reconstructionism, Dominion Theology, Christian Millenarianism, Apocalyptic Catholicism, and Christian Identity, to which most violent activists can be linked.[6] The textual sources used include both parts of the Bible, most notably Gideon, from the book of Judges and the Phineas story from the book of Numbers, and movement manifestos and writings. Perhaps the most prolific and infamous author is Rev. Michael Bray of the Reformed Lutheran Church in Bowie, Maryland, who was the author of *Ethics of Operation Rescue* and *A Time to Kill*, the latter of which provides biblical, ethical, and historical justifications for the use of force in the case of antiabortion activism and which denounces Christian pacifism.[7] The question of whether he advocates the murder of doctors is posed in the appendix, and in response Bray answers: "No. We are not embarrassed about stopping short of advocating the slaying of government-approved childkillers. . . .We simply declare that the slaying of (even) government sanctioned child-killers is justified. . . ."[8]

. . .

There are numerous examples of the blurred and contingent boundaries between the three wings. While most mainstream antiabortion organizations and activists denounce violence publicly, such as Richard Doerflinger, assistant director of the Office of Prolife Activities of the National Conference of Catholic Bishops (NCCB), others (including the NCCB itself) have indirectly justified the bombing of clinics by blaming them on the very existence of the clinics themselves.[9] In another example of the overlap between mainstream and extremist antiabortion activists, and support of the latter by the former, California-based Baptist minister Wiley Drake signed a letter of support for James Kopp on the Army of God Web site following his murder of Dr. Barnett Slepian. Yet this did not prevent him from later becoming vice president of the mainstream Southern Baptist Convention.[10] While overlap between mainstream and extremist organizations and activists is rare, it is more common that violent or extremist activists have relationships and associations with militant ones or receive support from them.

. . .

The first recorded incident of antiabortion violence was an arson attack on an Oregon abortion clinic that occurred in March 1976, three years after the *Roe v. Wade* decision and the legalization of abortion. The perpetrator of the first attack was Joseph C. Stockett, who was convicted and imprisoned for two years.[11] . . . Antiabortion violence increased in the following two years, with four arson attacks in 1977 and three arson attacks and four bombing in 1978.[12] The following year, on February 15, 1979, the first abortion clinic to open post-*Roe*, located in Hempstead, New York, was the target of an arson attack by Peter Burkin.[13] Burkin was tried and acquitted of attempted murder and arson and found not guilty of arson and reckless endangerment by reason of insanity.[14] Up until this point all attacks been perpetrated by individuals and had targeted clinics, but in 1982 the first attack on an individual took place, as did the first appearance of the Army of God. Using the Army of God moniker, Don Benny Anderson, Wayne Moore, and Matthew Moore kidnapped abortion provider Dr. Hector Zevallos and his wife in Granite City, Illinois. The victims were not killed and were released after a week, and Anderson was caught and convicted for kidnapping as well as three unrelated clinic bombings in Florida and Virginia.[15]

Attacks increased significantly in 1984, with twenty-five bombings and arson attacks that year alone; in fact, 1984 was named the "Year of Fear and Pain" by Joseph Scheidler's Pro-life Action Network.[16] Among the string of attacks were more appearances by the Army of God. Michael Bray, author of *A Time to Kill* and suspected author of the *Army of God Manual*, along with Thomas Eugene Spinks and Kenneth William Shields, carried out eight bombings in Virginia, D.C., Maryland, and Delaware, using the Army of God moniker in the Virginia attack.[17]

. . .

The 1990s was the most violent period of antiabortion activism. . . . The first attack of the 1990s was also the first assassination of an abortion provider, that of Dr. David Gunn by Michael Griffin on March 10, 1993, in Pensacola, Florida.[18] It was in response to Gunn's murder and Griffin's trial that Paul Hill issued his "Defensive Action Statement" with its argument for "justifiable homicide," signed by Hill, Bray, and thirty-two others.[19] The statement read:

> We, the undersigned, declare the justice of taking all godly action necessary to defend innocent human life including the use of force. We proclaim that whatever force is legitimate to defend the life of a born child is legitimate to defend the life of an unborn child. . . .[20]

. . .

Soon after the murder of Gunn, in August 1993, Rachelle "Shelly" Shannon, an Oregon housewife, committed a series of arson and acid attacks on clinics and wounded Dr. George Tiller of Wichita, Kansas, in an attempted assignation.[21]

Because Tiller was one of the few to practice so-called late-term abortions, a particular target of mainstream, militant, and extremist antiabortion activists, he was a frequent target of enmity, threats, and attacks before he was eventually killed by Roeder in 2009. In 1981 Tiller was the target of the forty-five-day "Summer of Mercy" protest organized by Operation Rescue as well as oppositional legal strategies.[22]

. . .

The following year, on July 29, 1994, Hill applied his justifiable homicide argument and assassinated Dr. John Britton and James Barrett at The Ladies Center clinic in Pensacola, Florida.[23] Michael Bray, who had been released from prison in 1989, served as public spokesperson for both Shannon and Hill.[24] That same year defrocked Catholic priest and founder of Life Enterprises Unlimited Fr. David Trosch sent a letter to Congress promising a period of "massive" killing of not only abortion providers, abortion rights groups, women's rights groups, and the manufacturers of intrauterine devices and the morning-after pill but also the president, the U.S. attorney general, and Supreme Court justices, thus bringing the battle to the government and back to the courts where *Roe* was decided.[25] The anti-government enmity, strategy, and threat was shared by Missionaries to the Preborn leader Matthew Trewhella in his call for the formation of militias at the United States Tax Payers Party convention in Wisconsin and the organization of firearms training for activists.[26] The year ended in December with attacks on two Brookline, Massachusetts, abortion clinics in which two people were killed and five wounded by John Salvi.[27]

. . .

On April 7, 2009, soon after the inauguration of Barack Obama, the U.S. Department of Homeland Security Threat Analysis Division, originally formed in the wake of 9/11, issued the report *Rightwing Extremism: Current Economic and Political Climate Fueling Resurgence in Radicalization and Recruitment.* The report argued that the economic downturn, the election of the first African American president, gun-control legislation, and returning military veterans presented "unique drivers for rightwing radicalization and recruitment," including both organized and lone wolf attacks.[28] Although focused on hate-based racist and antigovernment groups and widely criticized by the right as a liberal attack on conservatives, its publication was followed by several attacks, including the murder of Dr. George Tiller by Roeder in May 2009.

. . .

In response to both Republican and Tea Party (as well as some "Blue Dog" Democrat) pressure and liberal democrat fears of losing the health care vote, the abortion provision was removed from the health care bill (H.R. 4872) when Obama signed the Patient Protection and Affordable Care Act and Health Care and Education Reconciliation Act of 2010 in March 2010. Less than a month later Roeder was sentenced to fifty years in prison for the murder. While justice was served to Roeder for the crime, the fact that the abortion provision was taken out of the bill following the murder and prior to the vote as well as the increasing overlap of the mainstream, militant, and extremist wings of the antiabortion movement around this issue raises some serious questions. First, if abortion is legal, but abortion rights, provision, and access are scaled back or limited in response to pressure that includes violence, does this mean that violence has become more legitimate than the law on abortion or that terrorism influenced the democratic process? Second, if the mainstream antiabortion movement fails to condemn terrorism or even benefits politically from the threat and pressure of extremism and violence, are they complicit? Finally, what do these developments and relationships say about the distinction between mainstream, militant, and extremist antiabortion activism? These are questions that demand answers and, as the debate and battle over abortion develops and transforms, research and analysis.

Notes

1. "Coalition Letter to Congress," Stop the Abortion Mandate, July 22, 2009, http:// stoptheabortionmandate.com/prep/coalition/coalition-letter-to-con gress/.
2. [Dallas A. Blanchard, *The Anti-Abortion Movement and the Rise of the Religious Right: From Polite to Fiery Protest* (New York: Twayne Publishers, 1994)], 56.
3. [Christopher Hewitt, *Understanding Terrorism in America: From the Klan to Al Qaeda* (London: Routledge, 2003)], 58.
4. [Jeffrey Ian Ross, *Political Terrorism: An Interdisciplinary Approach* (New York: Peter Lang, 2006)], p. 157.
5. Blanchard, *Anti-Abortion Movement*, 58.
6. [Frederick Clarkson, "Anti-Abortion Bombings Related," *Intelligence Report* Summer 1998]; [Mark Juergensmeyer, *Terror in the Mind of God: The Global Rise of Religious Violence* (Berkeley: University of California Press, 2001)], 24–30; and [Patricia Baird-Windle and Eleanor J. Bader, *Targets of Hatred: Anti-Abortion Terrorism* (New York: Palgrave, 2001)], 237–38.
7. Clarkson, "Anti-Abortion Bombings Related"; Juergensmeyer, *Terror in the Mind of God,* 21.
8. Quoted in Baird-Windle and Bader, *Targets of Hatred*, 237–38.
9. Blanchard, *Anti-Abortion Movement*, 100.
10. SPLC, "Assassin Supported by Baptist Official Is Convicted," *Intelligence Report*, no. 125 (Spring 2007).
11. NAF, "History of Violence," 2008, http://www.prochoice.org/about _abortion/ violence/history_violence.html.
12. Ibid.
13. [Dallas A. Blanchard and Terry J. Prewitt, *Religious Violence and Abortion: The Gideon Project* (Gainesville: University Press Florida, 1993)], 185.
14. NAF, "History of Violence."
15. [Frederick Clarkson, "Anti-Abortion Movement Marches on after Two Decades of Arson, Bombs, and Murder," *Intelligence Report*, no. 91 (Summer 1998)]; and Blanchard and Prewitt, *Religious Violence and Abortion*, 188–89).
16. Clarkson, "Anti-Abortion Movement Marches On."

17. Blanchard and Prewitt, *Religious Violence and Abortion*, 195.
18. Hewitt, *Understanding Terrorism in America*, 41; Clarkson, "Anti-Abortion Movement Marches On"; Juergensmeyer, *Terror in the Mind of God*, 136.
19. SPLC "The Signers," *Intelligence Report*, no. 91 (Summer 1998).
20. Quoted in ibid.
21. Juergensmeyer, *Terror in the Mind of God*, 21 and 136.
22. "Doctor's Late-Term Case Set for Trial," *Washington Times*, March 15, 2009.
23. Juergensmeyer, *Terror in the Mind of God*, 21.
24. Ibid., 21.
25. Clarkson, "Anti-Abortion Bombings Related."
26. [Martin Durham, *The Christian Right, the Far Right and the Boundaries of American Conservatism* (Manchester: Manchester University Press, 2000)], 99.
27. [Carol Mason, *Killing for Life: The Apocalyptic Narrative of Pro-Life Politics* (Ithaca: Cornell University Press, 2002)], 66.
28. United States Department of Homeland Security, Threat Analysis Division, *Rightwing Extremism: Current Economic and Political Climate Fueling Resurgence in Radicalization and Recruitment*, April 7, 2009.

47

The Rhetoric of Slavery in the Pro-Life Discourse of US Bishops

Bryan N. Massingale

Bryan Massingale, professor at Fordham University and Roman Catholic priest, is a leading figure in theological ethics. This excerpt is taken from a longer essay that examines and critiques three arguments by Catholic prolife activists that seek to draw parallels between slavery and abortion: the movement to frame the antiabortion movement as a "new abolitionism"; the idea that denial of fetal personhood is the equivalent of the denial of personhood of enslaved peoples; and the refutation of the claim that one can be personally opposed to a moral evil and yet legally support it. This excerpt focuses on the attempt to compare the infamous *Dred Scott* decision about the rights of African Americans as citizens and prolife claims of fetal personhood.

A survey of the U.S. bishops' statements on the Church's pro-life stance and the struggle against abortion reveals a tendency to draw comparisons with and make parallels between the evil of African slavery in the United States and the practice of terminating fetal life. . . .

As early as 1976, in the aftermath of the 1973 *Roe v. Wade* U.S. Supreme Court decision legalizing the procuring of an abortion, leaders in the U.S. hierarchy noted what they considered to be parallels with the American

Source: Bryan M. Massingale, "A Parallel That Limps: The Rhetoric of Slavery in the Pro-Life Discourse of U.S. Bishops," in *Voting and Holiness: Catholic Perspectives on Political Participation*, ed. Nicholas P. Cafardi (Mahwah, NJ: Paulist, 2012), 158–77.

experience of slavery. In his testimony before Congress on behalf of a constitutional amendment protecting unborn human life, Cardinal Terence Cooke, then archbishop of New York, connected *Roe v. Wade* with the 1857 *Dred Scott* Supreme Court decision concerning slavery. He called both decisions "mistaken and ill-considered" and further declared that each manifested "an equal disregard for human life."[1]

This essay explores and critiques the parallels drawn between the struggles against slavery and abortion in the pro-life discourse of the U.S. Catholic hierarchy. In doing so, my intent is neither to undermine nor challenge the justified concern of the Church's leadership for human dignity and the protection of life. I do not believe, however, that this cause is helped by mistaken, imprecise, misleading, or even offensive lines of argument. Such argumentation, in fact, weakens the case that the bishops seek to make on behalf of our faith.

. . .

An Equivalent Denial of Personhood

[One] way in which slavery is invoked in Catholic and episcopal pro-life discourse is by stating that it, like abortion, reflects a denial of the very personhood of a class of human beings. We see this comparison reflected in Cardinal Cooke's remarks at this essay's beginning. . . . A brief resume of the Dred Scott decision helps to appreciate the force of this appeal.

Writing for the six-justice majority in *Dred Scott*, Chief Justice Roger B. Taney argued that persons of African descent in the United States did not enjoy legal freedoms, rights, and protections under our Constitution since the authors of the document—being products of the prevailing social consensus—could not have deemed them to be full and equal members of the human race. Thus the Court held:

> [Negroes] were at that time considered as a *subordinate and inferior class of beings*, who had been subjugated by the dominant race and, whether emancipated or not, yet remained subject to their authority, and *had no rights or privileges but such as those who held the power and the Government might choose to grant them*.
>
> They had for more than a century before been regarded as being of an inferior order, and altogether unfit to associate with the white race, either in social or

political relations; *and so far inferior that they had no rights which the white man was bound to respect*; and that the Negro might justly and lawfully be reduced to slavery for his benefit. He was bought and sold, and treated as an ordinary article of merchandise and traffic, whenever a profit could be made by it. . . .[2]

The argument made by certain pro-life advocates, then, is that just as the *Dred Scott* decision was an official rejection of the personhood of African slaves— now rightly considered a profoundly tragic mistake—so the *Roe* decision likewise tragically and wrongly denies the personhood of unborn human beings. As the Illinois Right to Life Committee declares, both decisions are "an *equivalent* denial of personhood for two different categories of human beings, slaves and unborn children."[3]

This equivalence argument is forthrightly made by leading Catholic prelates. Archbishop Timothy Dolan of New York provides a notable example, rooted in an explicit comparison with *Dred Scott*:

Tragically, in 1973, *in Roe v. Wade*, the Supreme Court also strangely found in the constitution the right to abortion, thus declaring an entire class of human beings—now, not African Americans, but pre-born infants—to be slaves, whose futures, whose destinies, whose very right to life—can be decided by another "master." These fragile, frail babies have no civil rights at all.[4]

. . .

The claim is that both African slaves and unborn lives are subject to legal decisions and folk practices that deny their full human status. "Equivalence" is the key term in this appeal. The success of the appeal turns upon an "equivalent" loss or denial of personhood. The argument is that just as we now reject the monstrosity of denying the personhood of black people, so we should now be filled with a similar revulsion at legal denials of personal status for the unborn.

Yet the claim to equivalence is the weakness of this appeal. For the essence of slavery lies not in a denial of personhood, but in the ownership of persons. American slavery was the state- and religious-sanctioned ownership of human beings, maintained through coercion and other brutal practices, for the purpose of exploited labor and unjust enrichment.[5] The acknowledgment of the enslaved community's "personhood" is evidenced both in common social practices and in the *Dred Scott* legal decision so often cited to support this supposed equivalence.

The Enslaved as Persons in Common Practice. Slave owners indisputably recognized that the enslaved were persons possessing sentience and independent volition. Why else would slave insurrections be feared, unsupervised gatherings be forbidden, harsh punishments be meted out, fugitive laws be passed, or armed posses be necessary if the enslaved did not possess a freedom and will that could be—and often was—at odds with that of their masters?[6] In addition, the enslaved were baptized and catechized. These practices demonstrate not only an acknowledgment of personhood, but also an admission that the enslaved possessed a human "soul" destined for eternal salvation.[7]

Moreover, slave masters had sexual relationships with their slaves, though such intercourse was often exploitative for the gratification of carnal pleasure or the increase of the master's slave population.[8] Such couplings, however, acknowledge—albeit in abusive ways—a common, shared humanity. This personhood is further conceded through the practice of enslaved women being charged with rearing and even nursing the white children of a plantation household. Infrequently, slave masters also entered into marriage-like relationships with an enslaved woman.[9] Even where such unions were legally and socially proscribed, the very prohibition acknowledged that the enslaved could freely choose to love—an unquestionable quality of personhood. Finally, slaves were at times emancipated by their owners. The very concept of manumission demonstrates that the underlying personhood of the slave was never seriously in question; slavery was a legal "fiction," not a metaphysical claim or theological status.

. . .

Indeed, the historical record shows that American society developed no consistent rationalization for the practice of African enslavement or ownership.[10] These justifications ranged from the effects of God's curse upon some of Noah's descendants, to the alleged intellectual inferiority of Africans established by so-called "scientific" evidence, to the argument that slavery was part of God's plan for the redemption of pagan Africa.[11] What made such rationalizations necessary, however, were the moral quagmires occasioned by the undeniable personhood of one's property. The implacable reality of the enslaved's consciousness and independent volition is what made slavery so ethically challenging and legally problematic.

While one can be opposed to abortion for many reasons, one has to concede that the personhood of the enslaved was commonly acknowledged and accepted in social practice. This differential treatment of enslaved and pre-born life undermines the argument that slavery and abortion both rest upon an equivalent denial of personhood. At the least, those who assert such an equivalence have to demonstrate that embryonic human life, from the "moment of conception," possesses the same degree of free volition, independent judgment, and sentient consciousness as did the enslaved Africans. Absent this, the equivalence argument fails.

The Legal Argument of Dred Scott: A Matter of Citizenship. It is true that the infamous Supreme Court *Dred Scott* decision stated that the enslaved were of a "subordinate and inferior class of beings." Such language would seem to give some support for those who claim a kind of equivalent denial of the personhood for both enslaved Africans and unborn lives.

However, a careful examination of *Dred Scott* leads to a more complex understanding of the intent of this ruling. The legal question involved the right of a fugitive slave, Dred Scott, to challenge his return to his master after being captured in a free state. In other words, did this runaway slave have the legal standing to pursue a case in the judicial system? In deciding this question, the Court specifically declared that the constitutional question before it was not one of personhood, but rather, citizenship:

> The only matter in issue before the court, therefore, is whether the descendants of such slaves, when they shall be emancipated, or who are born of parents who had become free before their birth, are citizens of a state, in the sense in which the word "citizen" is used in the Constitution of the United States. And this being the only matter in dispute in these pleadings.[12]

. . . It is in this connection that the Justices made their tragic reference to Africans being of "an inferior class of beings." The relevant citation follows, responding to the question of whether Africans or their descendants were "citizens":

> We think they are not, and that they are not included, and were not intended to be included, under the word "citizens" in the Constitution, and can, therefore, claim none of the rights and privileges which that instrument provides for and secures to citizens of the United States. On the contrary, they were at that time considered as a subordinate and inferior class of beings, who had been subjugated by the dominant race, and whether emancipated or not, yet remained subject to their authority, and had no rights but such as those who held the power and the Government might choose to grant them . . .
>
> In the opinion of the court, the legislation and histories of the times, and the language used in the Declaration of Independence, show, that *neither the class of persons* who had been imported as slaves, nor their descendants,

whether they had become free or not, were then acknowledged as a part of the people, nor intended to be included in the general words used in that memorable instrument.[13]

My intent in rehearsing this history is neither to defend nor excuse this abominable decision. Honesty compels us to admit, however, that while *Dred Scott*'s understanding of the enslaved's personhood is muddled and convoluted, the decision did not entail a denial of "personhood" or the human status of the enslaved, but the denial of the rights and status of citizenship. This is an important distinction, which makes the parallel or comparison with abortion inexact, to say the least. Indeed, the Court acknowledged that the enslaved and their descendants, whether emancipated or not, do constitute a "class of persons." Yet the Court held that such "persons" were not "citizens," and that therefore they were not entitled to petition the courts for a redress of grievances. My point is that the record seriously challenges the claims (1) that this decision turned upon a denial of personhood; and (2) that an equivalent denial is at play in the moral debate over legalized abortion.

Those who would argue for such an equivalence have to demonstrate that the current judicial system posits the personhood of unborn life "from the moment of conception," and yet denies the unborn fetus the rights of citizenship. Absent this, the equivalence argument fails.

Notes

1. "Statement of Terence Cardinal Cooke before the Subcommittee on Civil and Constitutional Rights of the House Committee on the Judiciary" (March 24, 1976). Available online at http://www.usccb.org/prolife/issues/abortion/roevwade/CookeTestimony76.pdf.
2. This decision is substantially reproduced in *The Annals of America*, vol. 8 (New York: Encyclopaedia Britannica, 1968), 440–49; emphases added.
3. Illinois Right to Life Committee, "Slavery Compared to Abortion." Online at www.illinoisrighttolife.org/SlaveryAbortion.htm; emphasis added.
4. Archbishop Timothy M. Dolan, "On the Front Lines for Life" (October 22, 2009). Available online at www.cny.org/archive/tdcolumn/tmd102209.htm.
5. This definition is my summary derived from the studies of Joe R. Feagin, *Systemic Racism: A Theory of Oppression* (New York: Routledge, 2006),19,

and Beverly Eileen Mitchell, *Black Abolitionism: A Quest for Human Dignity* (Maryknoll, NY: Orbis Books, 2005), 19.

6. For a comprehensive study of the fear of slave insurrections and rebellions, see John Hope Franklin and Loren Schweninger, *Runaway Slaves: Rebels on the Plantation* (New York: Oxford University Press, 1999).

7. Such admissions were common among Catholic prelates during the nineteenth century. See, for example, the letter of Bishop William Elder (Natchez, Mississippi), which speaks of the "high degree of sanctity" among properly catechized slaves ([Kenneth J. Zanca, ed., *American Catholics and Slavery, 1789-1866: An Anthology of Primary Documents* (Lanham, MD: University Press of America, 1994)], 237).

8. The sexual exploitation of female slaves by a plantation's master and teen-aged sons is a staple feature of the testimonies of freed slaves. See, for example, Douglass's indictment of the compromise of the enslaved sexual virtue ([Frederick] Douglass, *Narrative of the Life of Frederick Douglass, [An American Slave: Written by Himself* (New York: Barnes and Noble Classics, (1845) 2003], 100). Other testimonies to this can be gleaned from the masterful study of John W. Blassingame, *Slave Testimony: Two Centuries of Letters, Speeches, Interviews, and Autobiographies* (Baton Rouge: Louisiana State University Press, 1977).

9. Cyprian Davis details one such relationship between Michael Healy and a slave woman named Mary Eliza. Though they could not be legally married, they lived in a monogamous and apparently loving union. Among their children were three priests, who would play prominent roles in Catholic life: James, Patrick, and Alexander Healy. See [Cyprian Davis, *The History of Black Catholics in the United States* (New York: Crossroad, 1990)], 146–52.

10. [Mitchell, *Black Abolitionism*], 108.

11. Source documents for the justifications and defenses offered for African enslavement are found in Zanca, *American Catholics and Slavery*, 1–9; 191–216.

12. Excerpts of the *Dred Scott* decision cited in this section are taken from ibid., 54–56.

13. Emphasis added.

48

Framing Choice:
CPCs [Crisis Pregnancy Centers] and the Co-optation of Freedom

Ziad Munson

A sociologist with interests in religion and political violence, Ziad Munson analyzes how those working in crisis pregnancy centers (CPCs) attempt to coopt the abortion rights concept of choice by offering pregnant women more choices. He argues that while CPCs downplay overt religious messages, they are largely staffed by prolife Christian women who offer pregnant women the opportunity to "choose" Christianity rather than abortion. Munson notes the contradiction between CPCs' attempts to appear clinical and unbiased by focusing on scientific information about pregnancy and developing life in the womb, especially through the use of prenatal ultrasounds, and simultaneously refusing to share information about abortion services.

CPCs are pro-life social movement organizations that seek to attract pregnant or potentially pregnant women to convince them to carry their pregnancies to term. CPCs have existed since the beginning of the movement; the first were established in the late 1960s, before abortion was effectively legalized in the United States through the 1973 *Roe v. Wade* and

Source: Ziad Munson, "Religion, Crisis Pregnancies, and the Battle over Abortion," in *Religion in Disputes*, ed. Franz von Benda-Beckmann, Keebet von Benda-Beckmann, Martin Ramstedt, and Bertram Turner (New York: Palgrave Macmillan, 2013), 37–53.

Doe v. Bolton decisions of the Supreme Court. The number of CPCs has grown steadily since that time. Sometime in the mid-1990s, the number of CPCs operating in the United States surpassed the number of abortion providers. Today, there are approximately 2,900 CPCs spread throughout the country.[1] CPCs are often hard to spot in a community. They typically have ambiguous, generic names (e.g., Women's Counseling Center, A Woman's Concern, and Birthchoice), and are located in nondescript offices and storefronts. In some cases, CPCs are located adjacent to abortion clinics.

. . .

CPCs are significant in part because, through their existence and operation, they seek to wrest control over the frame of choice as it is applied to the abortion debate.[2] The pro-choice movement has long framed its position in terms of reproductive choice for women. Many pro-choice activists—and the vast majority of the pro-choice public—are not so much in favor of abortion as they are in favor of leaving reproductive decision-making to women themselves. Abortion rights as a matter of freedom of choice resonate powerfully with larger narratives of American individualism and individual freedom. The framing of the pro-choice position in these terms offers the pro-choice movement its most resonate ideological connection to the larger American public.[3] CPCs represent a significant threat to pro-choice ownership over this ideological frame. CPC activists believe that *they* are in the business of increasing the range of choices available to pregnant women, a belief they trace to cognitive, emotional, and practical foundations.

On a cognitive level, activists believe CPCs and their one-on-one counseling provide the information and data pregnant women need to make an informed decision about their pregnancy. They believe many abortions occur because pregnant women simply do not have the facts about fetal development, the mother–child bond, or the links many pro-life activists allege between abortion and breast cancer, posttraumatic stress disorder, and other medical problems.[4]

. . .

On a practical level, some activists also believe women resort to abortion because they do not have the basic material necessities for carrying a pregnancy to term. This is where the noncounseling services of the CPCs come into play. "We get accused of only caring about the baby and not the mother. So how do you help the mother?" asks Sharon, a 50-year-old Catholic activist. "Well, you provide her with maternity clothes, you take her to the doctors, you say you will help find a place for her to live if she's thrown out of her home or has no place to live." Providing such services is seen by such activists as an additional way in which they give women a meaningful choice between alternatives.

These cognitive, emotional, and practical elements of the CPC ideology come together to present a significant challenge to the pro-choice movement's ownership over the choice frame. They do so by denying the conflict between pro-life and pro-choice positions that has heretofore been accepted by partisans on both sides of the debate.

. . .

The choice being presented by CPCs is, of course, a carefully crafted one. For most CPCs, part of that crafting includes the downplaying or outright elimination of religious messages or themes. However, opening up the frame of choice also introduces the possibility of bringing religious faith to the table as yet another option pregnant women might choose. The co-optation of the choice frame thus dovetails with the Christian evangelical tradition of offering witness and an invitation to God's love. This is certainly the tradition in which many of the activists themselves are rooted.

. . .

The majority of CPC activists inform their work with a deep personal sense of religious faith. For them, this is the very basis of the dispute in the abortion debate. And once they have defined the relationships they develop with the women who come into the centers as one of expanding their range of viable choices, bringing religion into the tableau of options feels natural to many of them. Cindy, a 44-year-old activist and member of an independent church, puts it this way:

> I try to be very careful about how I come across, because you're not here to save everybody. You can plant the seed that they need the Lord, but you have to gauge how far you can go.

. . .

Faith is couched in terms of a choice, one that might help a pregnant woman in addressing the difficult issues she faces. Religious faith as an individual choice—analogous to the choice of what to do with a pregnancy—dovetails well with larger American understandings of religion. American religious exceptionalism is defined in large part by the range of religious options available to individuals.[5] This fact is reflected in religious conversion rates in the United States, which are the highest in the world (Barro et al., 2010). To choose one's faith, in the same way one might choose whether or not to continue a pregnancy, makes a great deal of sense in this cultural context. CPC activism thus co-opts their opponents' frame of choice in two senses: first, they put forth their activism as "merely" offering choices about pregnancy and, unofficially, choices about religion; second, in doing so, their work becomes a matter of simply presenting several more options in the dizzying array of choices available to every individual in the United States in all aspects of life (Schwartz, 2004).

The growth of CPCs has also been accompanied by a medicalization of the work they do and the arguments they make.[6] For many years now, CPCs have endeavored to look and operate more like medical clinics and less like social movement organizations. They accomplish this by adopting the aesthetic of many medical clinics, with sterile-looking office space, a front desk and waiting rooms, and so forth. Some have an assortment of color-coded manila folders clearly visible behind the receptionist or in an administrative area, mirroring the way in which many medical clinics store patient records. CPCs generally refer to the women who come into the centers as "clients" or even "patients" to underscore the medical presentation of the organization.

Beyond just these aesthetics, CPCs have introduced an array of services that blur the distinction between their centers and bona fide medical clinics. Offering pregnancy tests is, of course, the first step in this approach. However, some CPCs now offer prenatal and even early pediatric care, performed by nurses and physicians. Some also employ state-licensed social workers to conduct their one-on-one meetings with the pregnant women who come into the center. But perhaps the most potent symbol of the move by CPCs to medicalize their image and their work is the increasing focus on ultrasound machines.

Performing ultrasounds on pregnant women accomplishes several goals for the organizations. First, the grainy fetal images produced by the machines help humanize the fetus and, thus, underscore the larger message of the pro-life movement that abortions are really the killing of unborn children. It is a "proof" of the pro-life worldview. Activists certainly see ultrasounds as their most potent weapon. One clinic director believed that 85 percent of "abortion-minded" women who are shown their own ultrasound choose to carry their pregnancies to term.[7]

. . .

Religion is completely absented from this side of CPC work, and indeed this is one of the goals of the organizations. By medicalizing their look, their personnel, their equipment, and even their advice, CPCs are moving the abortion issue out of the realm of religious or political dispute and into the realm of the presumed impartiality and expert judgment of sophisticated machines and medical professionals.

. . .

Medicalizing CPCs thus has the potential to make abortion an issue over which regular citizens (or at least pregnant women who come into CPCs) are not authorized to have an opinion due to their lack of technical knowledge. CPCs thereby move the debate over abortion out of the realm of personal opinion or moral values and into the realm of depoliticized technocracy. . . . The medicalization of the abortion issue by CPCs seeks to once again remove abortion from the sphere of moral public debate to the specialized domain of "science," but to do so in ways that support and expand their commitment to ending legalized abortion.

The focus on science also stands in some tension to the rhetoric of choice the movement seeks to co-opt from the pro-choice movement. On the one hand, CPC activists argue, they are simply offering choices to women (choices not only about pregnancy but also—in many cases—about religious faith). On the other hand, they also argue that there really is no choice to be made, because the cold rationality of modern science can demonstrate conclusively that abortion is the killing of an unborn child. The movement seeks to have it both ways: not only to be advocates for true, fully informed choice, but also to demonstrate that scientific and medical expertise permit only one choice—continuing all pregnancies to term.

Notes

1. This number is particularly remarkable when compared to the fewer than 450 free-standing clinics that provide abortion services.
2. Social movement theory contains a vast literature on framing, which traces its origin to Goffman's classic *Frame Analysis* (1974). A summary and analysis of this literature is outside the scope of this chapter, but see Snow et al. (1986), Tarrow (1994), and Benford and Snow (2000) for overviews of this work.
3. Condit (1990) provides the most detailed analysis of how the pro-choice movement developed the choice frame, noting that the frame was largely responsible for retaining legalized abortion in the United States (albeit with significant caveats). Staggenborg (1991), Ferree et al. (2002), and Burns (2005) have all added to this study of the choice frame.
4. Such claims are not based on scientific evidence, but they continue to persist within the pro-life movement.

5. A significant portion of the literature in the sociology of religion has devoted itself to modeling American religious behavior within a rational choice framework that highlights religious affiliation as a choice rather than an ascribed characteristic. For a well-developed example of this approach, see Finke and Stark (2005).
6. For a theoretical review of the medicalization process using the abortion debate as an example, see Halfmann (2011).
7. There is no scientific study to back up this claim, but many CPC directors report similar patterns and the cultural place given to babies—and particularly images of babies—leaves little reason to be skeptical of such claims.

References

Barro, R. J., J. Hwang, and R. M. McCleary. "Religious Conversion in 40 Countries." *Journal for the Scientific Study of Religion* 49, no. 1 (2010): 15–36.

Benford, R. D., and D. A. Snow. "Framing Processes and Social Movements: An Overview and Assessment." *Annual Review of Sociology* 26 (2000): 611–639.

Burns, G. *The Moral Veto: Framing Contraception, Abortion, and Cultural Pluralism in the United States.* New York: Cambridge University Press, 2005.

Condit, C. M. *Decoding Abortion Rhetoric: Communicating Social Change.* Chicago: University of Illinois Press, 1990.

Ferree, M. M., W. A. Gamson, J. Gerhards, and D. Rucht. *Shaping Abortion Discourse: Democracy and the Public Sphere in Germany and the United States.* New York: Cambridge University Press, 2002.

Finke, R., and R. Stark. *The Churching of America, 1776–2005: Winners and Losers in Our Religious Economy.* New Brunswick, NJ: Rutgers University Press, 2005.

Goffman, E. *Frame Analysis: An Essay on the Organization of Experience.* Cambridge, MA: Harvard University Press, 1974.

Halfmann, D. "Recognizing Medicalization and Demedicalization: Discourses, Practices, and Identities." *Health* 16, no. 2 (2011): 186–207.

Schwartz, B. *The Paradox of Choice: Why More Is Less.* New York: Ecco, 2004.

Snow, D. A, E. B. Rochford, S. K. Worden, and R. D. Benford. "Frame Alignment Processes, Micromobilization, and Movement Participation." *American Sociological Review* 51, no. 4 (1986): 464–481.

Staggenborg, S. *The Pro-Choice Movement: Organization and Activism in the Abortion Conflict.* New York: Oxford University Press, 1991.

Tarrow, S. *Power in Movement: Social Movements and Contentious Politics.* New York: Cambridge University Press, 1994.

49

When There's a Heartbeat: Miscarriage Management in Catholic-Owned Hospitals

Lori R. Freedman, Uta Landy,

and Jody Steinauer

The research for this essay was conducted at the Bixby Center for Global Reproductive Health, University of California, San Francisco, where Lori Freedman is a sociologist and associate professor. Uta Landy, PhD, has been internationally active in medical education in family planning since 1985. Jody Steinauer, MD, PhD, is Director of the Bixby Center. This excerpt, which discusses the tensions that arise between ethical strictures in Catholic medical care facilities and physicians' legal and medical obligations to provide the best care for their patients, raises important questions about women's reproductive health and safety in a healthcare context where increasing numbers of hospitals are run by religious organizations that refuse to follow standards of care outlined by physicians and medical professional organizations.

Over the past decade, as Catholic hospitals have merged with and purchased nonsectarian hospitals around the United States, the lay press and legal journals have featured discussion about the impact of these mergers on patient care, particularly with regard to reproductive health.[1-5] The literature

Source: Lori R. Freedman, Uta Landy, and Jody Steinauer, "When There's a Heartbeat: Miscarriage Management in Catholic-Owned Hospitals," *American Journal of Public Health* 98, no. 1 (2008): 1174–8.

has focused on policies prohibiting tubal ligation, contraceptive services, emergency contraception, and abortion. Although other religiously owned and nonsectarian hospitals may also prohibit or limit some of these services, Catholic-owned hospitals are the largest group of religiously owned nonprofit hospitals, operating 15.2% of the nation's hospital beds,[6] and increasingly they are the only hospitals in certain regions within the United States.[7] The result is that Catholic and non-Catholic patients alike come to depend on these facilities for emergencies, childbirth, and routine procedures without knowing how some of their options are potentially curtailed.

. . .

Catholic-owned institutions and their employees must adhere to medical practice guidelines contained in the "Ethical and Religious Directives for Catholic Health Care Services" (hereafter called "the directives") written by the Committee on Doctrine of the National Conference of Catholic Bishops.[8] The directives state that abortion is never permitted. However, regarding emergency care during miscarriage management, the manual used by Catholic-owned hospital ethics committees to interpret the directives states that abortion is acceptable if the purpose is to treat "a life-threatening pathology" in the pregnant woman when the treatment cannot be postponed until the fetus is viable.[9] The experiences of physicians in our study indicate that uterine evacuation may not be approved during miscarriage by the hospital ethics committee if fetal heart tones are present and the pregnant woman is not yet ill, in effect delaying care until fetal heart tones cease, the pregnant woman becomes ill, or the patient is transported to a non-Catholic-owned facility for the procedure.

. . .

According to the generally accepted standards of care in miscarriage management, abortion is medically indicated under certain circumstances in the presence of fetal heart tones. Such cases include first-trimester septic or inevitable miscarriage, previable premature rupture of membranes and chorioamnionitis, and situations in which continuation of the pregnancy significantly threatens the life or health of the woman. In each instance, the physician must weigh the health impact to the woman of continuing the pregnancy against the potential viability of the fetus. Ideally, the physician then engages in a sensitive decisionmaking process with the patient. The physician reviews with the patient the risks of continuing the pregnancy and the likelihood of fetal survival, as well as management options that include "expectant management" (i.e., no intervention) and termination of pregnancy, with the physician often recommending a form of management.

The patient then chooses how to proceed; when fetal survival is no longer possible or when continuing the pregnancy involves significant risk, she may decide to terminate the pregnancy. For spiritual or psychological reasons, a patient may prefer to delay induction of labor or surgical uterine evacuation until there is no fetal heartbeat, even in cases in which the risk of expectant management to her health is great.

In general, this process of assisted decisionmaking is guided by informed consent or informed choice,[10] which requires that the patient understand all appropriate medical options, as well as the relevant risks and benefits of each, before choosing and consenting to a course of management. Informed choice and consent may be compromised when hospital policies restrict physicians from offering treatment options routinely available in other hospitals.

Overview of Catholic Policy

The standards of medical care put forth in the directives are at variance with those generally recognized in other medical settings, particularly regarding care at the beginning and ending of life. They were codified over 50 years ago to ensure strict obedience to Catholic principles by all employees of Catholic-owned hospitals, without local variation.[11] The directives sanction prenatal care and natural family planning but prohibit nearly all other reproductive services, including all other birth control methods, emergency contraception, infertility treatment, sterilization, and abortion.[8] In Catholic-owned hospitals, physicians must request approval to terminate a pregnancy for any indication from the ethics committee, which interprets and enforces the directives. Such consultations can be done quickly over the phone with an on-call representative of the committee, typically a priest or nun, if the medical situation is urgent. In theory, therefore, consultation with the ethics committee presents only a minor delay to urgent care. If the situation is not urgent, the committee convenes to discuss the matter and then offers its ruling.

An important qualification of the prohibition of abortion is made in Directive 47. Termination of pregnancy is permissible if the health of the mother is at risk:

> Operations, treatments, and medications that have as their direct purpose the cure of a proportionately serious pathological condition of a pregnant

woman are permitted when they cannot be safely postponed until the unborn child is viable, even if they will result in the death of the unborn child.[8]

The death of the fetus is therefore acceptable as a secondary consequence of actions intended to preserve the health of the pregnant woman. However, the manual of Catholic hospital ethics committees, used to help them interpret and apply the directives, warns, "The mere rupture of membranes, without infection, is not serious enough to sanction interventions that will lead to the death of the child."[6] By contrast, writing in a leading Catholic health journal, other Catholic health ethicists offer a more liberal interpretation of Directive 47: uterine evacuation is indicated if abortion is inevitable and delay will harm the pregnant woman.[12] Therefore, the former—and arguably more authoritative—source approves of uterine evacuation only after a woman becomes sick, and the latter approves of it as a measure to prevent sickness. . . .

Nontreatment, Delays, and Transport of Patients

Obstetrician–gynecologists working in Catholic-owned hospitals described cases in which abortion was medically indicated according to their medical judgment but, because of the ethics committee's ruling, it was delayed until either fetal heartbeats ceased or the patient could be transported to another facility. Dr P, from a mid-western, mid-sized city, said that at her Catholic-owned hospital, approval for termination of pregnancy was rare if a fetal heartbeat was present (even in "people who are bleeding, they're all the way dilated, and they're only 17 weeks") unless "it looks like she's going to die if we don't do it."

In another case, Dr H, from the same Catholic-owned hospital in the Midwest, sent her patient by ambulance 90 miles to the nearest institution where the patient could have an abortion because the ethics committee refused to approve her case.

> She was very early, 14 weeks. She came in . . . and there was a hand sticking out of the cervix. Clearly the membranes had ruptured and she was trying to deliver. . . . There was a heart rate, and [we called] the ethics committee, and

they [said], "Nope, can't do anything." So we had to send her to [the university hospital]. . . .

In residency, Dr P and Dr H had been taught to perform uterine evacuation or labor induction on patients during inevitable miscarriage whether fetal heart tones were present or not. In their new Catholic-owned hospital environment, such treatment was considered a prohibited abortion by the governing ethics committee because the fetus is still alive and the patient is not yet experiencing "a life-threatening pathology" such as sepsis. Physicians such as Dr H found that in some cases, transporting the patient to another hospital for dilation and curettage (D&C) was quicker and safer than waiting for the fetal heartbeat to stop while trying to stave off infection and excessive blood loss.

Dr B, an obstetrician–gynecologist working in an academic medical center, described how a Catholic-owned hospital in her western urban area asked her to accept a patient who was already septic. When she received the request, she recommended that the physician from the Catholic-owned hospital perform a uterine aspiration there and not further risk the health of the woman by delaying her care with the transport.

> Because the fetus was still alive, they wouldn't intervene. And she was hemorrhaging, and they called me and wanted to transport her, and I said, "It sounds like she's unstable, and it sounds like you need to take care of her there." And I was on a recorded line, I reported them as an EMTALA [Emergency Medical Treatment and Active Labor Act] violation. And the physician [said], "This isn't something that we can take care of." And I [said], "Well, if I don't accept her, what are you going to do with her?" [He answered], "We'll put her on a floor [i.e., admit her to a bed in the hospital instead of keeping her in the emergency room]; we'll transfuse her as much as we can, and we'll just wait till the fetus dies."

Ultimately, Dr B chose to accept the patient to spare her unnecessary suffering and harm, but she saw this case as a form of "patient dumping," because the patient was denied treatment and transported while unstable.

Circumventing the Ethics Committee

Some doctors have decided to take matters into their own hands. In the following case, the refusal of the hospital ethics committee to approve uterine evacuation not only caused significant harm to the patient but compelled a perinatologist, Dr S, now practicing in a nonsectarian academic medical center, to violate protocol and resign from his position in an urban northeastern Catholic-owned hospital.

> I'll never forget this; it was awful—I had one of my partners accept this patient at 19 weeks. The pregnancy was in the vagina. It was over. . . . I'm on call when she gets septic, and she's septic to the point that . . . she's 106 degrees. And I needed to get everything out. And so I put the ultrasound machine on and there was still a heartbeat, and [the ethics committee] wouldn't let me because there was still a heartbeat. This woman is dying before our eyes. I went in to examine her, and I was able to find the umbilical cord through the membranes and just snapped the umbilical cord and so that I could put the ultrasound—"Oh look. No heartbeat. Let's go." She was so sick she was in the [intensive care unit] for about 10 days and very nearly died . . . And I said, "I just can't do this. I can't put myself behind this. This is not worth it to me." That's why I left. . . .

From Dr S's perspective, the chances for fetal life were nonexistent given the septic maternal environment. For the ethics committee, however, the present yet waning fetal heart tones were evidence of fetal life that precluded intervention. Rather than struggle longer to convince his committee to make an exception and grant approval for termination of pregnancy, Dr S chose to covertly sever the patient's umbilical cord so that the fetal heartbeat would cease and evacuation of the uterus could "legitimately" proceed.

. . .

Given the prevalence of Catholic-owned health care today, these issues bring to light important policy questions about standards of medical practice and a patient's right to information. Patients entering a Catholic-owned hospital may be aware that abortion services are not available there, but few prenatal patients conceive of themselves as potential abortion patients and therefore they are not aware of the risks involved in being treated there; these include delays in care and in being transported to another hospital during miscarriage, which may adversely affect the patient's physical and psychological well-being.

References

1. Vitello P. Used to big losses, Schenectady is hit hard by plan for hospitals. *New York Times*. December 4, 2006:B1.

2. Sloboda M. The high cost of merging with a religiously controlled hospital. *Berkeley Womens Law J.* 2001; 16:140–156.

3. Labi N. Holyowned. Is it fair for a Catholic hospital to impose its morals on patients? *Time.* 1999;154(20):85–86.

4. Fogel SB, Rivera LA. Saving Roe is not enough: when religion controls healthcare. *Fordham Urban Law J.* 2004; 31(3):725–749.

5. Brooks P. Merge talk under way for Kingston's two hospitals. [Kingston, NY] *Times Herald-Record.* December 30, 2006.

6. *Catholic Health Care in the United States.* Washington, DC: Catholic Health Association; 2007.

7. Uttley L, Pawelko R. No strings attached: public funding of religiously sponsored hospitals in the United States. In: The Merger Watch Project. New York, NY: Family Planning Advocates of New York State; 2002:11–12.

8. Catholic Health Association. Ethical and religious directives for Catholic health care services. *Origins.* 2001; 31(9): 153, 155–163.

9. Cataldo PJ, Moraczewski AS. *Catholic Health Care Ethics: A Manual for Ethics Committees.* Boston, MA: National Catholic Bioethics Center; 2002.

10. Dickens BM, Cook RJ. Dimensions of informed consent to treatment. *Int J Gynaecol Obstet.* 2004; 85(3):309–314.

11. O'Rourke KD, Kopfen-Steiner T, Hamel R. A brief history. A summary of the development of the Ethical and Religious Directives for Catholic Health Care Services. *Health Prog.* 2001; 82(6):18–21.

12. deBlois J, O'Rourke KD. Care for the beginning of life. The revised Ethical and Religious Directives discuss abortion, contraception, and assisted reproduction. *Health Prog.* 1995; 76(7):36–40.

50

Double Effect, All Over Again:

The Case of Sister Margaret McBride

Bernard G. Prusak

Bernard Prusak is a professor of philosophy whose teaching and research focus on bioethics, Catholic moral philosophy, and Catholic social teachings. Prusak discusses an event that happened in 2009: the excommunication of a Sister of Mercy nun Margaret McBride who, in her capacity as the chair of the ethics committee at the Catholic hospital where she worked, authorized the abortion of an eleven-week-old fetus of a woman with acute pulmonary hypertension. Prusak analyzes the way in which the Catholic principle—known as double effect—that can render some pregnancy terminations legitimate was ruled by the local bishop as not having been applicable in this situation.

On its face, the highly publicized and much-discussed excommunication *latae sententiae*, "by the very commission of the act," of Sister Margaret McBride appears well-founded in the principles of Roman Catholic moral thought. In November 2009, the ethics committee, chaired by Sister McBride, of St. Joseph's Hospital in Phoenix, Arizona, permitted the abortion of an eleven-week-old fetus in order to save the life of its mother. This woman was suffering from acute pulmonary hypertension, which her doctors judged would prove fatal for both her and her pre-viable child.[1] The doctors accordingly advised that she have an abortion; the mother eventually and

Source: Bernard G. Prusak, "Double Effect, All Over Again: The Case of Sister Margaret McBride," *Theoretical Medicine and Bioethics* 32, no. 4 (2011): 271–83.

reluctantly agreed (she was also the mother of four children at home); and so too did the ethics committee, in what the hospital later described as a "tragic case" [2]. Yet, as Thomas J. Olmsted, the bishop of Phoenix, observed in a statement critical of the hospital and of Sister McBride, under the principles of Catholic moral thought, "While medical professionals should certainly try to save a pregnant mother's life, the means by which they do it can never be by directly killing her unborn child. . . . The direct killing of an unborn child is always immoral, no matter the circumstances, and it cannot be permitted in any institution that claims to be authentically Catholic" [2].

In support of this claim, Bishop Olmsted went on to cite both Pope John Paul II's encyclical *Evangelium Vitae*, which states that "direct abortion, that is, abortion willed as an end or as a means, always constitutes a grave moral disorder, since it is the deliberate killing of an innocent human being" [3, sec. 62]; and the United States Conference of Catholic Bishops' *Ethical and Religious Directives for Catholic Healthcare Institutions*, which states that "[a]bortion (that is, the directly intended termination of pregnancy before viability or the directly intended destruction of a viable fetus) is never permitted. Every procedure whose sole immediate effect is the termination of pregnancy before viability is an abortion" [4, sec. 45]. Bishop Olmsted might also have cited the *Catechism of the Catholic Church*, which states that "direct abortion, that is to say, abortion willed either as an end or a means, is gravely contrary to the moral law" [5, sec. 2271]. In a statement on the diocese's website, as well as in a statement to the media, Father John Ehrlich, the diocese's medical ethics director, put the point briefly, in language drawn from Paul's Letter to the Romans (3:8): "no one can do evil that good may come" [6].

All this is the stuff of an introductory ethics course at almost any Catholic college, as well as at many secular institutions. So too is the principle under which, according again to media reports [1], the ethics committee believed abortion to be permitted in this case: namely, what is often called, though the nomenclature did not appear until the twentieth century, the principle of double effect [7]. Textbook formulations of this principle, whose "ancestors . . . are the sixteenth- and seventeenth century commentators on Aquinas's theory of action" [8, p. 530], identity four conditions that must be satisfied for an action that has two effects, one of which is evil while the other is good, to be morally permissible. Joseph Mangan summarizes those conditions in an oft-cited discussion as follows [9, p. 43]:

(1) that the action in itself from its very object be good or at least indifferent;

(2) that the good effect and not the evil effect be intended;

(3) that the good effect not be produced by means of the evil effect;

(4) that there be a proportionately grave reason for permitting the evil effect.

The *Ethical and Religious Directives for Catholic Healthcare Institutions* gestures toward the principle of double effect (hereafter, PDE): "Operations, treatments, and medications that have as their direct purpose the cure of a proportionately serious pathological condition of a pregnant woman are permitted when they cannot be safely postponed until the unborn child is viable, even if they will result in the death of the unborn child" [4, sec. 47]. Yet, *pace* the ethics committee, the case in question does not appear to satisfy all the conditions of the PDE, in particular, the third condition, that the evil effect (here, the death of the fetus) may not be the means to the good effect (here, saving the life of the woman). Instead, in the case in question, the abortion appears to have been "direct" inasmuch as it was "willed . . . as a means," to use the language of *Evangelium Vitae* and the *Catechism*.

This case, then, appears to be different from operations in which the death of a fetus is an inevitable, secondary consequence. The paradigmatic example of such a case cited by most commentators, and likewise by the USCCB's Committee on Doctrine in a June 23, 2010, statement [10], is surgery to remove a cancerous but gravid uterus [11, 12]. In this case, it is claimed that the death of the fetus is not "directly intended"; instead, what is directly intended is the cure of a proportionately serious pathological condition. Such a case thus appears to fall clearly under section 47 of the *Ethical and Religious Directives* while the Phoenix case does not. For the Phoenix case appears to violate Paul's rule—named the "Pauline principle" by Alan Donagan [13]—that evil is not to be done that good may come.

. . .

As I have already noted, a commonly cited case is surgery to remove a cancerous but gravid uterus: more fully, hysterectomy against uterine cancer even when a woman is pregnant. (Whether it was a mistake to apply the PDE to this case is a disputed point in the literature,[2] but as I have also noted, the USCCB's Committee on Doctrine cites just this example in its defense of Bishop Olmsted.) This procedure is commonly thought to be permitted under the PDE since the object of the action—namely, that to which it is immediately directed, removing the cancerous uterus—is good or at least indifferent (condition 1); the action is done with the right intention of preserving the woman's life (condition 2); the death of the fetus (which is understood to be not yet viable *ex utero*) is only foreseen and does not figure as the means toward preserving the woman's life (condition 3); and preserving the woman's life is a sufficiently serious reason to go ahead with the action despite the harm that it will also bring about and for which the agent is then responsible, though in this case, not culpable (condition 4).

. . .

Hysterectomy against uterine cancer even when a woman is pregnant is commonly contrasted with fetal craniotomy in the course of labor gone tragically wrong.[3] This latter case is commonly thought *not* to be permitted under the PDE, as it appears not to satisfy the third condition, namely, that the evil effect (here, the death of the fetus) may not be the means to the good effect (here, saving the life of the woman). From this point of view, fetal craniotomy to save a woman's life, because it is done as a means, is the direct killing of an unborn child, and as such, gravely wrong. The customary, textbook interpretation of the PDE affirms the dictum that "he who intends the end intends the means." In other words, it regards as intended not only the good effect that one seeks, but the means to that effect, which is then independently evaluated as good or evil [17]. So a hysterectomy against uterine cancer is permitted even when a woman is pregnant, but an abortion when a woman's life is endangered by complications of labor, or for that matter by pulmonary hypertension, is forbidden. For, in the first case, the death of the fetus is, strictly speaking, not intended but only foreseen—it is a so-called indirect rather than direct abortion—whereas in the second case the death of the fetus is intended, since he who intends the end intends the means.

It has been suggested that the death of the fetus in the Phoenix case might likewise be categorized as an indirect abortion, or in other words, as only indirectly intended. (By the way, the point of this terminology of direct and indirect intention, as Warren Quinn has observed, appears to be to acknowledge the "linguistic impropriety in an agent's asserting, with a completely straight face, that a clearly foreseen harm or harming is quite *un*intended" [18, p. 335]. . . . .) Writing in *America*, Kevin O'Rourke noted that "the hospital's ethics committee identified the pathological organ as the placenta," which "produces the hormones necessary to increase the blood volume in pregnant women," and in this case, apparently "put an intolerable strain on the woman's already weak heart" [19, p. 16]. What the committee might have recommended, then, was removal of the organ in which the placenta is located, namely, the uterus, thereby making this case analogous to hysterectomy against uterine cancer even when a woman is pregnant. As a physician observed in a letter on O'Rourke's article, the committee might also have authorized, yet more precisely, removal of the placenta itself, "even though the procedure would indirectly result in the loss of the pregnancy" [20]. Inasmuch as the death of the fetus would not serve as the means to saving the life of the woman—inasmuch as removing the placenta would do so—this procedure, too, might be cast as analogous to hysterectomy against uterine cancer, and so thought to be permitted under the PDE.

Let us put aside, however, the medical question of the identity of the pathological organ. I think one lesson that we can draw from the Phoenix case is that cases that appear to fall clearly under this or that precedent might appear quite different after casuists have had a look. Another lesson, perhaps, is that casuistry's bad name is not altogether undeserved—at least insofar as it proceeds according to what has been called the geometric method, judging actions in view of whether they satisfy idealized, atemporal, and necessary conditions, and seeking to justify a controversial action by redescribing it in terms that satisfy the conditions in question [14, 21]. Whether O'Rourke has proceeded in this way is a separate question, but is it really the case that abortion in the Phoenix case would be morally justified if the doctors had intended to save the woman's life by removing the placenta, thereby indirectly aborting the fetus, but not morally justified if the doctors had intended to save the woman's life by directly aborting the fetus?

. . .

Casuistry, however, is vulnerable to degeneration into moral legalism, with prudence or practical wisdom giving way to rote application of rules under the guidance of "ethics experts."[4] Whereas the PDE should have what Keenan calls "a heuristic and confirming function" [14]—suggesting that, if a new case satisfies its conditions, there is reason to think that one can be as certain about it as earlier thinkers were about the paradigm cases—what happens instead, when moral legalism prevails, is that the PDE is invested with authority of its own and made into the up-or-down test of a case's morality. In other words, it is enshrined into, precisely, a principle. To put the point somewhat dramatically, the moral wisdom reflected in the PDE is replaced by an image of itself, the principle so derived, which poses the danger of distorting evaluations of new cases that do not satisfy this principle and that might better be resolved by looking to other cases and principles altogether.

Another principle within Catholic moral thought is the principle of choosing the lesser evil in circumstances where, however one acts, an evil is bound to occur [23]. There is no question here, it must be noted, of doing evil that good may come: in the circumstances appropriate to this principle, one is not free to do good, but only to choose between evils. It seems that the

Phoenix case involving Sister McBride is more congruent to the paradigm cases that gave rise to this principle than to the paradigm cases that gave rise to the PDE. That the principle of choosing the lesser evil has lately been obscured, for whatever reason,[5] is only more reason to look at it again. I think that the Phoenix case also indicates that there is reason for the United States Conference of Catholic Bishops to consider the incorporation of this principle, duly qualified, into the *Ethical and Religious Directives*. For purposes of helping prudence prevail, there is more work to be done than the PDE can do.

Notes

1. According to media reports, the doctors estimated the likelihood of death at "close to 100%" [1].
2. See Sulmasy [15]. Sulmasy claims that it was a mistake, originating in the early twentieth century, to apply the principle (which he prefers to call a rule) to the cases of the cancerous gravid uterus and tubal ectopic pregnancy. Yet he acknowledges that "the traditional view" is that "these are typical applications of the RDE [rule of double effect] (even paradigmatic instances of its use)."
3. For an instructive, though doleful, discussion of fetal craniotomy from a medical perspective, see Parikh [16].
4. Cf., e.g., R.M. Hare, who speaks witheringly of "some ecclesiastics and lawyers, who simply make the old casuistical moves without any attempt to justify them" [22, p. 70].
5. The explanation, to speculate a bit, may have to do with the more or less consequentialist interpretation of the fourth condition of the PDE, in terms of weighing good effects against bad effects. This interpretation was advanced in the twentieth century, in much qualified form, by so-called proportionalists. As the tradition of Catholic moral thought is antipathetic to consequentialism, more conservative representatives of the tradition reacted by magnifying the third condition of the PDE, with the result that any doing of evil became nearly unthinkable. For precision on the "consequentialism" of proportionalists, see Lisa Sowle Cahill [24]. . . .

References

1. Haggerty, Barbara Bradley. 2010. Nun excommunicated for allowing abortion. National Public Radio, May 19.
2. *The Arizona Republic*. 2010. Statements from the Diocese of Phoenix and St. Joseph's. May 15.

3. Pope John Paul II. 1995. *Evangelium vitae.*
4. Committee on Doctrine of the United States Conference of Catholic Bishops. 2001. *Ethical and religious directives for Catholic healthcare institutions.* 4th ed. USCCB.
5. *Catechism of the Roman Catholic Church.* 1997. 2nd ed. Washington, DC: United States Conference of Catholic Bishops.
6. Ehrlich, John. 2010. Abortion performed at St. Joseph's Hospital. *Respect for Life Newsletter, Diocese of Phoenix* 1(1).
7. Kaczor, Christopher. 1998. Double-effect reasoning from Jean Pierre Gury to Peter Knauer. *Theological Studies* 59: 297–316.
8. Boyle, Joseph M. Jr. 1980. Toward understanding the principle of double effect. *Ethics* 90: 527–538.
9. Mangan, Joseph T., S.J. 1949. An historical analysis of the principle of double effect. *Theological Studies* 10: 41–61.
10. Committee on Doctrine of the United States Conference of Catholic Bishops. 2010. The distinction between direct abortion and legitimate medical procedures. June 23.
11. Grisez, Germain G. 1970. Toward a consistent natural-law ethics of killing. *The American Journal of Jurisprudence* 15: 64–96.
12. Cavanaugh, T.A. 2006. *Double-effect reasoning: Doing good and avoiding evil.* Oxford: Oxford University Press.
13. Donagan, Alan. 1977. *The theory of morality.* Chicago: University of Chicago Press.
14. Keenan, James F., S.J. 1993. The function of the double effect principle. Theological Studies 54: 294–315.
15. Sulmasy, Daniel P. 2007. "Reinventing" the rule of double effect. In *The Oxford handbook of bioethics*, ed. Bonnie Steinbock, 114–149. Oxford: Oxford University Press.
16. Parikh, Mahendra N. 2006. Destructive operations in obstetrics. *Journal of Obstetrics and Gynecology of India* 56: 113–114.
17. Marquis, Donald B. 1991. Four versions of double effect. *Journal of Medicine and Philosophy* 16: 515–544.
18. Quinn, Warren. 1989. Actions, intentions, and consequences: The doctrine of double effect. Philosophy & Public Affairs 18: 334–351.
19. O'Rourke, Kevin. 2010. Complications. *America* 2: 15–16.
20. Keffer, J.H. 2010. The placenta is key. America 16: 28–29.
21. Jonsen, Albert R., and Stephen Toulmin. 1988. *The abuse of casuistry: A history of moral reasoning.* Berkeley: University of California Press.
22. Hare, R.M. 1993. Is medical ethics lost? *Journal of Medical Ethics* 19: 69–70.
23. Bretzke, James T., S.J. 2007. The lesser evil. *America* 26: 16–18.
24. Cahill, Lisa Sowle. 1981. Teleology, utilitarianism, and Christian ethics. *Theological Studies* 42: 610–629.

51

The Myth of Abortion as Black Genocide

Shyrissa Dobbins-Harris

Shyrissa Dobbins-Harris has her JD from the UCLA School of Law with a focus on critical race studies. We have excerpted a section from her law journal article that explains how the concept she calls "misogynoir," or "anti-Black misogyny," can be found in the historical treatment of Black women's bodies as well as in contemporary antiabortion activism. Dobbins-Harris addresses the often overlooked antiabortion discourses of the Nation of Islam and conservative figures in the Black church.

Misogynoir and Stereotypes of Blackwomen

The myth of abortion as Black genocide depends on denying Blackwomen their humanity and their agency to make medical decisions regarding their reproduction. The proponents of this myth rely heavily on misogynoir, which is anti-Black misogyny targeting Blackwomen. The term Misogynoir was created by queer Black feminist Moya Bailey who was searching for a term to correctly describe the particular brand of hatred (racialized sexism and sexist racism) aimed at fellow Blackwomen.[1]

. . .

Source: Shyrissa Dobbins-Harris, "The Myth of Abortion as Black Genocide: Reclaiming Our Reproductive Choice," *National Black Law Journal* 26 (2017): 85–127.

All non-Blackwomen can be perpetrators of misogynoir, and in perpetuating the myth of abortion as Black genocide, anti-choice activists rely on misogynoir to accuse Blackwomen of committing genocide.

The proponents of this myth sexualize racism by centering Blackwomen and their wombs as the site of genocide, without taking into account the actions of any male partners. As a result, they have mentally separated the Blackwoman from the fetus in her uterus. Now, there is a potential (and often actual) conflict between the interest of the Blackwoman (an actual person) and the embryo (who is being personified by anti-choice activists).[2] This is an illustration of maternal-fetal conflict, a predicament that Blackwomen have long been forced into since the times of their enslavement.[3]

The common stereotypes of jezebel and mammy are used as tools to justify the continued focus on the reproductive capabilities of Blackwomen. The jezebel stereotype paints some Blackwomen (particularly Blackgirls and young women) as promiscuous seductresses with insatiable sexual appetites.[4] This stereotype helped to normalize, and to some explain away, the rape of enslaved Blackwomen by their masters and other men. In 1859, an appellate court in Mississippi overturned a death sentence for a Black male slave convicted of raping an enslaved Blackgirl around 9 years old.[5] The legal basis for the decision was that the law did not recognize rape between slaves.[6] Despite the young age of the victim, the stereotypes of lewd and promiscuous Blackgirls and women kept her rape from being recognized by law.

Even after emancipation, Blackwomen were assumed to be naturally promiscuous and lewd, thus incapable of being legally raped.[7] As Dorothy E. Roberts, an American scholar and social justice activist writes, "The image of the sexually loose woman who is unrapable, who always consents, and who is therefore unprotected by the law, is a black woman."[8] Tracking the continued sexualization of Black bodies before, during, and after the end of chattel slavery showcases the continued sexualized violence that Blackwomen face and endure without legal recourse. After emancipation, Blackwomen were at continued risk of rape by their white employers privileged by a legal system that fails to see Blackwomen as sexual victims deserving of justice.[9] Even in modern times, for every one Blackwoman that reports her rape 15 others do not.[10] Further the over incarceration of Blackwomen puts them at greater risk for sexual violence within the prison system.[11]

On the other hand, some Blackwomen are labeled as mammies and pushed to fulfill a strong and desexualized matriarchal role. Mammies originated as overweight, often dark-skinned, Blackwomen who cared for their masters' and later their employer's children with selfless love.[12] Despite being literal property, the mammy is always loving to her white family and seems to genuinely care for them.[13] A common depiction of this non-threatening caricature is that of Aunt Jemima, the syrup brand character.[14] The mammy stereotype in its modern depictions transfers the previous affections for the master's family to her own Black family. Modern films that use this stereotype include The Help, Big Momma's House, and the entire Madea and Nutty Professor franchises.[15] The spirit of the mammy is reintroduced to Blackwomen when they are urged to think of their fetuses first, and themselves and their wants second, if at all.

Supporters of the Myth of Abortion as Black Genocide

Many Black religious leaders, in many Christian denominations as well as leaders of the Nation of Islam, preach that abortion by Blackwomen is contributing to genocide.[16] Baptist Pastor Childress has coined the phrase, "the most dangerous place for an African American is in the womb of their African American Mother."[17] Pastor Childress is the president of the Life Education and Resource Network (LEARN), the largest Black anti-choice group in the United States.[18] He also launched the website Blackgenocide.org in 2012 where he argues that abortion has caused 15.5 million deaths since 1973.[19]

The Nation of Islam (NOI) also holds strong anti-choice and anti-contraceptive views based both on theology as well as their understanding of government provided reproductive services. The NOI's views and theology are not that of Sunni or Shia Muslims and in fact are vastly different when it comes to race.[20] The NOI is a strictly Black organization and holds anti-white separatist ideals.[21] Further, NOI personifies God in their founder WD Fard, in direct contradiction to the more mainstream interpretations of the Quran that Sunni and Shia Muslims follow.[22] They also uphold Elijah Muhammad as another and recent prophet of God, despite Muhammad's proclamation that he was the final prophet of God.[23]

The "prophet" Elijah Muhammad preached strict paternalism over Blackwomen and girls in his religious organization. Female members recall feeling safe in the presence of their NOI brothers noting, "[t]hey would not allow you to walk at night by yourself. If you came to a meeting you could rest assured that someone would take you home."[24] This paternalism also functioned to limit premarital sex of Blackwomen in the Nation. One male member recalled ". . . Bein[g] chaperoned was there to benefit them. You know to eliminate this (sexual advances by men)."[25]

The NOI's separationist ideology included the formation of a separate moral code for its followers. Abortion and contraception fell outside of this code and, to the NOI, were racist attacks used by the white majority against the Black race.[26] Speaking to Dominican college students, the current leader Luis Farrakhan remarked that, "Once you get pregnant, this womb of yours, sisters, is sacred. That's where God operates, in your womb . . . the next scientist to overcome disease, the next leader to lead the people to their destiny will come from your womb . . . so the protection of your womb is critical . . ."[27]

Farrakhan's remarks illuminate the elevated status belonging to that of unborn Black fetuses. The assumption that the Blackwoman could only make the assumedly male "next leader" or "scientist to overcome disease" speaks to the misogynoir underlying Farrakhan's treatment of Blackwomen. He argues that God, the most supreme being in NOI theology, operates inside the womb of pregnant Blackwomen, suggesting that those same Blackwomen are not good enough to be the great leaders or scientists for their own communities. Farrakhan's remarks are following in Elijah Muhammad's teaching that Blackwomen's bodies are the "field" of the nation, and were commonly represented in cartoons in *Muhammad Speaks*, the NOI paper.[28]

The NOI leader's remarks also rely heavily on the mammy and jezebel stereotypes of Blackwomen. He appeals to the possibility of future success for the current fetus, in hopes that these possibilities will be enough to convince Blackwomen not to abort. During the twentieth anniversary of the Million Man March in 2015 Farrakhan preached,

> Now it is your body. You can do with it as you please, but it would be so tragic if the next Sitting Bull[29] was aborted . . . It would be tragic, if the next Malcolm X or Martin Luther King or Moses or Abraham or Jesus was flushed away. You don't know who your child is going to be.[30]

Farrakhan's rhetoric first offers the choice of abortion, painted as a selfish act, then appeals to the self-sacrificing mammy to persuade her to give birth instead. He also assumes that the fetuses in jeopardy of termination could be great and righteous leaders, on the converse these fetuses could also be the next Yakub.[31] This possibility isn't discussed because Farrakhan and his believers would rather persuade women towards birth instead of providing them information and agency to choose their own pregnancy outcomes.

Instead of believing that a pregnant Blackwoman could herself become the next savoir, Farrakhan transfers all of his hopes for the Black race to her presumably male fetus. By sidestepping the wealth of potential that is Blackwomen, even those who have unplanned pregnancies and abortions, Farrakhan is further relying on misogynoir to pressure women to conform to his anti-choice ideals.

. . .

Blackwomen have always been champions of reproductive choice, and have worked tirelessly to create a better world for those that choose birth and their babies. The myth of abortion as Black genocide has been, and still is, continually used to diminish the revolutionary work of Blackwomen. But their response to this myth and its propaganda showcase the ingenuity and perseverance of Blackwomen. One American feminist historian wrote about Blackwomen in slavery, saying "those who encounter oppression through the body, the body becomes an important site not only of suffering but also . . . resistance."[32] This resistance is longstanding, and has culminated in a focus on Reproductive Justice, encompassing more than just the right to "choose" abortion.

. . .

By attacking the misogynoir of anti-choice activists, Blackwomen continue to assert their agency over themselves, and their communities. Not only can a race divided not flourish, but any movement that fails to center those members at the margins will inevitably reproduce the same oppressions that they claim to want to end. By trusting and empowering Blackwomen to make their own reproductive decisions, anti-choice activists can shift their considerable resources to more worthwhile and non-oppressive causes to ensure the thriving of the Black race.

Notes

1. Kesiena Boom, *4 Tired Tropes That Perfectly Explain What Misogynoir Is- And How You Can Stop It*, EVERYDAY FEMINISM (Aug. 3, 2015), http://www.everydayfeminism.com/2015/08/4-tired-tropes-misogynoir/.
2. Anti-choice activists such as Pastor Childress and Dr. Aveda King believe that personhood begins at contraception. I believe that every woman has a right to make her own medical decisions. Penny Starr, Alveda King on *'Black Lives Matter'—'From Conception to Natural Death'*, CNS News (Jan. 8, 2015, 6:36 PM), http://www.cnsnews.com/news/article/penny-starr/

alveda-king-black-lives-matter-conception-natural-death. I believe the ability to make and exercise these reproductive decisions is crucial to self-determination of women and girls. There is not a conceivable point where I personally believe that this right can be diminished or should be limited for the interest of the fetus. According to Guttmacher Institute, two-thirds of abortions occur at eight weeks or earlier, with ninety-one percent of abortions occurring within the first thirteen weeks. Fetal viability is widely accepted to be between twenty-two and twenty-four gestational weeks, and even at this point I don't believe that a woman's ability to terminate her pregnancy should be abridged by legislation. See *Induced Abortion in the United States: September 2016 Fact Sheet*, GUTTMACHER INST., Guttmacher.org.

3. [Dorothy Roberts, KILLING THE BLACK BODY: RACE, REPRODUCTION, AND THE MEANING OF LIBERTY (1997)], at 39.

4. David Pilgrim, *Jezebel Stereotype*, FERRIS STATE UNIV. (2012).

5. A. Leon Higginbotham, Jr., Essay, *What Took Place and What Happened: White Male Domination, Black Male Domination, and the Denigration of Black Women*, Wash. Post (1995).

6. Id.; . . . Patricia A. Broussard, Black Women's Post-Slavery Silence Syndrome: A Twenty-First Century Remnant of Slavery, Jim Crow, and Systemic Racism—Who Will Tell Her Stories?, 16; J. GENDER RACE & JUST. 373, 381 (2013); accord ENCYCLOPEDIA OF RAPE 235 (Merril D Smith ed. 2004).

7. Higginbotham, *supra* note [5].

8. Dorothy E. Roberts, *Rape, Violence, and Women's Autonomy* 9 UNIV. PA. LEGAL SCHOLARSHIP REPOSITORY 359, 365 (1993).

9. Id. at 366.

10. Bureau of Justice Statistics Special Report. Hart and Rennison, 2003, U.S. DEPT. OF JUSTICE.

11. "[A]n African American woman is eight times more likely than a European American woman is to be imprisoned." Amnesty Int'l, *Women in Prison: A Factsheet 2*, http://www.prisonpolicy.org/scans/women_prison. pdf.

12. Jim Crow Museum of Racist Memorabilia, *The Mammy Caricature*, FERRIS STATE UNIV.

13. Id.

14. Id.

15. Big Momma's House and the Madea and Nutty Professor franchises further the desexualization of Black Matriarchs by allowing men in drag to portray these roles (Martin Lawrence, Tyler Perry, and Eddie Murphy respectively). Hilary Christian, *There's Nothing Funny in the Misogynoir of Crossdressing Instagram 'Comedians.'* FOR HARRIET, http://

www.forharriet.com/2015/09/theres-nothing-funny-in-misogynoir-of. html#axzz4c19acTvH.

16. Pastor Clenard H. Childress Jr. is a Baptist Pastor, while Dr. Alveda King is an Evangelist Christian. L.E.A.R.N. Nebraska [Black Genocide, http:// www.blackgenocide.org/abortion.html]; see also Evangelist Alveda C. King, http://www.priestsforlife.org/staff/alvedaking.htm; Kathryn Joyce, *Abortion as 'Black Genocide': An Old Scare Tactic Re-Emerges*, Political Res. Associates (April 29, 2010).

17. Thomas D. Williams, *Black Pastor Tells NAACP Abortion is Racist Genocide*, BREITBART (Jul. 20, 2015).

18. Id.

19. See Gerard M. Nadal, Black Genocide and Planned Parenthood, Coming Home (Feb. 1, 2010) (depicting a graph originally provided by Rev. Childress of LEARN, the largest anti-choice Black organization in the United States).

20. Unlike the NOI, which is focused on only Black members, Sunni and Shia followers are of many different races and ethnicities. "[I]n religious writings the dominant normative view echoed the Koran's insistence that religiosity took precedence over ethnic or racial background." James Jankowski, *Islamic Views of Ethnicity and Race-Bibliography*, J. RANK SCI. & PHILOSOPHY.

21. *Nation of Islam*, Southern Poverty L. Ctr.

22. Religious News Service, *Muslims See Contrasts with Nation of Islam Tents of Farrakhan's Group Have Historically Different From Mainstream Islam's. Publicity of Upcoming Million Man March Accents Distinctions.*, L.A. TIMES (Oct. 14, 1995).

23. Id.

24. Edward E. Curtis IV, BLACK MUSLIM RELIGION IN THE NATION OF ISLAM, 1960–1975 121 (2006).

25. Id.

26. Donald T. Critchlow, INTENDED CONSEQUENCES: BIRTH CONTROL, ABORTION, AND THE FEDERAL GOVERNMENT IN MODERN AMERICA 142 (1999).

27. *Nation of Islam Leader Warns Against Abortion*, DOMINICA NEWS ONLINE (Dec.5, 2012, 7:39AM).

28. Curtis, *supra* note [24]. On the other hand, some Blackwomen found the reverence for their reproductive capacities comforting. One member, Lorraine Muhammad explained, "The value that the Nation put on women, I haven't found that anywhere else. The minister talks about the value of the woman and the value of your womb and to hear that come from a man—it's one thing to hear that from a woman but to hear that from a man is different. There is continual upliftment. Sometimes you

find it hard to believe how valuable you are. It's overwhelming to believe how powerful we are as individuals." Dawn-Marie Gibson & Jamilah Kari, WOMEN OF THE NATION: BETWEEN BLACK PROTEST AND SUNNI ISLAM 139 (2014).

29. Sitting Bull was a Hukpapa Lakota Chief who united all the Lakota tribes in a struggle for survival in the Great Plains against American military power and manifest destiny. West Film Project & WETA, New Perspectives on the West, PBS (2001).

30. Penny Starr, *Farrakhan on Abortion: 'It Would Be So Tragic If the Next' MLK or Jesus 'Was Flushed Away'*, CNS News (Oct. 12, 2015 2:39 PM).

31. In NOI theology Yakub is the father of the devil and the evil scientist responsible for creating the white race through inbreeding and infanticide. Eric Pement, *Luis Farrakhan and the Nation of Islam: Part Two*, 26 CORNERSTONE 32–36 (1997).

32. Stephanie M. H. Camp, CLOSER TO FREEDOM: ENSLAVED WOMEN AND EVERYDAY RESISTANCE IN THE PLANTATION SOUTH 94 (2004).

52

#BlackBabiesMatter:

Analyzing Black Religious Media in Conservative and Progressive Evangelical Communities

Monique Moultrie

Monique Moultrie is a professor of Africana studies and religious studies at Georgia State University and has published and lectured on sexuality and the Black church, womanist sexual ethics, critical race theory, and ethnographic approaches to the study of religion. In this piece, Moultrie focuses on the common claim about the sacrality of life that appears in two different streams of Black digital media associated with the Black Lives Matter hashtag campaign. She examines the differences between the Black conservative Christian prolife emphasis on Black Babies Matter and progressive religious supporters of Black Lives Matter who emphasize the ongoing struggle to have the sacredness of Black lives and Black bodies recognized, respected, and protected from violence.

This article begins its interrogation of the sacrality of black life by juxtaposing those who contend that Black Babies Matter as pro-birth-oriented, religiously motivated activists with those opponents asserting Black Lives

Source: Monique Moultrie, "#BlackBabiesMatter: Analyzing Black Religious Media in Conservative and Progressive Evangelical Communities," *Religions* 8, no. 11 (2017): 255. https://doi.org/10.3390/rel8110255.

Matter who present an intersectional pro-life approach. The comparison of views relies on womanist cultural analysis as its main methodology to analyze and interpret digital media and explore its ramifications for African American Religion.[1]

Digital Media and African American Religion

. . .

Philosopher of religion Terrence Johnson contends that the Black Lives Matter movement emerges from an African American religious context as it "inherits its call to '(re)build the Black Liberation movement' from the Black Church's historical role in developing a theology of liberation based on social justice" (Johnson 2016). He is clear that is he not indicating any causality from the Black Church to the Black Lives Matter movement; instead, he is positing that they share vocabulary, songs, and even political ideology such that the basic building blocks for what defines justice and what it means to be human are found in black churches. This is contestable given the cognitive dissonance many black millenials have with black religiosity and especially black Christianity. Yet, when one looks at activism regarding Black Lives Matter from black persons claiming a religious identity, this is not as specious a claim.

Demographically, one can make a claim that African Americans who do not eschew Christianity are a part of the digital religion population that syncs new media with their religious lives. According to a Pew Center study, 40% of 18–29-year-old African Americans who use the Internet use Twitter (compared to 28% of younger whites) and there is a noticeable six percentage point difference among black youth using social networking sites like Facebook compared to whites (Pew Research Center 2014). Given the statistic that black Protestants have retained more millenials than any other racial demographic, it is reasonable to presume that these millenials are media oriented and invested in the cultural practices and rituals that Sorett described (Lee 2015).

This would make digital media significant for black Protestant meaning making. Scholars contend that the Black Lives Matter movement has decentered the black church as the site for meaning making and solutions to the injustice of the world. Analysis of religious media associated with the movement supports this assertion, as this is certainly not the call to return to the black church's status quo. Instead, activists on both the left and right are expanding the church and the message of Christianity's involvement through their activism.

. . .

Conservative Religious Actors Utilizing Digital Religion

. . .

Rev. Clenard Childress, a New Jersey Pastor and founder of BlackGenocide.org calls the Black Lives Matter movement the best thing that happened to the "anemic black pro-life movement" (Cunningham 2015). Childress has regularly supplied protesters from his two hundred–member New Jersey congregation as they see Black Lives Matter protests ripe for the anti-abortion message. He specifically recruits other black pastors for this type of activism, as he believes Christians have a moral duty to inform the community of systematic targeting of black communities through eugenics and population control. Childress primarily utilizes digital media like the All Black Lives Matter project circulating through Historically Black Colleges and Universities' campuses to advance his cause. His website, BlackGenocide.org, is his gift to the anti-abortion movement, as it is a multi-media mural presentation of his views comparing black abortion to genocide.

Childress argues that the Black Lives Matter movement has given his cause a way of beginning a conversation with younger blacks, and this is also true of Rev. Alveda King's outreach through the Priests for Life organization. While both Childress and King used imagery and tactics connecting their cause with the Civil Rights movement, both see in the Black Lives Matter movement an opportunity to make an impact on a cause that they feel religiously called to pursue. In Alveda King's 23 March 2015 blog post "Why All Lives Matter," she opens with an image of a fetus with the caption "Black Lives Do Matter! Hands Up-Don't Abort," which she attributes to the www.AfricanAmericanOutreach.org website, which is an arm of her organization, Civil Rights for the Unborn. The blog makes comparisons between the Ferguson police department scheme to disproportionately issue tickets against blacks to Planned Parenthood's "systematic" targeting of minorities.[2]

. . .

Perhaps the most successful and notable digital activist utilizing religious media to offer alternatives to the Black Lives Matter movement is Ryan Bomberger, the founder of the Radiance Foundation, an organization devoted to "creatively affirm(ing) that every human life has purpose."[3] He is the creative force behind the 2010 billboard campaigns from TooManyAborted.com that sought to expose the disproportionate impact of abortion on the black community by naming black children an endangered species and calling the womb the most dangerous place for black children.

. . .

Theological Framings for Black Babies Matter Campaigns

These conservative Christian activists share similar Biblical and theological framings that condition their responses to contemporary social issues like abortion or even civil rights protests. Common ground is typically found in the sacredness of human life, which for conservatives begins at conception. This article does not offer a thorough juxtaposition between the theological justifications for and against abortion.[4] Instead, it looks more narrowly at the specific rationales for sacrality of human life debated from religious media activists on each side.

Evangelical ethicist David Gushee wrote a substantive treatise on the sacredness of human life, and his argument is instructive for exploring how these black conservative activists understand abortion or even the taking of black lives by the police. Gushee begins with evangelical definitions for sanctity of human life that parallels some of the digital media statements by black conservative Black Babies Matter activists. He summarizes the literature by stating that human life is sacred because it is precious to God (based on Psalms 116:15), because humans are created in God's image (based on Genesis 1: 26–27), and because God also took human nature in the form of Jesus (based on John 1:1, 14).[5] Gushee admits that debates on the sacredness of human life are often waged over abortion and that the theology of creation depends heavily on biblical rationale. His text provides similar logic to what is espoused by activist groups. Unlike activists, Gushee acknowledges that the biblical base for being pro-life is disputable because there is no "explicit condemnation of abortion" in the Bible, but this acknowledgement comes with significant biblical support for the pro-life position found in biblical affirmations that God is creator of every human, that fertility is a part of God's plan, children are thus gifts from God, and finally that even in the development process, God is present and providential (Gushee 2013, p. 357).

These views on the sacredness of human life are shared by most of the religious activists on the conservative and progressive side. Yet, conservatives often go a step further to insist that this sacredness begins at the moment of conception, whereas progressives attribute sacredness and human life to a live birth. Particularly popular among conservatives is the proof they find in Psalm 139:13–16, which states, "For you created my inmost being; you knit me together in my mother's womb. I praise you because I am fearfully and wonderfully made . . . My frame was not hidden from you, when I was made in the secret place, when I was woven together in the depths of the earth. Your eyes beheld my unformed body." Activists like Rev. Alveda King argue that this scripture speaks of the unborn child as a person with whom God is interacting, and activist Ryan Bomberger states that this scripture shows just how purposeful every life is to God, with no child being unplanned.

. . .

Prominent in their rhetoric is that Black Lives Matter proponents must care about black life from the "womb to the tomb," as Rev. Alveda King reminds her audiences that "everybody's civil rights count" (Heretik 2017). The rationale behind this logic is that every person carries the image of God, and this begins in the womb. Thus, every black zygote, embryo, or fetus is already a part of God's plan and deserving of respect expected of all persons.

. . .

This results in a pro-birth doctrine that many conservative activists like Ryan Bomberger are happy to accept, while opponents contend that this is a myopic view that limits these justice-oriented organizations' full capacity to work on behalf of the black community. The debate around the Black Lives Matter movement has amplified this tension as lines are drawn with antagonists within the conservative movement questioning the Black Lives Matter movement's commitment to black life in light of its perceived silence on the disproportionate number of black abortions performed annually.[6]

. . .

Theological Framings for Progressive Participation in Black Lives Matter Campaigns

[P]rogressive religious activists . . . share similar biblical and theological framings that motivate their actions in the digital and physical world. They also share a common belief in the sacredness of human life, but for progressive religious activists, this sacrality does not end after conception but mandates working on the behalf of the sacred nature of black life throughout its stages of development. They share David Gushee's consensus on the sacred nature of human life, but they mediate his perspective through the lenses of black liberation theologies. Black and womanist theologies often link the sacredness of human life to a consideration of the full humanity of blacks that are lived out in a belief that God cares about the full thriving of black life.

Rev. Willis Johnson, a pastor of Wellspring United Methodist church in Ferguson, offers one of the most succinct depictions of Black Lives Matter and theology of creation:

> Yes, black lives do matter, and yes, they matter because there's a God who believes that all life is sacred. While this has racial implications and tension an economic reverberation, there's a historical record of a system and a culture that are violent toward black people at any given time . . . So there is a God who is a God of all the oppressed. There's a God who cares, and there's a sacredness of person because we're all created in the image of God. (Francis 2015, p. 23).

Belief that God's image is imprinted on all life meant that as religious activists they needed to be concerned with the racial and economic realities of black people.

Womanist theologian Kelly Brown Douglas contends that according to an African worldview, all is sacred because it is connected to the creator God who is sacred. She remarks that God intends for black bodies to be cherished and respected because biblical scripture teaches that God looked out at creation and it was good. Beyond this basic building block for sacredness of human life in womanist theology, she states that this good creation requires that black bodies be free from human constraints that prevent them from being who God created or threatens their life. Thus, "black life has meaning beyond the images constructed by the narratives of a stand-your-ground culture" (Douglas 2015, pp. 150–51). Thus, as laborers for justice, progressive religious activists are encouraged to resist anything or anyone that threatens the fullness of black life.

In essence, to be fully black is to be fully human and the "quest for black people to be seen as *fully* human is a significant component of this movement for racial justice" (Francis 2015, p. 56). The daily dehumanization that occurs with inadequate education, health care, policing, disproportionate imprisonment, sexism, homophobia, transphobia, etc. threaten the capacity to be fully human and fully created as God intended. Thus, Black Lives Matter religious activists push back against stereotypes and discrimination and shows God's love and God intentions in the world. This action is imbued with their liberation theological determination that full humanity involves a more just notion of humanity that desires God's freedom to be manifest in the lives of all. Progressive religious activists are making plain a womanist ethic of incarnation that envisions black bodies as made from the same substance of God; thus, black humanity cannot be divorced from the God incarnate (Turman 2014, p. 161).

. . .

Nyle Fort, a young seminarian activist, organized a commemoration of the "conversations and words of black people who have been murdered by vigilantes or police officers" at Riverside Church; despite its physical locale, the service was live-streamed, tweeted, and catalogued on YouTube for a much wider audience (Wright 2017, p. 167; Blackmon 2015). Rev. Traci Blackmon preaches the first word commemorating Amadou Diallo. She reminds the audience that they are all gathered because of the failure to acknowledge the holy in one another, and she refused to just focus on the interruption of Diallo's life but instead will concentrate on his incarnation.

This echoing of his sacredness and humanity is also represented in Fort's closing sermon commemorating Sean Bell who was murdered on his wedding day. . . . Fort concludes with an invitation for all listeners to marry the movement for justice. He vows to "love black people unapologetically; unlearn systems of oppression of patriarchy, homophobia, capitalism, militarism, and white supremacist theologies; stand alongside my transgender brothers and sisters against trans-antagonism and violence; organize within my community; take care of my elders and to inspire a generation . . . and to not simply preach love with my lips, but to practice love with my life" (Fort 2015). These commitments have been demanded since the enslavement of Africans on American soil and have been a part of secular and religious black liberation efforts. Yet, progressive religious activists' focus on the combined sacredness of creation and the full humanity of blacks presents an opportunity to "pray with our feet until there is no more blood in our streets" (Francis 2015, p. 128).

Notes

1. Womanist cultural analysis describes the merging of womanist methodology and cultural studies to analyze digital media from the perspective of the black producers and consumers of media. This methodology includes a close reading of the texts (in this case, Twitter, Facebook, and blog posts) while being sensitive to their articulated religious perspectives. I would like to acknowledge Toni Bond Leonard, one of the founding mothers of reproductive justice, for her assistance in preparing this article.
2. (King 2015). Rev. Alveda King garners a lot of traction with her statements because of her use of statements from her uncle, the civil rights icon Dr. Martin Luther King, Jr. Yet, she is also notable from her funded position as an African American outreach activist with the largely white organization Priests for Life.
3. The Radiance Foundation states that its mission is to be an "educational, faith-based, life–affirming organization" utilizing "creative ad campaigns, powerful multi-media presentations, fearless journalism, and compassionate community outreaches," http://www.theradiancefoundation .org/about/.
4. This would require a vast comparison and even if just narrowing down perspectives from the Protestant black Christian perspective, this still leaves hundreds of years of debates. For a more thorough analysis of Catholic and Protestant views on abortion, see Castuera (2017).
5. (Gushee 2013, p. 30). Gushee's definitions of the sacredness of human life are taken from evangelicals and Catholic Christians before he provides his own historically and theologically researched definition that is useful for this discussion.
6. Although white women currently make up the majority of abortion patients at 39%, black women are disproportionately represented in the abortions received, with black women representing 28% of abortions performed while constituting only roughly 13% of the total population. See Jerman et al. (2016).

References

Blackmon, Rev. Traci deVon. 2015. 7 Last Words: Strange Fruit Speaks: "Mom, I want to go to college". Video.

Castuera, Ignacio. 2017. A Social History of Christian Thought on Abortion: Ambiguity vs. Certainty in Moral Debate. *American Journal of Economics and Sociology* 76: 121–227.

Cunningham, Paige Winfield. 2015. 'Black Babies matter': The black anti-abortion movement's political problems. *The Examiner*, September 28.

Douglas, Kelly Brown. 2015. *Stand Your Ground: Black Bodies and the Justice of God*. Maryknoll: Orbis Books.

Fort, Rev. Nyle. 2015. 7 Last Words: Strange Fruit Speaks: "I love you (too)". Video.

Francis, Leah Gunning. 2015. *Ferguson & Faith: Sparking Leadership & Awakening Community*. St. Louis: Chalice Press.

Gushee, David. 2013. *The Sacredness of Human Life: Why an Ancient Biblical Vision Is Key to the World's Future*. Grand Rapids: Eerdmans Publishing, Co.

Heretik, Jack. 2017. Dr. Alveda King Praises Trump for Leading Civil Rights for the Unborn. *Washington Free Beacon*, July 17.

Jerman, Jenna, Rachel K. Jones, and Tsuyoshi Onda. 2016. *Characteristics of U.S. Abortion Patients in 2014 and Changes Since 2008*. New York: Guttmacher Institute.

Johnson, Terrence. 2016. Black Lives Matter and the Black Church: Responding to Religion and Black Lives Matter. Berkley Forum, October 19.

King, Alveda. 2015. Why All Lives Matter. March 23. Available online: http://www.priestsforlife.org/ africanamerican/blog/index.php/why-all-lives-matter.

Lee, Morgan. 2015. Why Black Churches are Keeping Millenials. *Christianity Today*, January 30.

Pew Research Center. 2014. African Americans and Technology Use—A Demographic Portrait.

Radiance Foundation. 2016. No, You Don't Have to First Solve the World's Other Injustices to be Pro-Life. February 12.

Turman, Eboni Marshall. 2014. *Toward a Womanist Ethic of Incarnation: Black Bodies, the Black Church, and the Council of Chalcedon*. New York: Palgrave Macmillan.

Wright, Almeda. 2017. *Spiritual Lives of Young African Americans*. New York: Oxford.

53

Muftis in the Matrix:

Comparing Online English- and Arabic-Language Fatwas about Emergency Contraception

L. L. Wynn and Angel M. Foster

L. L. Wynn (PhD, Princeton University) is a professor at Macquarie University in Sydney, Australia, who has published on issues of reproductive health technologies, sexuality, and religion. Angel Foster, who has her DPhil in Middle Eastern studies from the University of Oxford, teaches at the University of Ottawa. These two researchers have co-written numerous articles and coedited several books about sexuality and reproductive health in the Middle East and North Africa. This essay investigates the growing world of virtual, online *fatwas* addressing legal aspects of sexual practices, contraception, and abortion for Muslims worldwide. Wynn and Foster show that these *fatwas* are directly relevant for all English-speaking observant Muslims, including the increasing numbers of Muslims in the United States.

"Emergency contraception" (EC) refers to an array of medications and devices that can be taken after sexual intercourse to reduce the risk of pregnancy. This class of postcoital contraception includes pills of different

Source: L. L. Wynn and Angel M. Foster, "Muftis in the Matrix: Comparing Online English- and Arabic-Language Fatwas about Emergency Contraception," *Journal of Middle East Women's Studies* 14, no. 3 (2018): 314–32.

types and the intrauterine device (IUD). EC offers a last chance to prevent pregnancy after sexual assault or unprotected or underprotected consensual sex. Since none of the methods of EC interrupt an established pregnancy, they are not abortifacient (Trussell 2012, 28). Moreover, most EC pills use the same hormones or materials found in regular oral contraceptive pills. However, EC is widely misunderstood to be equivalent or related to abortion, and many global debates about this reproductive health technology have hinged on this misunderstanding.

. . .

In this article we examine English- and Arabic-language "cyberfatwas," or fatwas posted on the internet issued by Islamic religious experts and consumed by a global online readership (Bunt 2003, 136–37) about EC. These cyberfatwas offer a lens onto current debates around contraception, reproduction, and sexuality among Muslims who produce and rely on such material globally. New technologies provide key moments for articulating contemporary concerns around sexuality and reproduction. We found English-language fatwas more conservative with regard to the use of EC than Arabic-language fatwas. The significant differences in the ways that the English- and Arabic-language fatwas discuss the technology suggest that local debates and the concerns of non-Muslim religious constituencies influence the opinions of Muslim communities in different locations. Our findings illustrate how the relationship to and understanding of EC as a new technology was framed by orientations to and understandings of existing related technologies.

. . .

Cultural and Social Controversies

. . .

In the United States and parts of the world influenced by the Vatican, debates around EC have often turned on definitions of when "life" begins—whether at fertilization or at implantation (Wynn and Trussell 2006, 313). In contrast, near consensus exists within Sunni and Shi'a Islam that the soul is infused with "life" after fertilization and implantation and that nonpermanent methods of contraception, including oral contraceptive pills and IUDs, are permissible within the marital relationship (Dardir and Ahmed 1981; Roudi-Fahimi 2004). By Islamic jurisprudent analogy, EC pills would presumably be similarly defined, but there were no documented fatwas about EC in the early years of dedicated product availability in the Arab world (Wynn et al. 2005, 42).

To determine whether this situation has changed, in 2016–17 we reviewed online fatwas in English and Arabic regarding EC. We selected these two languages because Arabic and English are the most dominant languages of the online fatwa websites. We conducted a systematic search of these fatwa databases and other online resources for any formal rulings or theological commentaries on EC that might be influencing Muslims who turn to online sources in Arabic or English seeking moral guidance on the use of this reproductive health technology.

Fatwas and Fatwa Websites in Perspective

Fiqh is the Arabic term for Islamic jurisprudence: the interpretation of shari'a (divine Islamic law) by expert jurists over hundreds of years following the methods and rules of recognized schools of legal thought and practice (*madhahib*). This entails forms of reasoning, analysis, and interpretation that apply the Quran (the Muslim holy book as revealed to the Prophet Muhammad) and hadith (the recorded sayings and actions of the Prophet Muhammad) to analogous situations and contexts. A fatwa is a nonbinding interpretation by a religious expert (a *mufti*), usually but not always produced in response to a question or concern of believers (and sometimes state authorities). Fatwa authors typically draw on and reason with relevant Islamic jurisprudence.

. . .

Prior to the internet, Muslims seeking guidance could ask their local imam or mufti for advice about applying Islamic law in their lives, and in some countries these rulings are issued by government religious institutions and have legal weight in family court (Wynn 2016, 553). But Muslims increasingly turn to the internet for information about religious interpretations to guide their actions. Websites sometimes dubbed "fatwa banks" are a popular resource that emerged in the late 1990s (Bunt 2003, 124–30). These sites are technologically sophisticated, and many offer newsfeeds and searchable fatwa databases. Most of these sites are bilingual or multilingual. For example, Islam Q&A (founded by Sheikh Muhammed Salih Al-Munajjid, a Palestinian-born sheikh raised and residing in Saudi

Arabia) offers fatwas in Arabic, Urdu, English, French, Spanish, Japanese, Indonesian, and Uyghur. Over time these sites have evolved from primarily English-language-dominated to offering more content in Arabic and other languages, mirroring developments on the internet more broadly. However, a fatwa in one language can be quite different from a fatwa in another language on the same website about a similar issue.

. . .

The sites are diverse, representing different schools of jurisprudence, social movements, and national perspectives. For example, Egypt, Saudi Arabia, and Malaysia have fatwa websites that articulate state-sanctioned versions of Islam. Other websites are complex transnational collaborations, which can be hard to categorize in terms of nationality or a particular school of Islamic jurisprudence. For example, IslamOnLine.net is registered in Doha, Qatar, by Sheikh Yusuf Qaradawi. It was launched in the United States and by 2003 was staffed by about a hundred Egyptians, many of them graduates and students of Egypt's al-Azhar University (Bunt 2003, 147–48). IslamOnLine.net has a "scholar database" with entries from all over the world. Its experts write in different languages and issue opinions according to their areas of expertise and linguistic ability. Some religious figures, moreover, write for multiple websites. For example, Ebrahim Desai, a South African mufti, not only founded the askimam.org fatwa website but also writes for IslamOnLine, as do scholars from North America and many other places. These online fatwa databases thus represent a sophisticated transnational phenomenon of religious cybercosmopolitanism, a digital phenomenon that reflects the cosmopolitanism of Islam.

. . .

English-Language Fatwa Themes on EC

. . .

Mechanism of Action

Four of the eight English-language fatwa sites discussed EC's mechanism of action. Two of these declared that EC causes an early abortion because of a postfertilization mechanism of action and thus that EC, like abortion itself, is forbidden in Islam except under particular circumstances. One additional fatwa called EC an "early abortion" but did not specifically discuss the mechanism of action. For example, on a previously popular fatwa website now defunct but archived on web.archive.org (daruliftaa.com, which described itself as the "Institute of Islamic Jurisprudence"), a reader asked: "I have been under the impression that in Islam it is forbidden to use the morning after pill as it is an abortive method of birth control. A friend recently argued that it was not, and that it is permissible to use it. Could you please provide a detailed response as to what the majority of scholars say regarding this issue?" In response, Mufti Muhammad ibn Adam of Leicester, United Kingdom, analogized the pill to the IUD. His ruling hinged on the mechanism of action of EC pills: if the pills work to prevent fertilization, he said, then they are permissible like other forms of nonpermanent contraception, but if they prevent implantation of a fertilized egg, then this constitutes an early abortion, and they can be used only under specific circumstances. He cited other jurisprudence experts who, he said, considered the IUD a "device of abortion" because of a potential postfertilization mechanism of action (Adam n.d.).

In contrast, two of the English-language fatwas that discussed mechanism of action said that EC was a contraceptive, not an abortifacient, and thus permissible even if there was a postfertilization mechanism of action. Abukhadeejah.com is a self-proclaimed pacifist, Salafist website that asserts the importance of "upholding rulers," even unrighteous ones, and claims that "modern-day insurgencies" come from the Shiʿa. The fatwa on this site likened EC to withdrawal, a contraceptive method employed by the Prophet Muhammad.

. . .

Extramarital Sex

Two of the eight English-language websites mentioned extramarital sex as an issue to be factored into a consideration of EC's permissibility in Islam. Both of these were in response to questions about whether it is religiously permissible for pharmacists to provide the drug. For example, an unnamed mufti on Islamweb writes:

> Contraceptive pills are permissible if there is a necessity and provided that both spouses agree to it and that the wife is not harmed by using it, and on the condition that its use does not lead to permanent birth control. Similarly,

selling these pills is also permissible, but if in general the people of a given country use these pills to commit Zina (fornication or adultery) or . . . it is known that a particular person wants to use it for this purpose, then it is not permissible to sell it to them or to whoever wants to use it for this purpose. This applies to both Muslim and non-Muslim buyers. (Islamweb 2009)

Arabic-Language Fatwa Themes on EC

. . .

Mechanism of Action

The mechanism of action of different modalities of EC is the most dominant theme on Arabic-language websites, although these posts do not always respond to a question. Posting on the website Aslein.net, self-described as "The source of religion, the source of jurisprudence," Ahmed Muhammad Kanaan states that even if EC worked to prevent implantation of a fertilized egg, this would not constitute a forbidden technology because ensoulment of the fetus does not occur before forty days after fertilization (Aslein.net 2007). This is the only Arabic-language fatwa to specifically mention ensoulment, a concept more often employed in discussions of the permissibility of abortion than in discussions of contraception.

Islamic jurisprudence debates around when life begins have historically focused not on fertilization versus implantation but on the concept of ensoulment, that is, the point at which a fetus is "infused with life" (Wynn et al. 2005, 42). There is no uniform theological position on the timing of ensoulment among schools of Islamic jurisprudence (Bowen 1997, 163–65). On fatwa.islamweb.net, a self-described moderate website for Muslims and non-Muslims who want to know about Islam, a doctor asks for a fatwa about how to treat a woman who has had extramarital sex and takes EC afterward. The doctor states that she or he does not know whether EC prevents implantation into the uterus of a fertilized egg and wonders if it is sinful to provide these pills and if taking them constitutes causing an abortion. In response, the unsigned fatwa (this website does not name muftis) states:

No, there is no resemblance, because if pregnancy is established then EC pills fail to have any ability to end that pregnancy, even when using the loop [IUD] as emergency contraception, first a pregnancy test should be done. As for abortion pills, they work after pregnancy is established. Accordingly, it is known that these [EC] pills prevent pregnancy and they are not considered to kill the fetus and thus no forgiveness need be sought. (Islamweb 2011)

Extramarital Sex

Like the English-language websites, the question of whether EC availability facilitates extramarital sex is also a concern, coming up in two of the five Arabic-language fatwas. In both cases it is in response to a specific question. The website Islamic-fatwa.com is described as a fatwa network answering people's questions since 2005, with an archive of over seventy-five thousand fatwas, and run by Ahmed al- Hajji al-Karaday, a Kuwaiti mufti and member of the Jurisprudence Committee (*hay'at al-ifta'*). A questioner states that she committed unlawful sexual intercourse without penile penetration and took emergency contraceptive pills the same day. She subsequently took two pregnancy tests, both positive. After consulting a doctor, she took abortion pills and got a negative result on a third pregnancy test; the arrival of her period followed. She tells the mufti that she has repented and now wants to know if she did wrong in taking the pills, noting that she did not know whether she was actually pregnant and thus had induced an abortion, particularly since there was no penetration and she had taken EC pills immediately afterward. The mufti responds stating that God in his grace and generosity had sheltered her from pregnancy, and urges her to now repent, stay away from men who are not her relatives, and pray that God sends her a husband. He does not mention EC or abortion pills in any way, despite the question (Islamic-fatwa.com 2013).

. . .

Conclusion

English-language online fatwas about EC are significantly more likely to rule that EC is not religiously acceptable, whereas no Arabic-language online fatwas state that EC is forbidden to Muslims. In contrast, Arabic-language questions to online fatwa sites are proportionally more concerned about whether EC will facilitate illicit sex among the unmarried and whether contraceptives pose health risks to women.

These findings may reflect the broader global concerns about EC's mechanism of action. In the United States and in Catholic-majority countries, debates about EC have often centered on whether EC only prevents fertilization of the egg or whether it can prevent the implantation of a fertilized egg in the uterus. As we have seen in this review of English- and Arabic-language fatwas, a postfertilization mechanism of action appears to be a nonissue for Arabic-speaking experts in Islamic jurisprudence. . . .

This analysis of online cyberfatwas pertaining to EC has implications for new reproductive technologies beyond current Islamic jurisprudence. Online religious advisers are shaping a global Islamic discourse around technology and bodies and creating vocabulary for talking about interpretive possibilities. Given the anonymity of the internet, lay users in turn decide what to adopt or reject of the nonbinding advice offered, with few social consequences. The differential interpretations and understandings of EC in Arabic and English fatwas show that the so-called global *umma** is differentiated in its interpretative practices and priorities. However, the religious interpretations of contraception and abortion in these cyberfatwas are as a whole significantly more flexible than in Western conservative Christian contexts.

References

Adam, Muhammad ibn. n.d. "The Morning-After Pill." web.archive.org/web /20150708123257/http://www.daruliftaa.com/node/5407

Aslein.net. 2007. "Ruling on inserting an IUD into a woman." January 27. www .aslein.net/archive/index .php/t-5492.html

Bowen, Donna Lee. 1997. "Abortion, Islam, and the 1994 Cairo Population Conference." *International Journal of Middle East Studies* 29, no. 2: 161–84.

Bunt, Gary R. 2003. *Islam in the Digital Age: E-Jihad, Online Fatwas, and Cyber Islamic Environments.* London: Pluto.

Dardir, Ahmed M., and W. Ahmed. 1981. "Islam and Birth Planning: An Interview with the Grand Mufti of Egypt." *Popular Science* 2: 1–5.

---

*Eds.: Umma refers to the global Islamic community.

Islamic-fatwa.com. 2013. "Repentance from Adultery." Fatwa 65046. November 6. www.islamic-fatwa.com/fatwa/65046

Islam Q&A. 2000. "Ruling on Selling Contraceptive Measures." Fatwa 10101. October 5. islamqa.info/en/10101

Islamweb. 2009. "A Muslim Pharmacist Selling the Morning-After Pills to Non-Muslims." Fatwa 130134. December 14.

Islamweb. 2011. "Ruling on Taking Emergency Contraceptive Pills." Fatwa 165765. October 20. fatwa.islamweb.net/fatwa/index.php?page=showfatwa&Option=FatwaId&Id=165765

Roudi-Fahimi, Farzaneh. 2004. "Islam and Family Planning." Population Reference Bureau MENA Policy Brief

Trussell, James. 2012. "Emergency Contraception: Hopes and Realities." In *Emergency Contraception: The Story of a Global Reproductive Health Technology*, edited by Angel M. Foster and L. L.Wynn, 19–38. New York: Palgrave Macmillan.

Wynn, L. L. 2016. ""Like a Virgin": Hymenoplasty and Secret Marriage in Egypt." *Medical Anthropology* 35, no. 6: 547–59.

Wynn, L. L., Angel M. Foster, Aida Rouhana, and James Trussell. 2005. "The Politics of Emergency Contraception in the Arab World: Reflections on Western Assumptions and the Potential Influence of Religious and Social Factors." *Harvard Health Policy Review* 6, no. 1: 38–47.

Wynn, L. L., and James Trussell. 2006. "The Social Life of Emergency Contraception in the United States: Disciplining Pharmaceutical Use, Disciplining Sexuality, and Constructing Zygotic Bodies." *Medical Anthropology Quarterly* 20, no. 3: 297–320.

54

Abortion and Religion after *Dobbs*

Margaret D. Kamitsuka and
Rebecca Todd Peters

In this chapter, the editors of *Abortion and Religion* offer a brief reflection on *Dobbs v. Jackson*, the Supreme Court ruling that was issued as the book was in production. We direct readers to find more resources on the overturning of *Roe v. Wade* at this book's companion website: https://abortionreligionreader.com/.

On June 24, 2022, the Supreme Court of the United States overturned almost fifty years of precedent for legal access to abortion care in the United States. The *Dobbs v. Jackson* decision is expected to impact access to abortion for the 58 percent of women of reproductive age in the United States living in at least twenty-nine states hostile to abortion rights.[1] Some states are now seeking to force women to bear children as well as to punish people who have abortions or even a suspected abortion, potentially making it a capital offense.[2] *Dobbs* also ignited a firestorm of legal debate because it "set aside the rule of stare decisis" in overturning *Roe*. For some constitutional scholars, the very legitimacy of the Court "is at stake."[3]

The opinion of the Court penned by Justice Samuel Alito shocked many people for a number of reasons,[4] including for its covert nod to prolife views, widely espoused by conservative evangelical and Catholic Christians and written into the Mississippi "Gestational Age Act," which was the case heard by the Supreme Court. *Dobbs* states that

> the Court considers whether a right to obtain an abortion is part of a broader entrenched right that is supported by other precedents. . . . What sharply

distinguishes the abortion right from the rights recognized in the cases on which *Roe* and *Casey* rely is something that both those decisions acknowledged: Abortion is different because it destroys what *Roe* termed "potential life" and what the [Mississippi] law challenged in this case calls an "unborn human being."[5]

From the start, the *Dobbs* decision changed the status of the prenate, moving it front and center in the Court's deliberation.[6]

The view that "abortion presents a profound moral question"[7] or that terminating a pregnancy means killing an unborn human being are not necessarily exclusively prolife positions. Legal scholar Judith Thomson famously argued that one can be justified in terminating a pregnancy even when conceding the personhood of the fetus, based on the principle that no one has the right to demand extraordinary life support from another person without their consent.[8] However, *Dobbs* did not just affirm the moral seriousness of abortion but went further to affirm the notion that the State has a "legitimate interest" in "protecting the life of the unborn"[9] in whatever way the State sees fit. Moreover, *Dobbs* adopts the language of "unborn child," found in the Mississippi Act.[10] *Dobbs* heightens the importance of that term by including sections of historical legal codes that use "unborn child" or related phrases about pregnancy.[11]

Alito references the diversity and "conflicting" nature of beliefs on abortion. However, the fact that he felt entitled to remove a right with which the American public had lived for a half century strongly suggests his intention for the Court to throw legal weight behind the view held "fervently" by some believers—namely, "that a human person comes into being at conception and that abortion ends an innocent life."[12]

There are significant questions and concerns raised by the *Dobbs* decision. Students and scholars of ethics, theology, gender, law, and religion who have benefited from this book will want to probe more deeply into the explicit and implicit religious viewpoints and political ideologies *Dobbs* asserts or implies. We offer these three points as a place to begin further study.

The Originalism of *Dobbs* and White Christian Nationalism

Several Justices on the Court are noted for their philosophy of originalism, the doctrine of abiding by the so-called original intention of America's founding fathers. While originalism may spring from respect for the noble principles enshrined in the Constitution, scholars have noted the history of its use having an ignoble effect. Originalist appeals to the Constitution have been used to deny rights to persons or groups not in the purview of or presenting a concern for that document's white, male drafters, such as enslaved people. The nineteenth-century *Dred Scott* Supreme Court ruling "was the first major originalist ruling, claiming to find its defense of slavery and its assertion that even free Black people could not be citizens in the original intent of the founders."[13]

Critics of originalism also fear that its proponents will make common cause with Christian biblical literalists, or that the latter will throw their support behind originalism because it is deemed to uphold societal structures they find more amenable to their fundamentalist views on procreation and sexuality (e.g., no contraception, no abortion, no same-sex marriage). The jury is still out on those entanglements.[14]

Beyond the fundamentalist Christian attraction to originalism, another disturbing intersection may be at work. When America was founded, the laws intentionally put power in the hands of white, male landowners—only 16 percent of the population.[15] The extent to which eighteenth-century US lawmakers saw themselves as also enshrining Christian principles is a question for historians. Christian nationalists today do read Christianity back onto the documents of the new nation, even claiming them to be "divinely inspired."[16]

Important work is underway on the long and tortured history of using Christianity to offer moral legitimation and authority to political leaders, particularly for consolidating and exerting power over the lives of people who are marked as others.[17] Christian nationalism is on the rise in the United States.[18] Christian white supremacy groups continue to work overtly and covertly to harass, attack, and disenfranchise people they see as a threat, directing particular attention at those who are BIPOC,[19] immigrants, Jewish, Muslim, and other religious minorities. The insurrection at the Capitol on January 6, 2022, revealed the extremism of white Christian nationalists acting on their belief that America should revert to being a white Christian nation.[20]

There are troubling questions about how *Dobbs* is situated in the history of the intersections of originalism and white Christian nationalism. In what ways does *Dobbs*'s originalism harbor a covert dog whistle that functions to encourage increasingly militant white Christian nationalist groups?[21] What parallels do you see between originalism and biblical literalism and how might those parallels influence how you think about the logic of *Dobbs*?

Dobbs and Conservative Christian Claims of Fetal Personhood

The claim in Christian prolife circles—evangelical and Catholic—that personhood begins at conception is ubiquitous. While this position is largely a product of the nineteenth century, it has severe implications for religious governance (e.g., abortion at any stage incurs the penalty of instant excommunication in Roman Catholicism). Debates about the moral status of the prenate command a large swath of scholarly literature as well.[22] Some scholars are unconcerned that the Court may be harboring a bias toward a conservative Christian position and effectively imposing it on broad segments of the population—secular people, many Christians, and adherents of other religions—who hold different views on gestational development and personhood status. These conservative scholars are willing to take Alito at his word that the Court's "decision is not based on any view about when a State should regard prenatal life as having rights or legally cognizable interests."[23] These scholars consider that "*Dobbs* offers an opportunity to Americans who will now be forced to discuss the morality and law of abortion on the state level."[24] The upheaval in and danger for the lives of pregnant people— now without access to adequate healthcare for contraception, miscarriage, or abortion—seems to be a subordinate concern of these scholars.

Several questions arise regarding morality and the status of the prenate. When *Dobbs* declares the "profound wrongness" of *Roe*,[25] should one interpret that statement as a moral judgment also on the wrongness of ending any pregnancy? In what ways does a presupposition of personhood (with legal rights) from conception underlie *Dobbs* so that it functionally codifies—and essentially canonizes—a conservative Christian position?

Dobbs's Originalism and Buttressing Patriarchal Authority

Conservative Christianity is noted for its affirmation of a gender binary— under the guise of maleness and femaleness as God's intended creation— and a patriarchal gender hierarchy. As Russell Moore, past President of the Ethics & Religious Liberty Commission of the Southern Baptist Convention, has argued, "Patriarchy is good for women, good for children, and good for families."[26] When Pope John XXIII wrote "within the family, the father stands in

God's place. He must lead and guide the rest by his authority," he encapsulated the notion of gender hierarchy in official Catholic social teachings.[27]

The framers of the Constitution were neither evangelical Christians nor Roman Catholics, but their world epitomized a binary gender hierarchy. Women were notably absent in the process of framing the Constitution. In 1776, Abigail Adams wrote gently but pointedly to her husband John, who would participate in the Constitutional Convention the next year, "Do not put such unlimited power into the hands of the husbands. Remember all men would be tyrants if they could."[28] Neither he nor the other framers listened. It took until the women's rights convention at Seneca Falls in 1848 to propose a revised "Declaration of Independence": "We hold these truths to be self-evident: that all men and women are created equal."[29] Seneca Falls was a product of its times and did not speak to all inequalities and oppressions. It represents the complicated and evolving nature of our democracy and the continued need for vigilance in political empowerment.[30]

As of 2022, there is no Equal Rights Amendment to the Constitution, which failed to be ratified in 1972, the year before *Roe*. Now there is neither ERA nor *Roe*. The Justices who wrote the *Dobbs* dissenting opinion see the implications in saying, "With sorrow—for this Court, but more, for the many millions of American women who have today lost a fundamental constitutional protection—we dissent."[31]

Without rehearsing the gains and setbacks for women's rights, the questions that loom large at this historical moment are: To what extent does *Dobbs*'s defense of the "unborn human being" function to suppress the rights of women and pregnancy-capable people, effectively denying them equality and liberty before the law? As we engage in the vigilant work of political empowerment for women, what role can and should religion play in our democracy?

Notes

1. Elizabeth Nash, "State Abortion Policy Landscape: From Hostile to Supportive," *Guttmacher Institute* (August 29, 2019).
2. Elissa Spitzer, "Some States Are Ready to Punish Abortion in a Post-Roe World," CAP (June 24, 2022).
3. "'Abortion Is Just the Beginning': Six Experts on the Decision Overturning Roe," *New York Times*, Opinion (June 24, 2022).

4. In one poll taken before the *Dobbs* ruling, "only one in three (33%) of . . . voters think SCOTUS is likely to overturn *Roe*." Hart Research Associates and ALG Research, "Memorandum" (November 12, 2021), https://bit.ly /3QhzvUm.

5. *Thomas E. Dobbs, State Health Officer of the Mississippi Department of Health* v. *Jackson Women's Health Organization,* Supreme Court of the United States, 4. Concurring opinions were written by Justices Thomas and Kavanaugh and Chief Justice Roberts. A dissenting opinion was written by Justice Elana Kagan.

6. Prenate is Peters's term for the developing products of conception as long as it remains inside the body or uterus. See her discussion in this book, p. 6.

7. *Dobbs v. Jackson*, p. 8.

8. Judith Jarvis Thomson, "A Defense of Abortion," *Philosophy & Public Affairs* 1 (1971): 47–66.

9. *Dobbs v. Jackson*, 8.

10. Ibid., 7.

11. Ibid., 98. E.g., "quick with child" (98), "being with child" (111).

12. Ibid., 1.

13. Michael Waldman, "Originalism Run Amok at the Supreme Court," Brennan Center for Justice (June 28, 2022). See the essay by Brian Massingale in this volume.

14. Peter J. Smith and Robert W. Tuttle, "Biblical Literalism and Constitutional Originalism," *Notre Dame Law Review* 86 (2011): 693–764.

15. Jane Hampton Cook, "How Did John Adams Respond to Abigail's 'Remember the Ladies?'" *Journal of the American Revolution* (August 18, 2020).

16. Andrew L. Whitehead and Samuel L. Perry, *Taking America Back for God: Christian Nationalism in the United States*, updated ed. (New York: Oxford University Press, 2022), xi.

17. Willie James Jennings, *The Christian Imagination: Theology and the Origins of Race* (New Haven: Yale University Press, 2010).

18. Kathrine Stewart, "Christian Nationalists Are Excited About What Comes Next," *New York Times* (July 5, 2022).

19. BIPOC: Black, Indigenous, People of Color.

20. Philip Gorski, "White Christian Nationalism: The Deep Story Behind the Capitol Insurrection," *ABC News* (January 13, 2021).

21. Robert Spitzer, "Originalism, History, and Religiosity are the Faults of Alito's Reasoning in Dobbs," *History News Network* (May 29, 2022).

22. This book gives some examples in Part 4.

23. *Dobbs*, quoted in M. Cathleen Kaveny, "Dobbs and Fetal Personhood," *Religion and Politics* (July 19, 2022).

24. Ibid.

25. *Dobbs v. Jackson*, 64.

26. Russell D. Moore, "After Patriarchy, What? Why Egalitarians Are Winning the Gender Debate," *Journal of the Evangelical Theological Society* 49, no. 3 (September 2006): 576.

27. John XXIII quoted in Christine E. Gudorf, "Encountering the Other: The Modern Papacy on Women," *Social Compass* 36, no. 3 (1989): 297.

28. Cook, "How Did John Adams Respond to Abigail's 'Remember the Ladies?'"

29. Elizabeth Cady Stanton, "Seneca Falls Declaration (1848)," http://www .digitalhistory.uh.edu/disp_textbook.cfm?psid=1087&smtID=3.

30. Tammy L. Brown, "Celebrate Women's Suffrage, but Don't Whitewash the Movement's Racism," ACLU (August 24, 2018).

31. Elana Kagan, dissenting opinion, *Dobbs v. Jackson*, 60.

Index

Page numbers in *italics* denote figures and tables.
For Arabic surnames, initial hyphenated articles (al-) are disregarded in alphabetization.